Bedside Cardiology

Bedside Cardiology

Second Edition

Jules Constant, M.D.

Associate Clinical Professor of Medicine, State
University of New York at Buffalo School of Medicine;
Physician in Medicine, Buffalo General Hospital, Buffalo

Little, Brown and Company

Boston

To Elizabeth, my wife

The second edition of *Bedside Cardiology,* like the first, is designed not only for those who wish to learn how to diagnose cardiac disorders by means of history and physical examination, but also for those who have a phonocardiograph and pulse amplifier available. Since these diagnostically useful instruments are also necessary for the development of skills in auscultation and pulse recognition, I would encourage their incorporation into all teaching programs, even for self-training in the private office.

In order to reach both the medical student who wishes to learn the basic facts and skills and the cardiologist trainee, the asterisk method of the first edition is again used here. An asterisk (*) placed in front of a question tells you that it is for the advanced student or of interest only to a cardiologist or trainee in cardiology. For the medical student a glossary is provided to define words or lesions that may be new to those in the first two or three years of medical school. Any word referred to in the glossary is set in **boldface** in the text.

The question-and-answer format (Socratic method) has been continued, since it has found wide acceptance among students, who tell me that it serves as a stimulus to clear thinking, as well as allowing the text to be turned into programmed learning by covering up the answer on either a first or second reading. In this edition, material for the cardiologist has been presented as much as possible in straight narrative form under the subheading: *Note.*

This edition had to be enlarged, in part because of the tremendous advances made in the ability to diagnose cardiac abnormalities in the past six years. This revision has required entirely new chapters, such as those on systolic time intervals and abdominal murmurs and major additions made necessary by relatively newly discovered entities such as the ballooned valve syndrome and hypertrophic subaortic stenosis. Advances in diagnostic techniques such as echocardiography have brought new aspects of these entities to our attention.

To make the book more useful for the cardiologist in training, it has been further enlarged by the addition of many new illustrations, including actual phonocardiograms and photographs that illustrate basic methods.

The first edition was designed for those in their fourth year of medical school or on the graduate level. This edition can also be used by students in the first three years of medical school, since the glossary that has been added defines or describes most of the lesions or conditions mentioned in the non asterisk sections of the book.

J. C.

Acknowledgments

For their criticisms of the manuscript and for their donation of many of the phonocardiograms and illustrations, I would like to thank Dr. Antonio C. deLeon, Jr., Washington, D.C.; Dr. Charlotte Friedland, Mexico City; Dr. Joseph Murgo, Fort Sam Houston, Texas; Dr. William Nasser, Indianapolis; Dr. Sudhaker Reddy, Dr. Rosemarie Salerno, and Dr. Leonard Shaver, Pittsburgh; Dr. Narasimha Ranganathan, Toronto, Canada; Dr. Pravin Shah, Rochester, New York; Dr. Peter Vlad, Buffalo, New York; Dr. Charles Woolley, Columbus, Ohio; Dr. Samuel Zoneraich, New York; Dr. Willard Harris, Los Angeles, California; and Dr. Allan Adelman, Toronto, Canada.

Contents

Bedside Cardiology

The Evolving Checklist in History-Taking

GENERAL ADVANTAGES OF A CHECKLIST

Medical students have traditionally learned to take histories by memorizing a standard check-list, and have been warned that it must not be used in front of a patient. We have long maintained that this method of interrogation can be a major cause of poor diagnosis and that in sheer exasper-ation at the inefficient way in which the usual history is taken, we may ultimately turn to com-puterized questionnaires.

At the inception of our elective training program in cardiology, we could not allow students to do any actual patient workups because teaching each one how to take the detailed history we required for a cardiac diagnosis was too laborious. Finding that even our residents needed con-stant repetition to memorize all the questions relevant to a differential diagnosis of heart disease, we drew up a general checklist from which they could determine that they had at least asked the important questions.

Although we were surprised at how good a history could be taken with this aid, we were frus-trated to find that residents did not know what subsequent questions to ask if the patient responded affirmatively to a more general question. This prompted us to extend the questionnaire to incor-porate, at least on the important items, questions to be asked when the patient says yes.

While we were constructing this detailed questionnaire, it became apparent that we could teach cardiological diagnosis to students by listing the questions under the differential diagnosis. For example, if the patient admitted to having edema, an asterisk could be placed beside that ques-tion, indicating that the student should turn to a separate sheet outlining the differential diagnosis of edema by headings, under which are further questions to elicit each possible cause.

As we learned more about the relation between symptoms and diagnoses, the checklist evolved. For example, when we learned that excess perspiration is found in almost all patients with pheo-chromocytomas, this went into our new checklist on the sheet for "If the Patient Says Yes to Hypertension" as a question under the subtitle "Pheochromocytoma."

Many residents were highly resistant to the idea of reading questions to patients, mainly object-ing because patients might consider them incompetent or their memories faulty. The image of the physician as an omniscient, godlike figure would, they feared, be lost on a patient watching someone reading questions to him like a clerk in a bank. This argument we found to be unsup-ported by the results of actual practice; in fact, just the opposite impression seems to be conveyed to the patient. We have solicited patient opinion and have noted that a patient may not even recall a few days later that a checklist was used. The commonest reaction we have found is delight in encountering the first physician who cared enough about them to try to get a good history. They occasionally expressed amazement at the tremendous amount of thought that must have gone into the preparation of such a detailed questionnaire. It cannot be overemphasized that if patients notice it at all, they are only favorably impressed with the physician's thoroughness.

A second argument against the checklist is that it prevents one from noticing a patient's facial expression that may reveal the true meaning behind the answer. This implies that the physician's eyes are glued to the questions, which is unnecessary since one may easily keep a finger on the place as one looks up at the patient during questioning. Thus it is a matter of how rather than whether to use a checklist.

The third objection is that the list gives the patient no opportunity to be spontaneous or to associate freely. On the contrary, one of the checklist's strengths is that should the patient wish to enlarge on a point or go to another complaint spontaneously, one's organized line of questioning may be safely disturbed. Merely by noting where he is on the checklist, when the patient is finished with his "free association," the physician can immediately go on from where he left off. Without a checklist, a physician may object to a patient's getting off the subject for fear he may forget his place on his memorized list.

Most practicing physicians who hear about our using a checklist object that on such sheets there is often not enough room to write down all the details in case the patient says yes to a question. Further, since there is no way of knowing how lengthy the history of the present illness will be, enough room may not be allowed. Physicians often say that they have a "thousand" sheets of a checklist made up when they first went into practice which cannot be used because it is not applicable to what they have since learned.

Our residents never make this objection because our histories are written on separate blank sheets. This is the only way to make history form flexible because there is only a slight relationship between the headings on the checklist and the way in which the final history may be written up. In actual fact it is conceived of as a "reminder list" rather than as the traditional checklist that merely requires a check or a yes or no answer after each question. When a physician learns new questions to ask or new differential diagnoses, he only has to make up one new "reminder list" or merely add a word or two to the present one. We believe a checklist with a place beside each question for the answer is very unsatisfactory because it does not allow for evolution or for changes in organization.

Now let us enumerate some of the other advantages of a reminder list for the physician to use in his office, not only for cardiology but also for a complete workup if so desired.

1. No negative findings need be written down. If the checklist has been followed, you know which questions have been asked. This makes the final history much shorter and easier to read.
2. No errors of omission in history-taking need ever be made twice. If in retrospect one missed a diagnosis because a certain question was not asked, it goes down on the checklist for all future history-taking.
3. You may utilize new information from reading and lectures on how to make diagnoses as efficiently as a computer by merely putting into your checklist any new symptom that for the first time you have learned is part of a certain diagnosis. You are in effect programming your own computer by the built-in memory in your checklist. Thus the reminder list grows with your increase in knowledge.
4. There is no feeling of insecurity on leaving the bedside that you may have forgotten to ask something.
5. You can actually take a history much faster because there is no hesitation while you try to recall your place in your memorized medical school checklist. This is especially true if the patient rambles. If your histories are longer with a written checklist, then your mental checklist was inadequate. The checklist presented in this chapter is not actually as long as it appears at first glance. Many questions are repeated under different headings in order to complete a differential diagnosis.

6.   It helps the physician who must, in the first visit at least, take a good chief complaint history. If, for example, the patient complains of chest pain, in the checklist presented here one turns to a sheet headed "If the Patient Says Yes to Chest Pain," where the complete differential diagnosis of chest pain is found and serves as an organized outline for the present illness.

ADVANTAGES OF A CHECKLIST IN A TEACHING PROGRAM

1.   The teacher may merely insert into the checklist any idea in history-taking that he wishes to stress. For example, we like to teach the student to ask about *trepopnea,* i.e., breathing difficulty or other discomfort on lying in certain positions in bed but not due to heart failure. We feel that this helps him to distinguish between true left ventricular failure orthopnea and other causes of requiring more than one pillow to rest comfortably. We therefore merely insert the word *trepopnea* under the appropriate heading, which would be "Left Ventricular Failure," and because it is a new word, we may put the explanation in brackets after it. The student earns it because he sees this repeatedly every time he takes a history.
2.   Symptoms can be organized under their etiologies, so that the student learns to associate the two. He thus learns medicine from using the reminder list.
3.   With the checklist a student's very first history can be almost as meaningful as the experienced physician's because every question is given meaning by the heading under which it is placed. For example, he asks about orthopnea under "Left Ventricular Failure Symptoms," and about fatigue under "Low Output Symptoms."
4.   Those who wish to use their workups for research on symptoms in relationship to disease will be assured that in all the histories all the pertinent questions are asked.

So far we have made up a checklist only for cardiac disease, but we hope that it will serve as an example of what can be done in every form of history-taking, whether by the general practitioner or subspecialist. Each physician ought to make one to fit his own needs, and his list should evolve with his knowledge. The cardiologist should use the checklist presented here only as a "starter" upon which to build his own.

When the development and use of checklists are taught in medical schools, the result may be a generation of better diagnosticians who can perhaps compete successfully with the ever-threatening computer.

A "starter" cardiovascular checklist follows (see footnote).

GENERAL ORIENTATION

1.   Name, address, telephone number, age, occupation, and marital status.
2.   In order to decide if the cardiovascular problem is congenital or acquired, and if the patient is aware of the problem, ask when he was first told of heart trouble or murmur.
3.   If hospitalized, why?

+ before a question indicates that when a patient answers yes, follow-up questions are available on the page number given in parenthesis.

Boldface type indicates that the term is explained in the Glossary.

4.   Chief complaints or worst symptoms? When did each begin?
5.   If patient has been referred for a consultation, what problems are expected to be solved or clarified?

HEART FAILURE POSSIBILITIES

Symptoms of High Left Atrial Pressure

+1.   Dyspnea on exertion (DOE) (on the level or on climbing either hills or steps)? If not, is it because the patient is too limited in his exertion by either chest or leg pains? (P. 10.)

+2.   Orthopnea (because of dyspnea, the patient must raise head and shoulders in order to sleep)? (P. 11.)

+3.   Paroxysmal nocturnal dyspnea (PND)? (P. 12.)

4.   Pulmonary edema (sudden shortness of breath [SOB] and wheezing or cough at rest in the daytime)?

5.   Cardiovascular symptoms in pregnancy? Which trimester? (Dyspnea in the first trimester is a recognized phenomenon of uncertain etiology; in the last trimester, it may be cardiac or due to a high diaphragm.)

6.   Chest tap with needle? Site and appearance of fluid?

7.   Therapy with digitalis, diuretics, low-salt diet? Their effect? Dose? For how long?
Digitalis toxicity:
a) Gastrointestinal: diarrhea, anorexia, nausea, vomiting?
b) Muscle: severe weakness. [12] ?
c) Cerebral: dizziness (such as vertigo or loss of balance), hallucinations, or irritability?
d) Visual: blurring or inability to focus? Needs change of glasses? Color illusions?
e) Cardiac: palpitations, skipping, or "flip-flops"?
Diuretic side effects:
a) Weakness due to hypokalemia?
b) Muscle cramps or pains due to low intracellular potassium or magnesium?
Were any potassium retaining agents or supplements used? How were potassium supplements tolerated? How was low-salt diet tolerated? Was it strict?

8.   Were drugs taken that could precipitate borderline failure, i.e., propranolol, quinidine, reserpine, or guanethedine?
Note: For all positive drug histories in the checklist, ask about the dose of each drug, for how long the drug was taken, about whether it helped or had side effects, and why it was stopped.

9.   Cough or wheeze on exertion or assuming a supine position? (May mean high left atrial pressure of early failure.)

Symptoms of Peripheral Congestive Failure or Pseudo Right Heart Failure[1]

+1.   Peripheral edema? Maximum and minimum weight? Reason, if known, for any weight gain or loss. (P. 13.)

---

[1] Conventionally called *right heart failure,* though the right ventricle has not actually "failed." These symptoms or signs result from a high venous pressure and peripheral edema, which are almost always caused by left-sided myocardial or valvular damage alone. The right ventricle rarely fails except in severe pulmonary stenosis, severe pulmonary hypertension, or with a massive pulmonary embolus. **Tamponade** causes a biventricular failure, due mainly to restriction of diastolic filling.

2.   Abdominal swelling? (If this occurs before orthopnea or dyspnea, consider tamponade.)
3.   Upper abdominal pain, especially on exercise? (This suggests increased stretch of liver capsule due to hepatomegaly.)
4.   Bending or stooping discomfort? (Suggests hepatomegaly.)

Low Output State Possibilities

1.   Weakness and fatigue? Afternoon nap necessary? On drugs that could cause weakness, e.g., digitalis, diuretics, propranolol, or tranquilizers? Is there psychoneurotic basis (relation to family, spouse, work supervisor)?
2.   Coldness of extremities? For how long?
3.   Excess perspiration? (A common sign of failure in infants; if recent in an adult and not due to hyperthyroidism or neurosis, it suggests severe failure. With hot hands, it suggests thyrotoxicosis; with cold hands, it suggests psychoneurosis or heart failure.)
4.   Insomnia due to hyperpnea on going to sleep or dozing (**Cheyne-Stokes** respiration)? Ask spouse if she noticed this.
5.   Nocturia with polyuria (due to daytime failure corrected at rest)?

FIXED OUTPUT STATE POSSIBILITIES

+1.   Syncope, faintness, or dizziness. (P. 14.)
+2.   Chest pain or tightness. (P. 15.)

CHAMBER ENLARGEMENT POSSIBILITIES

1.   Trepopnea (certain positions in bed cause discomfort not due to heart failure)?
+2.   Palpitations or awareness of heartbeat? (P. 17.)
3.   Told of an enlarged heart? When first told? If yes, was it after an ECG or x-ray? If x-ray in hospital, was it portable?
4.   X-ray examination, fluoroscopy, or barium swallow? When and where were first and last ones done?

PAST CARDIAC SURGERY

1.   Date and place of surgery? Type of operation? Name of surgeon?
2.   Heart failure or other cardiac symptoms before surgery? Which symptoms were helped and for how long?
3.   Catheterized before or after surgery? Told about the results of the studies?
4.   Complications after surgery: embolic phenomenon, infections, or other?
5.   What treatment after surgery (anticoagulants, digitalis, or diuretics)? For how long?

ETIOLOGIES

Rheumatic Heart Disease Possibilities

History of Rheumatic Fever

1. Chorea ("St. Vitus' dance"), twitches, or clumsiness for a few months in childhood? Epistaxis? Frequent sore throats? Tonsillectomy and adenoidectomy? When?
2. Growing pains, i.e., *nocturnal* pains or aches in the legs? (Arthritis or other joint involvement in the daytime suggests rheumatic fever.)
3. Was the diagnosis of rheumatic fever based merely on fever and murmur, or were there actually red, swollen, painful joints? Hospitalized?
4. Therapy: aspirin, steroids, prophylactic penicillin, prolonged bed rest?
5. Family history of rheumatic fever? (This is almost as suggestive of a rheumatic origin to a patient's murmur as a history of rheumatic fever in the patient.)
6. Scarlet fever or any rash with joint pains?

History of Rheumatic Heart Disease

1. Murmurs heard on previous examination (school, pre-camp, operations, hospitalizations, insurance, Army)?
2. Cardiac catheterization results. When and where was it done?

Complications of Rheumatic Heart Disease

1. In the presence of mitral disease:
   a) Hemoptysis? Is it mixed or pure? Quantity, color, frequency? (If with dyspnea or pleuritic pain, consider pulmonary infarction. If from submucosal bronchial veins, the blood is dark, and it is usually due to high left atrial pressure in mitral stenosis.)
   b) Hoarseness without obvious upper respiratory infection? (This is Ortner's syndrome, due to the pressure of a large left atrium on an enlarged pulmonary artery, which in turn may press on peribronchial lymph nodes to compress the recurrent laryngeal nerve. Dysphagia and right posterior chest pains occur only if left atrial enlargement is extreme, due to chronic mitral regurgitation [5].)
   c) Winter bronchitis or wheezing?
   d) Ruptured chordae tendineae (suggested by sudden worsening of dyspnea, orthopnea, or PND)?
   e) Embolic phenomena: hematuria, pleurisy, unilateral weakness?
2. In the presence of aortic stenosis: angina, syncope, or dyspnea (a classic triad)?
3. In the presence of aortic regurgitation: nocturnal angina, awareness of large pulsations in arms, neck, or chest?
4. In the presence of bacterial endocarditis:
   a) Fever and night sweats (enough to require change of pajamas)?
   b) Tooth extraction or cleaning or other possible cause of bacteremia?
   c) Prolonged treatment with penicillin or other antibiotic?
   d) Embolic phenomena (due to bacterial endocarditis or venous stasis), pleurisy, hemoptysis, phlebitis, hematuria, back pain, petechiae, tender finger pads or cerebrovascular accident (unilateral weakness paralysis or speech difficulty)?
5. Epilepsy (increased incidence with mitral stenosis)?
6. Irregular palpitations with onset of dyspnea? (Suggests atrial fibrillation.)

ISCHEMIC HEART DISEASE POSSIBILITIES

+1.   Chest pains or tightness? (P. 15.)

2.   Previous myocardial infarction? If yes, what were symptoms and hospital course? What was patient told about the site and severity? Did failure develop afterwards? Did angina disappear afterwards? Put on long-term anticoagulants, special diet, or drugs?

3.   When was the first and last ECG taken? What was the patient told about it?

4.   Risk factors:
   a) *Major:* Hypertension, high cholesterol or triglycerides, smoking over 20 cigarettes a day, or family history of either infarction or angina at an early age.
   b) *Minor:* Diabetes, artificial or premature menopause, gout, intermittent claudication or sedentary occupation.
   High- or low-cholesterol diet or drugs?

5.   Marked postprandial somnolence? (Suggests severe hyperlipidemia.)

HYPERTENSIVE HEART DISEASE POSSIBILITIES

+1.   Hypertension? (P. 18.)

HIGH OUTPUT FAILURE POSSIBILITIES

1.   Anemia:
   a) Ever told of anemia? Pins and needles? Bleeding from menorrhagia, hemorrhoids, or ulcers (causing occult blood or melena)? Is anemia being treated?
   b) Marrow or metabolic disorders: upper gastrointestinal surgery in the past (causing vitamin B_{12} deficiency), sickle cell disease in self or family, contact with lead or radiation?

2.   Thyrotoxicosis: heat intolerance, weight loss, polyphagia, diarrhea, excessive sweating, frequent stools, polyuria, nervousness, irritability, restlessness, or muscle weakness on climbing? Thyroid surgery or treatment? Goiter?

3.   Beriberi: peripheral neuritis, syncope on exercise in hot weather, alcoholism with poor eating habits while drinking, occupation bartender, diet fads, upper gastrointestinal surgery in the past? Marked daily or weekly fluctuation of symptoms?

COR PULMONALE POSSIBILITIES

1.   Chronic obstructive pulmonary disease (COPD): Pulmonary function tests? Easier to breathe leaning forward? Smoking history? Told of emphysema? Chronic cough and sputum?

2.   Asthma, wheezing, or dyspnea relieved by bronchodilators?

3.   Ever work with beryllium or in a soft or hard coal mine?

4.   Syncope on exertion, emotion, or exposure to cold air? (Suggests primary pulmonary hypertension.)

5. Pulmonary emboli? History of phlebitis? Marked diuresis with diuretics? On contraceptive pill? Ever experience sudden dyspnea at rest, with palpitations, pleurisy, faintness, cold sweat, or hemoptysis? Recurrent stabbing groin pain [14]? Recent trauma or surgery?
6. History of lung infiltrate or tuberculosis?
7. Primary pulmonary hypertension? **Raynaud's phenomena** [18]? (Occurs in about a third of patients with primary pulmonary hypertension.) Phenformin treatment for diabetes [6].

PERICARDITIS OR **TAMPONADE** POSSIBILITIES

1. Chest trauma, pacemaker in the right ventricle, recent heart surgery or myocardial infarct, radiation to chest in past few months, renal failure, cancer, lymphoma, leukemia, myxedema, scleroderma, contact with tuberculosis, or recent viral infection?
2. Chest pain on motion, swallowing, or deep breathing?
3. Joint symptoms? (With face rash, suggests possible lupus erythematosus; with rash on limbs or body, suggests rheumatic fever.) On drugs that would produce lupus erythematosus syndrome (procainamide, hydralazine, penicillin, isoniazid)?
4. Past history of pericarditis? (In about a fourth of cases, idiopathic pericarditis is recurrent.)
5. Dyspnea on exertion (DOE)?
6. Edema or abdominal swelling preceding dyspnea? Abdominal swelling before edema?
7. Does the DOE stop immediately when the patient stops moving?

MYOCARDITIS AND OTHER HEART DISEASE POSSIBILITIES

1. "Collagen" disease: Raynaud's phenomenon, dysphagia, rheumatoid arthritis, tight skin, epistaxis?
2. Rheumatoid spondylitis: pain in the hip, sciatic region, or low back? Does the pain awaken patient in the early morning hours? Morning back stiffness? Pain increased on coughing? (Suggests aortic regurgitation in a small percentage.)
3. Diphtheria or syphilis history?
4. **Carcinoid heart disease:** diarrhea, bronchospasm, and flushing of the upper chest and head that lasts from minutes to days?
5. Parasitic disease (trichinosis or Chagas'): rare meat? Foreign travel?
6. Atrial myxoma: embolic phenomena, recurrent fevers, arthralgias, or skin lesions of a vasculitis type? Paresthesias in hands? Pulsations in neck (giant A waves, as in tricuspid stenosis)? Syncope or faintness?
7. Hemochromatosis: history of diabetes, especially if insulin resistant, skin color changes? Liver failure and enlargement symptoms: upper abdominal pain, sexual impotence, or gynecomastia? Arthritis?
8. Sarcoidosis: syncope (due to complete atrioventricular block)? Known bundle branch block? Abnormal chest x-ray? Cough? Kidney stones or eye symptoms?
9. **Hypertrophic subaortic stenosis:**
    a) Family history of sudden death?
    b) Angina or syncope after but not during exercise?
    c) Intermittent murmur?
    d) Symptoms worse on digitalis?
10. Amyloid heart disease: postural hypotension with peripheral neuropathy, skin plaques?

CONGENITAL HEART DISEASE POSSIBILITIES

1. Growth and development? (Compare with siblings.)
2. Mother's pregnancy:
    a) Drugs? (Stilbestrol in pregnancy has been linked to **transposition of the great vessels.**)
    b) Rubella in the first trimester? (Suggests **patent ductus arteriosus, ventricular septal defect** or **atrial septal defect, tetralogy of Fallot,** supravalvular aortic stenosis, or pulmonary artery stenosis. Deafness and cataracts are the common noncardiac lesions.)
    c) Viral illness? (In the last trimester, may produce myocarditis in newborn.)
3. Family history:
    a) Congenital heart or murmur in family?
    b) Diabetes? (Suggests complete transposition of the great vessels if with high birth weight.)
4. Cyanosis: When did it begin? (If cyanosis was present either from birth or within a few days of birth, it suggests transposition of the great vessels.) Was it delayed for years and associated with palpitations? (Suggests **Ebstein's anomaly,** especially if with little DOE. If delayed until adolescence or middle age, also suggests atrial septal defect with **Eisenmenger's reaction** [syndrome].) Does it occur only with crying or feeding or warm bath? Only with syncope? (Suggests **tetralogy.**) **Differential cyanosis** and **clubbing?** (P. 27.) (Suggests patent ductus arteriosus with Eisenmenger's syndrome, especially if there is unexpectedly little dyspnea on exertion.)
5. Frequent phlebotomies?
6. Syncope or faintness? On exposure to cold or only on effort or excitement (suggests **primary pulmonary hypertension**)? With straining after a long sleep and with cyanosis? (Suggests **tetralogy of Fallot.**) At rest? (Suggests tetralogy of Fallot or **atrioventricular block.**) Only with effort? (Suggests severe aortic stenosis, pulmonary stenosis, or primary pulmonary hypertension.)
7. Angina? (Suggests severe aortic stenosis, pulmonary stenosis, or primary pulmonary hypertension.)
8. Exact day the murmur was first heard? (Stenotic murmurs are heard in newborn nursery; left-to-right shunt murmurs are delayed at least a few weeks.) Was it discovered by physician who had seen the patient before or by a physician seeing the patient for the first time?
9. Frequent pneumonias? (Suggests either large left-to-right shunts with increased pulmonary blood flow, or severe pulmonary stenosis with decreased pulmonary blood flow.)
10. Squatting or knee-chest position frequent? (Suggests decreased pulmonary flow due to tetralogy of Fallot or, more rarely, due to tricuspid atresia.)
11. Headaches, epistaxis, leg fatigue or aches after exercise, cold legs, or claudication? (Suggests **coarctation.** Epistaxis alone suggests pulmonary stenosis or rheumatic fever.)
12. When and where was cardiac catheterization done? What were parents told of findings?
13. Dysphagia? (Consider coarctation, with the right subclavian artery passing behind the esophagus.)
14. Awareness of pulsations in the neck? (Consider coarctation, aortic regurgitation, thyrotoxicosis, or the venous pulsations of giant A waves in primary pulmonary hypertension or severe pulmonary stenosis.)

15.   Strokes? (Consider emboli from endocardial fibroelastosis if patient is an infant; or from idiopathic cardiomyopathy if patient is a child. May be due to paradoxical emboli or cerebral abscess if patient is cyanotic. Somnolence with cyanosis suggests cerebral abscess.)

16.   Hoarseness? (Suggests primary pulmonary hypertension or large patent ductus arteriosus [10].)

17.   Excessive sweating? (Sign of failure in infants.) Asthmatic attacks in newborn? (Suggests pulmonary edema.)

18.   Surgery? When, where, and by whom? What were the symptomatic results?

19.   Mental retardation? (Consider **Down's syndrome** or supravalvular aortic stenosis.)

20.   Swelling, pain, warmth, and tenderness of lower extremities? (Hypertrophic osteoarthropathy suggests patent ductus arteriosus with Eisenmenger's syndrome.)

21.   Did symptoms begin with severe retrosternal or upper abdominal pain with marked dyspnea? (In a young adult, this suggests a ruptured **aneurysm**, ruptured **sinus of Valsalva**, or acute infarction.)

22.   Recurrent bleeding from the nose, lips, or mouth, with hemoptysis or melena, multiple cerebral symptoms such as dizziness and visual disturbances, and a family history of epistaxis? (This is hereditary hemorrhagic telangiectasis or Rendu-Osler-Weber disease and suggests a pulmonary arteriovenous fistula, especially if the patient is cyanotic.)

23.   Has the mother been aware of the infant's heart beating against the chest wall, or of the vibrations of a thrill?

24.   Weakness and incoordination? (Suggests the cardiomyopathy of Friedreich's ataxia or muscular dystrophy.)

FOLLOW-UP QUESTIONS

If Patient Says Yes to Dyspnea on Exertion

Orientation

1.   What does the patient mean by DOE? (Some confuse it with weakness.)
2.   When did it begin? Did it suddenly become worse after being the same for years? (If rheumatic heart, consider atrial fibrillation, ruptured chordae tendineae, or acute infarction due to coronary embolus or thrombus.)

Severity

1.   How far can patient walk on a level at a fast, normal, or slow rate before DOE?
2.   Has it made him walk more slowly?
3.   How far does patient walk up a hill or up steps before DOE occurs?

Etiology

1.   Failure:
   a) Effect of digitalis, diuretics, low salt, or cardiac surgery?
   b) Does the patient also have classic orthopnea, or PND, or cough and wheeze on exertion or on assuming a supine position?

2. Angina equivalent:
   a) Does it last as long as angina (2—20 minutes)?
   b) Is it associated with chest tightness or pain?
   c) Is it unresponsive to digitalis?
   d) Does it come on at rest?
3. Arrhythmias:
   a) Ever told of an abnormal rhythm?
   b) Did the dyspnea begin suddenly one day and persist (e.g., as if from a persistent arrhythmia)?
   c) Does it occur with palpitations or begin and end suddenly while resting?
4. Anxiety or unknown cause:
   a) Ever had "nervous breakdown" or need for tranquilizers?
   b) If dyspnea occurred in pregnancy, in which trimester?
   c) Ever told of overbreathing? Does patient ever find himself overbreathing?
   d) Associated with numbness, tingling, dizziness, pain near apex of heart, and cold perspiration? (This suggests Da Costa's syndrome or **neurocirculatory asthenia** [11].)
   e) Is it relieved by rest, by a few deep breaths, or by further exertion?
   f) Are there good days without any shortness of breath?
   g) Worse if upset, and helped by sedatives?
5. Pulmonary disease or dysfunction:
   a) Associated with much weight gain?
   b) Asthma? Ever wheeze? Told of asthma? More difficulty breathing out than in? Helped by bronchodilators?
   c) Chronic obstructive pulmonary disease: easier to breathe leaning forward, smoking history, told of emphysema, chronic cough with sputum, had pulmonary function tests?
   d) Pulmonary embolism: SOB, faintness or syncope combined with either palpitations, hemoptysis, general chest or pleuritic pain, cold sweats, or phlebitis?
   e) Pneumothorax: sudden dyspnea and pleuritic pain of chest wall or shoulder, without radiating into the arm, but with dry cough?
6. Anemia: ever told of anemia or any bleeding from menorrhagia, hemorrhoids, or ulcers, either occult or with melena? Sickle cell disease, bone marrow, or metabolic disorders? Pins and needles? History of gastrectomy? Treatment for anemia such as vitamin B_{12} or iron?

If Patient Says Yes to Orthopnea

Orientation

1. When did it begin?
2. Spontaneous, or patient told by physician to use more pillows?

Severity

1. How many pillows needed?
2. How soon after patient lies flat is dyspnea noted?

Etiology

1. Cardiomegaly: Is the discomfort actually due to patient's feeling heartbeat on bed when lying on left side?
2. Musculoskeletal, chest wall, or neurological disorders:
    a) Is the discomfort lying flat due to neck or shoulder-girdle pain, backache, or dizziness?
    b) Does chest or only the head have to be on pillow?
3. High left atrial pressure:
    a) Dyspnea whether patient lies on back, left side, or right side?
    b) Improved by digitalis or diuretics?
    c) Does dyspnea occur if patient slips off pillows accidentally?
    d) Does dyspnea begin within a half-minute of lying flat?
    e) Associated with classic PND?
4. Markedly decreased vital capacity:
    a) Not completely free of dyspnea at any chest elevation? (Often seen in severe mitral stenosis.)
    b) Dyspneic for less than a minute supine, then is all right? (Suggests pulmonary hypertension.)

If Patient Says Yes to Paroxysmal Nocturnal Dyspnea

Orientation

1. When did PND first begin?
2. How frequent (number of times per night, week, month, or year)?
3. Longest and shortest time between attacks?

Is It Due to Left Ventricular Failure?

1. How long after patient is asleep does it occur? (It usually takes about 2—4 hours for tissue fluid to enter and fill the intravascular space enough to raise a high left atrial pressure.) Heavy or light sleeper? (If light sleeper, it is likely to occur sooner after falling asleep and it may not be as severe.)
2. What must patient do to get rid of it? (If from left ventricular failure, the patient must dangle or get out of bed.)
3. How long does it last? Shortest and longest time? (It takes at least 10—30 minutes for redistribution of fluid into extravascular space.)
4. Is it accompanied by cough? If with sputum, is it frothy or pink? Which starts first, the cough or SOB? (Chronic bronchitis patients may be awakened by a cough.)
5. Wheezing? (Demonstrate what is meant by this.) Is there a history of asthma in the family? Is it relieved by treatment for asthma?
6. Does it ever occur during the day when sitting or walking? (This suggests that you are not dealing with true left ventricular failure PND.)

7. Related to amount of work or fatigue during the day?
8. Effect of digitalis, diuretics, or low-salt diet?
9. Does patient awaken for some other reason (postnasal drip, nocturia, palpitations, or trepopnea) and then notice the dyspnea?
10. Chest pain or tightness with PND? (If so, it is nocturnal angina.)

If Patient Says Yes to Peripheral Edema

Orientation

When first noted?

Severity

1. Shoes too tight because of it? Does edema extend up to knees?
2. Effect of digitalis, diuretics, and low-salt diet? When did treatment begin?
3. Gone in the morning?

Etiology
1. Cardiac:
    a) Helped by digitalis? (Edema may be decreased by diuretics or low-salt diet, no matter what the etiology.)
    b) Other symptoms of low output or high left atrial pressure?
    c) Edema preceded dyspnea by days, weeks, or months? (This suggests constriction or tamponade, especially if abdominal swelling preceded the edema.)
2. Stasis or obstructive edema: obesity or pregnancy, tight panty girdle, varicose veins, or phlebitis history? Unilateral? Is collar becoming tight and face swollen (superior vena cava obstruction)?
3. Hormonal:
    a) Premenstrual: associated with breast fullness, headache, and mood changes?
    b) On estrogen or contraceptive pills?
    c) Aldosteronism: hypertension, weakness, tetany or paresthesias?
    d) Myxedema: voice change, dry skin, absent sweating, cold intolerance, unusual sluggishness, weight gain, sleepiness, menorrhagia, diminished hearing, watery or puffy eyes. Treated for hyperthyroidism? Effect of thyroid hormone? No help from digitalis? Results of thyroid tests?
4. Lymphatic obstruction: foot fungus, prostatic carcinoma symptoms?
5. Intermittent idiopathic edema of women: emotionally labile, unrelated to menses, history of diabetes or large babies, history of menstrual disorders?
6. Drug-induced: antihypertensives such as guanethidine, hydralazine, or *Rauwolfia* derivatives? Antirheumatics such as phenylbutazone or indomethacin?
7. Renal: facial and hand edema, worse on awakening? History of renal disease?
8. Cirrhosis: history of alcoholism? Hepatitis or jaundice with abdominal pain? Anorexia, fatigue, weakness, ascites? Bleeding from varices? (If polycythemia vera is present, consider hepatic vein thrombosis as a cause of ascites [Budd-Chiari syndrome].)

If Patient Says Yes to Syncope, Faintness, or Dizziness

Orientation

1. What does the patient mean by "dizziness"?
2. When did it first occur?
3. How often does it occur?
4. Longest and shortest time between episodes?

Etiology

1. Epilepsy:
   a) How long was patient unconscious?
   b) Was mind clear or foggy after attack? Prodrome or aura before attack?
   c) Did attack ever start with twitch of an extremity?
   d) Sore tongue or incontinence after attack?
   e) History of head trauma?
   f) Family history of convulsions?
   g) If attack was observed, were convulsions seen?
2. Orthostatic due to peripheral autonomic fault:
   a) Relation to body position?
   b) History of diabetes or sympathectomy or of using antihypertensive agents?
   c) Other autonomic disturbances: impotence, sphincter disturbances, peripheral neuritis, is worse in hot weather, or worse if fatigued? Absence of sweating? Only during pregnancy?
   d) Prodrome of faintness?
3. Excess bleeding: piles, black stools, history of anemia, menorrhagia, anticoagulants plus trauma to abdomen (ruptured spleen)?
4. Vertebral-basilar insufficiency (syncope not a feature): vertigo, tinnitus, diplopia, dysarthria, dysphagia, unilateral or bilateral transient blindness, face, arm, or leg weakness, numbness and tingling, "drop attacks" (sudden loss of postural tone without losing consciousness)?
5. Subclavian steal: the symptoms in (4) occur with arm movements and occasionally syncope, nausea, fatigue, and headaches [3, 19]? Post Blalock-Taussig operation? Claudication of hand and arm [7]?
6. Carotid insufficiency (syncope may occur): unilateral blindness, weakness or paresthesias, dysarthrias or aphasias (duration few minutes to few hours)?
7. Hysterical: never occurs when alone, associated paresthesias of hands or face (suggestive of hyperventilation), never injured self despite absence of prodrome, always with dyspnea and chest pains (as occasionally in hyperventilation)?
8. Vasovagal: Preceded by nausea or "sinking feeling" in epigastrium? Associated with acute fear or anxiety? Skin wet after attack? Pallor before or after attack? Associated with tight collar or head turning?
9. Hypertrophic subaortic stenosis: post-tussive, postural, or occurs immediately after cessation of exertion?
10. Adam-Stokes attacks:
    a) Flushed after, subjective or objective?
    b) Ever told of slow pulse?
    c) Unrelated to exertion?

11. Pulmonary embolism: preceded by light-headedness, with or without dyspnea [9, 15]?
12. Cough syncope, with strenuous cough [1]?
13. Intermittent obstruction from left or right atrial myxoma: syncope on changing chest position, Raynaud's phenomenon [17], intermittent fevers?

If Patient Says Yes to Chest Pain or Tightness

Orientation

1. When did it first begin?
2. Under what circumstances?
3. How often does it occur? Longest and shortest time between episodes?

Site

1. Have the patient point to the site and to where it radiates. Is site typical for angina, i.e., retrosternal, in the neck or the jaw, across the upper chest, and radiating to the left arm inner surface? Is it atypical but still possibly anginal, i.e., in the xiphoid, upper chest, triceps, biceps, pectorals, upper paravertebral area, and radiating down the right arm, with a heavy feeling in the arm, or localized pain in the wrist, elbow, or even right shoulder, or both?
2. Is there more than one primary site?
3. Is the pain very likely not angina, i.e.,
   a) Does it increase with inspiration?
   b) Does it last too long, i.e., over a half hour? (This may be due to infarction if it occurs only once, but is noncardiac if frequent.)
   c) Does it last only a few seconds, i.e., is it just a short stab, or are there repeated short stabs?
   d) Does it radiate down the lateral aspect of the arm?
   e) Does it start under the left breast and radiate laterally into the axilla and back?
   f) Is it brought on by a sudden arm movement or chest movement?
   g) Does it usually disappear when patient lies down? (Increased venous return aggravates angina.)

Character

Sticking or stablike, burning, aching, squeezing, tightness or pressure, superficial as if in skin or deep inside, tearing? Severity: mild, moderate, or severe.

Anginal Equivalent

Does patient have DOE or at rest that lasts 2–20 minutes and is not helped by digitalis?

Precipitating Causes

Effect of exertion (arm or leg), cold air, emotion, food, changing weather, sexual activity, lying on left side? Are there palpitations, i.e., awareness of heartbeat with the pain? (Some angina occurs only with arrhythmias.) Is it nocturnal? Hypertension? On tachycardia-producing drugs such as atropine or hydralazine?

Associated Signs or Symptoms

1.   Pallor?
2.   Dyspnea?
3.   Flatulence, nausea, or vomiting?
4.   Sweating?

Relieving Factors

1.   Relieved by rest or sedatives?
2.   Relieved or worsened by nitroglycerin? If not relieved, what dose was used? (A large dose may increase angina.) How is the nitroglycerin stored? (It will absorb onto paper.) Side effects from nitrates severe?
3.   Relieved by long-acting vasodilators, surgery, anticoagulants, antithyroid treatment, quinidine or propranolol low-fat or reducing diet, or exercise program?

Etiology

Coronary disease

1.   General indications of coronary disease:
     a) Does dyspnea accompany pain?
     b) Risk factors: diabetes, hypertension, sedentary life, artificial menopause, high cholesterol level, gout, **intermittent claudication,** heavy smoking, previous infarction or family history of cardiovascular disease? Did the infarct initiate the chronic pain, or eliminate it for a time?
     c) Emotional tensions at home or at work?
2.   Unstable angina: (May signify impending infarction.)
     a) Without apparent cause, is pain coming more frequently, with less provocation, lasting longer, or occurring at rest in the past few days or weeks?
     b) Is pain associated with sweating, faintness, or dyspnea for first time?
     c) Prinzmetal's variant (angina inversa), often nocturnal pain, commonly coming only at rest and relieved by exertion?

Noncoronary causes

1.   Congenital absence of pericardium: relieved by changing position in bed, brought on by lying on left side, lasts few seconds or minutes?
2.   Esophagitis: burning pain, brought on by eating or by lying down, acid reflux into mouth (water brash), relief with antacids? Hiatal hernia seen on x-ray?
3.   Root neuritis: past history of herpes zoster or back injury? Nitroglycerin relief wears off in a few minutes? Relieved or precipitated by certain movements of chest or arms? Herniated cervical disc: pain radiates to radial side of hand?
4.   Scalenus anticus or thoracic outlet syndrome: paresthesias and pain along ulnar distribution, aggravated by abduction of arm, lifting a weight, working with hands above shoulders, sleeping on side, or turning head? Pain more or less continuous [2, 16]?
5.   Costochondritis and myositis or local neuritis: local tenderness? Pressure in the area brings on the pain? (Angina following myocardial infarction can occur with local tenderness in trigger area.) Etiology suggested by a history of:
     a) Herpes zoster?

b) Chest injury?

c) Tietze's syndrome (painful swelling of costal cartilage [13]): worse on coughing? Unilateral or localized to one costochondral junction? Helped by salicylates [13]?

d) Gout: history of attack of gout with first episode of pain or preceding chest pain by many years? No radiation from anterior chest? Relieved by colchicine and not by nitrates? Lasts from minutes to days [8]?

6. Fixed output state: history of murmur or valve disease suggesting severe valvular stenosis or pulmonary hypertension?

7. Limited coronary flow or oxygen supply not due to coronary disease or fixed output: history suggesting anemia or arrhythmias?

8. Ballooned or prolapsed mitral valve syndrome: associated with light-headedness, fatigue, and palpitations, fleeting or lasting hours?

Diagnostic Tests

1. Electrocardiogram, resting and with exercise? Type of exercise test and results?
2. Coronary angiograms and result?

If Patient Says Yes to Palpitations

Orientation

1. When did they first begin? Shortest and longest duration? Shortest and longest time between episodes?
2. How much does it bother the patient, i.e., will he still need medical treatment if assured that it is harmless?

Types and Rates of Tachycardia

Distinguish paroxysmal tachycardia from premature contractions

1. Continuous or only occasional strong beat? Is it regular or irregular?
2. Ever told of abnormal rhythm? When was last ECG?
3. Ask patient to tap out the rate and rhythm.

Distinguish ectopic tachycardia from sinus tachycardia

1. Sudden onset and end? (Atrial tachycardias may start suddenly, but often end gradually because of sinus tachycardia following them. Atrial tachycardias occasionally end with short, sharp pain.)
2. Onset with rest, sitting quietly in chair? Ever awakened by it?
3. Always with exercise? (Suggests a sinus tachycardia.)
4. Pulsations in neck come and go? (A giant A wave of pulmonary hypertension or tricuspid stenosis disappears with atrial fibrillation.)
5. Do any maneuvers either by patient or physician sometimes stop it?

Do palpitations point to any chamber or great-vessel enlargement?

Site of palpitations? (Have patient point with one finger, or you point with finger to various places on chest wall and ask if beat felt there.)

What is its relationship to cardiac output and coronary filling?

1.   Does it cause dyspnea, oliguria, faintness, or angina?
2.   Does it cause polyuria? (Only with supraventricular tachycardia, with rate probably over 110 and lasting over 15 minutes.)
3.   Does it cause fatigue for many hours after it is over? (Common with supraventricular tachycardias.)

Etiology

1.   Much tea, coffee, alcohol, or tobacco? Any known precipitating factors?
2.   Drug: on digitalis? Dose and type? On diuretics without potassium-retaining agents? On tachycardia-producing drugs, such as hydralazine, or anticholinergic ulcer drugs?
3.   Thyroid disease? (See p. 7 for questions.)
4.   Flushing, headache, or sweating with it? (Suggests pheochromocytoma.)
5.   Changed or helped by drugs or vagal stimulating maneuvers?
6.   Told of abnormal ECG? (**Wolff-Parkinson-White** syndrome.)

If Patient Says Yes to Hypertension

Orientation

1.   When first told? Under what circumstances was it discovered?
2.   Has treatment been taken regularly? What drugs and dose?

Etiology

1.   Renal: previous kidney infection or nephritis, back injury or sport in which back injury may have occurred, frequency or nocturia, polyuria, prostatism, kidney x-rays, renal calculi, gout?
2.   Essential hypertension:
     a) Family history of hypertension?
     b) At what age first told? (Essential hypertension usually does not manifest itself before the fourth decade.)
3.   Coarctation: cold legs or intermittent claudication, nosebleeds, shoulder-girdle pain; angio-cardiograms?
4.   Pheochromocytoma: flushing with pounding headaches, dizziness, sweating, palpitations, nausea, chest pain, and paresthesias? Weight loss? Elevated blood sugars?
5.   Eclampsia: edema, hypertension, albuminuria, or convulsions in pregnancy?
6.   Aldosteronism: episodic or continual weakness, tetany, polyuria (mostly nocturnal), polydipsia, or headaches?
7.   Cushing's syndrome: hirsutism, corticosteroid intake, easy bruising, slow wound-healing, acne, muscle weakness, kidney stones, emotional lability or depression?
8.   Hormonal: on contraceptive pills?

Severity

1.   Past blood pressure reading?
2.   Visual problems, convulsions, coma, strokes, headaches, dyspnea on exertion, orthopnea, PND, epistaxis, or angina?

3.   X-ray or ECG abnormalities known?

4.   Amount and success of medical or surgical therapy? Side effects of treatment: muscle aches and cramps (from electrolyte imbalance), weakness, sleepiness, postural hypotension, nausea, nasal stuffiness, impotence, or palpitations?

NEW YORK HEART ASSOCIATION FUNCTIONAL AND THERAPEUTIC CLASSIFICATION [4]

The functional classification refers to fatigue, dyspnea, or angina. The original classification is too long to memorize, and a simplified one follows.

Class 1   Asymptomatic. (There is no Class 0 or classification for a patient with a normal heart.)
Class 2   Symptoms on ordinary exertion.
Class 3   Symptoms on less than ordinary exertion.
Class 4   Symptoms at rest.

The therapeutic classification also refers only to patients with abnormal hearts.

Class A   No restriction.
Class B   Severe effort restricted.
Class C   Ordinary effort moderately restricted.
Class D   Ordinary effort markedly restricted.
Class E   Confined to chair.

REFERENCES

1. Aaronson, D. W., Rovner, R. N., and Patterson, R. Cough syncope: Case presentation and review. *J. Allergy Clin. Immunol.* 46:359, 1970.
2. Adson, A. W. Surgical treatment for symptoms produced by cervical ribs and the scalenus anticus muscle. *Surg. Gynecol. Obstet.* 85:687, 1947.
3. Conrad, M. C., Toole, J. F., and Janeway, R. Hemodynamics of the upper extremities in subclavian steal syndrome. *Circulation* 32:346, 1965.
4. Criteria Committee, N.Y. Heart Association. *Diseases of the Heart and Blood Vessels: Nomenclature and Criteria for Diagnosis* (6th ed.). Boston: Little, Brown, 1964. P. 114.
5. DeSanctis, R. W., Dean, D. C., and Bland, D. F. Extreme left atrial enlargement. *Circulation* 29:14, 1964.
6. Fahlen, M., et al. Phenformin and pulmonary hypertension. *Br. Heart J.* 35:824, 1973.
7. Folger, G. M., Jr., and Shah, K. D. Subclavian steal in patients with Blalock-Taussig anastomosis. *Circulation* 31:241, 1965.
8. Frank, M., DeVries, A., and Atsmon, A. Gout simulating cardiac pain. *Am. J. Cardiol.* 6:929, 1960.
9. Fred, H. L., Willerson, J. T., and Alexander, J. K. Neurological manifestations of pulmonary thromboembolism. *Arch. Intern. Med.* 120:33, 1967.
10. Hornsten, T. R., Hellerstein, H. K., and Ankeney, J. L. Patent ductus arteriosus in a 72-year-old woman. *J.A.M.A.* 199:148, 1967.

11. Jarcho, S. Functional heart disease in the Civil War (Da Costa, 1871). *Am. J. Cardiol.* 4:809, 1959.
12. Lely, A. H., and vanEnter, C. H. Non-cardiac symptoms of digitalis intoxication. *Am. Heart J.* 83:149, 1972.
13. Levey, G. S., and Calabro, J. J. Tietze's syndrome: Report of two cases and review of the literature. *Arthritis Rheum.* 5:261, 1962.
14. McIntyre, K. M., Belko, J. S., and Sasahara, A. A. Pulmonary embolism: Premonitory signs and recurrence after vena cava ligation. *Arch. Surg.* 98:671, 1969.
15. Oster, M. W., and Leslie, B. Syncope and pulmonary embolism. *J.A.M.A.* 224:630, 1973.
16. Riddell, D. H., Kirtley, J. A., Jr., Moore, J. L., and Goduco, R. S. Scalenus anticus symptoms: Evaluation and surgical treatment. *Surgery* 47:115, 1960.
17. Skanse, B., Berg, N. O., and Westfelt, L. Atrial myxoma with Raynaud's phenomenon as the initial symptom. *Acta Med. Scand.* 164:321, 1959.
18. Walcott, G., Burchell, H. B., and Brown, A. L., Jr. Primary pulmonary hypertension. *Am. J. Med.* 49:70, 1970.
19. Williams, C. L., Scott, S. M., and Takaro, T. Subclavian steal. *Circulation* 28:14, 1963.

I
Inspection and Palpation

2
Cardiac Clues from Physical Appearance

EYES

1. How does **infective endocarditis** affect the eyes?
   ANS.: a) Hemorrhages and petechiae of the conjunctiva (due to bleeding tendency plus minute emboli). Evert lids to see these lesions.
   b) Oval hemorrhages near disk with white spot in center (Roth's spots).

2. Which cardiac condition besides hypertensive heart disease is associated with papilledema?
   ANS.: Hypoxic **cor pulmonale**. Here, it is due to high cerebrospinal fluid pressure with little elevation of jugular pressure.

3. With which cardiac lesions are cataracts associated?
   ANS.: It may be part of the rubella syndrome, in which a **patent ductus arteriosus** (PDA) and pulmonary artery (not valve) stenosis are the most common cardiac lesions. Deafness and mental deficiency due to microcephaly or slow rate of growth may coexist.

4. With which cardiac lesion is the pinpoint pupil of heroin addiction seen?
   ANS.: Tricuspid regurgitation (TR) due to infective endocarditis.

*5. Which cardiac abnormalities are associated with **hypertelorism**?
   ANS.: a) Pulmonary stenosis (PS), especially with an atrial septal defect (ASD) and also in **Noonan's syndrome** and multiple lentigines syndrome [4].
   b) **Hurler's disease**, or gargoylism, with mitral regurgitation.

6. Which kind of arcus (circumferential light grey ring around iris) is associated with hypercholesterolemia or coronary disease?
   ANS.: A thick band that
   a) Begins inferiorly, and
   b) Leaves a rim of iris peripherally.
   Note: The usual "arcus senilis" that is not necessarily associated with hyperlipidemia or coronary disease begins superiorly and extends to the rim of the iris.

---

*indicates material that is for electives or fellows in cardiology, or concerns rare phenomena, of interest primarily to cardiologists.

Boldface type indicates that the term is explained in the Glossary.

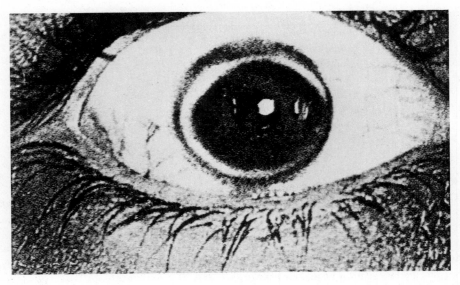

Courtesy Ayerst Laboratories

This type of arcus is a thick band of yellowish material surrounded by peripheral pigment and suggests a high serum cholesterol. It is not an arcus senilis, which has little known significance.

7.   Which cardiac lesions are common with the epicanthus of **Down's syndrome?**
      ANS.:   **Endocardial cushion defects,** especially of the complete variety.

8.   Which cardiac lesions should you suspect in the presence of an Argyll Robertson pupil (reacts to accommodation but not to light)?
      ANS.:   Luetic aortic aneurysm, or aortic regurgitation (AR) with coronary ostial stenosis.

*9.   What cardiac condition besides thyrotoxic heart disease can be associated with exophthalmos?
      ANS.:   Advanced congestive failure with high venous pressure and weight loss. The stare is probably due to the lid retraction caused by the strong sympathetic tone accompanying low cardiac output and exaggerated by the slight proptosis.
               Note: Severe TR can even cause systolic pulsation of the eyes. A pulsatile exophthalmos also may be caused by a carotid-cavernous sinus arteriovenous fistula, in which case a murmur can be heard over the eyeball.

*10.   What cardiac lesions should you suspect if you see a tremulous iris (iridodonesis)?
      ANS.:   This suggests Marfan's syndrome, in which the iris is not properly supported by the lens because of dislocation or weakness of the suspensory ligament. The cardiac lesions seen are aneurysms of the aorta or pulmonary artery, and myxomatous degeneration of the aortic or mitral valve, with consequent regurgitation.

11.   What are the retinal signs of various degrees of **arteriosclerosis?**
      ANS.:   Grade 1: Light reflex has increased width.
               Grade 2: Crossing deficits (arteriovenous nicking and right angles).
               Grade 3: Copper-wire arteries (red of artery slightly brownish due to thick walls).
               Grade 4: Silver-wire arteries (no red at all, only a whitish light reflex).

12. What are the retinal signs of different degrees of hypertension?
    ANS.: Grade 1: Generalized attenuation (arterio/venous ratio less than 2:3).
    Grade 2: Focal constriction.
    Grade 3: Hemorrhages and exudates.
    Grade 4: Papilledema.
13. What is the significance of **xanthelasma**?
    ANS.: Some (but not all) patients with xanthelasma have hypercholesterolemia [12].
*14. What cardiac conditions are associated with blue scleras?
    ANS.: a) Osteogenesis imperfecta with its fractures is associated with AR.
    b) Marfan's syndrome is associated with great-vessel aneurysms and mitral or aortic valve regurgitation.
    c) Ehlers-Danlos syndrome, with its hyperelastic, fragile skin, hyperextensible joints, and kyphoscoliosis, is associated with ASDs, tetralogy of Fallot, or regurgitant valves.

SKIN

General

1. Where should you look for tendon **xanthomas**? What do they signify?
    ANS.: Achilles tendon, extensor tendons of hands, plantar tendons on the sole, and patellar tendons. Usually, they indicate type II hyperlipoproteinemia (high cholesterol level).
*2. What cardiac diagnosis is associated with the smooth, glossy, drum-tight skin on the fingers seen in scleroderma?
    ANS.: Scleroderma may be associated with myocardial fibrosis or cor pulmonale due to pulmonary fibrosis.
3. What is the shoulder-hand syndrome?
    ANS.: It is a sympathetic abnormality of the left (occasionally both) upper extremities in which painful abduction of the shoulder is associated with swollen, painful hands and fingers. It is caused in some unknown way by myocardial infarction, often following infarction by several months. It has become rare now that long periods of complete immobility are no longer part of the treatment of infarction.

Skin Temperature

1. Which conditions that affect the heart can cause warmer-than-normal skin?
    ANS.: a) Thyrotoxicosis.
    b) Severe anemia.
    c) Beer drinker's acute **beriberi** [7].
2. What cardiac conditions are suggested by cold hands or feet?
    ANS.: a) If moist, they suggest anxiety and may explain chest pains, palpitations, and fatigue as due to **neurocirculatory asthenia** (Da Costa's syndrome).
    b) If only the feet are cold, and the patient has a history of **intermittent claudication**, peripheral arterial obstruction with poor collateral circulation is suggested.

c) If relatively recent in onset (few weeks to a few years), a low output state is suggested.

Note: The cold hands of the low output state can become warm when palmar erythema (liver palms) develop, secondary to cardiac cirrhosis.

Skin Color

1.   How do you detect central versus peripheral **cyanosis** clinically? What is the significance of this?

ANS.:   Central cyanosis (blue or purple) is seen in warm areas. Have a nurse or colleague stand beside the patient and compare tongues. In black patients, the conjunctiva may show it. If the nails are cyanotic *and the hands are warm,* the cyanosis is central.

Peripheral cyanosis is seen in cool areas such as the nail beds, nose, cheeks, earlobes, and outer surface of the lips.

Note: In about 15% of patients with tetralogy of Fallot, in which the right ventricle (RV) has two outlets for systole, the pulmonary stenosis may be so mild that there is still a left-to-right shunt through the ventricular septal defect (VSD) into the pulmonary artery. These children will be acyanotic. Nevertheless, tetralogy of Fallot is the commonest cause of cyanosis at birth.

*2.   How can cyanosis be increased in a patient with tetralogy of Fallot if questionable cyanosis is present?

ANS.:   a) By exercising [6]. This increases the right-to-left shunt into the aorta by
  1) Dilating muscle and skin vessels and thus decreasing peripheral resistance.
  2) Causing a tachycardia and thus increasing resistance to flow into the pulmonary artery by making the heart smaller and narrowing the RV outflow tract.

b) By inhaling amyl nitrite or taking a hot bath. This decreases peripheral resistance and favors flow from the RV into the aorta.

c) By crying. This increases pulmonary resistance and causes more RV blood to go out the aorta.

3.   How should you test for **clubbing** if it is equivocal or mild?

ANS.:   a) Look for obliteration of the normal angle between the base of the nail and the proximal skin [8].

b) If you can feel the loose end of the nail root, clubbing is probably present. Your palpating finger must point in the same direction as the patient's finger, i.e., you should approach the nail bed from behind and feel the edge of the nail root floating free while you depress the distal portion of the nail with another finger.

Note: No matter how severe the cyanosis, clubbing is rare before 3 months of age.

The earliest sign of clubbing is probably the reduction or absence of the groove where the root of the nail slips under the skin. Moist, warm fingertips are often associated signs.

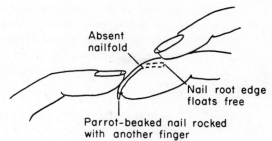

4. What is differential cyanosis and clubbing, and what is its significance?
    ANS.: If the hands are pink and the feet are blue, it means pulmonary hypertension with a right-to-left shunt via a PDA.

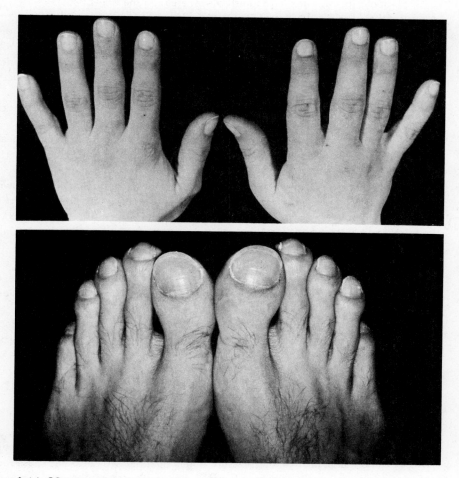

The feet of this 23-year-old man with a reversed shunt through a patent ductus were cyanotic and clubbed, while his hands were normal.

*5.   What is suggested by differential cyanosis and clubbing in which cyanosis and clubbing of the fingers are greater than that of the toes?

ANS.:   Complete transposition of the great vessels, with either a preductal coarctation or complete interruption of the aortic arch. Slightly less cyanosis of the left arm compared with the right favors coarctation rather than complete aortic interruption.

6.   What causes cyanotic cheeks?

ANS.:   The "malar flush" used to be considered a mitral facies. However, it can be seen in anyone with very low output and high pulmonary vascular resistance, high venous pressure, and loss of weight due to chronic heart failure (cardiac cachexia).

*7.   What should you suspect if the fingertips are red?

ANS.:   This is known as *tuft erythema* and may signify intermittent right-to-left shunts.

8.   What are the skin signs secondary to the small emboli of **infective endocarditis**?

ANS.:   Clubbing, splinter hemorrhages in the nails (not specific for emboli), and Osler's nodes (painful, tender, reddish brown areas on the finger pads).

9.   What is the cardiac significance of **Raynaud's phenomenon**?

ANS.:   It may presage primary pulmonary hypertension or a connective-tissue disease such as scleroderma (cardiac findings: myocardial fibrosis or **cor pulmonale**), disseminated lupus erythematosus (mitral valve vegetations or acute pericarditis as in Libman-Sacks syndrome), or polyarteritis (coronary artery obstruction and hypertension).

10.   What cardiac lesion is suggested by brownish, muddy pigmentation of the skin and signs of failure, such as loss of axillary and pubic hair?

ANS.:   Hemochromatosis with a cardiomyopathy due to iron deposits in the heart muscle, with secondary fibrosis.

*11.   With which cardiac condition is jaundice most likely to be associated?

ANS.:   a) Pulmonary infarction with reabsorption of pigment from broken-down red cells.
        b) High venous pressure due to severe TR, secondary to pulmonary hypertension.

*12.   What cardiac lesion is associated with multiple lentigines, i.e., multiple pigmented spots that, unlike freckles, begin at about age 6 and do not increase in number with sunlight?

ANS.:   Mild PS or hypertrophic subaortic stenosis [4, 14].

13.   With which cardiac conditions may you see facial flushing?

ANS.:   *a) Malignant carcinoid heart disease can cause a blotchy, cyanotic tinge, often associated with abdominal colic and bronchospasm. The cardiac lesions are fused tricuspid or pulmonary valves.
        b) If it occurs in the postsyncopal state, it suggests a **Stokes-Adams** attack. The high carbon dioxide levels resulting from the arrest cause marked vasodilation when circulation resumes.

Edema

1.   How should you elicit peripheral edema if it is slight?

ANS.:   Press for 10 sec with at least three fingers spread slightly apart, and feel for two hills between three valleys after release.

2.   What should you look for to rule out the heart quickly as a cause of peripheral edema?

ANS.:   A normal jugular venous pressure is incompatible with a cardiac cause for the edema unless diuretics have lowered venous pressure disproportionately to the relief of the edema.

Note: a) Only presacral edema may be present if the patient has been in bed for some time.

b) Peripheral edema is a common complaint in normal subjects, especially in women during their premenstrual periods or if they wear tight undergarments. It is expected in any obese subject and is probably due here to obstructed lymphatic drainage.

c) At least 10 pounds (4.5 kg) of body fluid must collect before pitting edema occurs.

EXTREMITIES

*1.   What cardiac lesion is suggested by short stature and cubitus valgus (medial deviation of the extended forearm)?

ANS.:   **Turner's syndrome**, with coarctation as a common abnormality.

*2.   Which extremity abnormalities are found with ASDs?

ANS.:   a) The thumb may have an extra phalanx ("fingerized thumb"), and it may lie in the same plane as the fingers, so that it is difficult to oppose thumb and fingers [1].

b) Distal radial and ulnar deformities, causing difficulty in supination and pronation.

Note: If (a) and (b) are present, it is the Holt-Oram syndrome, and the ASD is usually of the secundum type [5]. Pectus deformities of the sternum also occur [1].

3.   What hand and wrist signs suggest Marfan's syndrome with its possible cardiac abnormalities?

ANS.:   a) Thumb sign: When the fist is made over a clenched thumb, the thumb should not extend beyond the ulnar side of the hand. (False-positives occur in 1% of white children and 3% of black children.)

b) Wrist sign: When the wrist is encircled by the thumb and little finger (with light pressure), the little finger will overlap at least 1 cm in 80% of patients with Marfan's syndrome [15].

c) Fingers: Slender and long ("spider" fingers, or arachnodactyly).

Note: A forme fruste (incomplete form) of Marfan's syndrome with kyphoscoliosis, pectus carinatum (pigeon breast), and long extremities may occur in hemocystinuria, in which there may be thrombosing of intermediate-sized arteries, causing myocardial infarction.

*4.   Which is the only hand deformity ever correlated with rheumatic heart disease?

ANS.:   Ulnar deviation of the fourth or fifth fingers and flexion at the metacarpophalangeal joints. (This is Jaccoud's arthritis and is very rare.) The fingers can be moved freely into correct alignment [16].

*5.   What cardiac lesions are expected in an infant if the fingers are clenched, with the index finger crossing over the third finger?

ANS.:   This is characteristic of trisomy 16–18, in which a VSD or PDA is common. Also associated is double-outlet RV.

Note: The facies are abnormal, due to small mouth and jaw.

6.   Which is the commonest cardiac lesion associated with rheumatoid arthritic changes in the extremities?

ANS.:   Pericarditis and even occasional constriction.

*7.   What cardiac lesions are expected with polydactyly (an extra digit and often an extra toe),
      hypoplastic fingernails, and dwarfism?
      ANS.:   This is part of the Ellis-van Creveld syndrome (chondroectodermal dysplasia).
              About two-thirds of patients with this syndrome have an ASD or VSD and often
              an endocardial cushion defect of the complete atrioventricular canal type. A
              single atrium is also common.
                 Note: The upper lip of these patients is "tied" down to the alveolar ridge
              by multiple frenula. It is common among inbreeding communities, such as
              the Amish.

HEAD AND NECK

*1.   What cardiac abnormalities does neck webbing suggest?
      ANS.:   a) Turner's syndrome with coarctation, or
              b) **Noonan's syndrome**, or Ullrich's syndrome, with PS and, more rarely, hyper-
                 trophic cardiomyopathies [2, 10, 11, 13].
*2.   What is the facies of supravalvular aortic stenosis of the nonfamilial type?
      ANS.:   a) Broad, high forehead and puffy cheeks.
              b) Hypertelorism, strabismus, and sometimes epicanthal folds.
              c) Low ears.
              d) Upturned nose.
              e) Long upper lip and a wide mouth, with pouting, "cupid's-bow" lips.
              f) Hypoplasia of the mandible, with pointed chin and many dental abnormalities,
                 such as small teeth [2].
                 Note: These patients tend to have deep, somewhat metallic voices, are active,
              and have a happy outlook [9]. Some are mentally retarded.

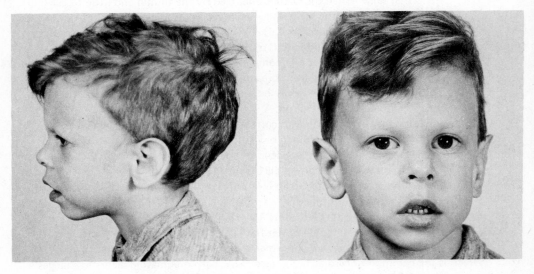

This boy with severe supravalvular aortic stenosis does not have all its facial characteristics; e.g.,
there is no hypertelorism or strabismus.

*3.   What is de Musset's sign? (Also called Musset's sign.)
       ANS.:   Head-bobbing movements secondary to the ballistic force of severe AR.
                Note: The sign was named after a patient, Alfred de Musset, a French poet
                whose nodding movements were described by his brother in a biography.
*4.   What is the facies of myxedema? What cardiac abnormalities are expected?
       ANS.:   a) Puffy lids and loss of outer third of the eyebrows.
                b) Scanty, dry hair and coarse, dry skin.
                c) Expressionless face and an enlarged tongue.
                Note: Myxedematous patients have **cardiomyopathies** due to increase in
                interstitial fluid and mucoid infiltration. They also have pericardial effusions.

CHEST AND RESPIRATION

1.   What cardiac abnormalities are suggested by a **pectus excavatum**?
       ANS.:   a) It may be **Marfan's syndrome**, with aortic or pulmonary artery aneurysms or
                   myxomatous degeneration of the mitral or aortic valve with regurgitation
                   (pectus carinatum, or pigeon breast, may also occur with Marfan's syndrome).
                b) It may be part of the straight back syndrome (see p. 270).
               *c) It may be **Noonan's syndrome**, with PS or occasionally with PDA.
2.   With what cardiac abnormality is a bilaterally increased anteroposterior chest diameter,
       sternal protrusion, and inspiratory indrawing of the lower ribs seen?
       ANS.:   Hyperkinetic pulmonary hypertension. (See p. 198 for explanation of types of
                pulmonary hypertension.) This is most commonly seen with a VSD [3].
3.   What should you suspect if only the left precordium bulges?
       ANS.:   An ASD with hyperkinetic pulmonary hypertension.
                Note: The RV never enlarges to the right; i.e., the right border of the heart on
                chest x-ray is never due to a RV, no matter how large it becomes.
4.   What should **Cheyne-Stokes** respiration suggest in a cardiac patient?
       ANS.:   Very low putput at rest.
5.   What is the significance of a short breath-holding time?
       ANS.:   It signifies either
                a) Chronic hyperventilation, or
                b) Poor psychophysical control of the breathing apparatus. The normal subject
                   (with his legs dangling) can hold his breath for 30 sec with a little encourage-
                   ment. Inability to hold it for at least 20 sec is abnormal and can explain
                   dyspnea on exertion.
                Note: Chronic hyperventilation may be either due to a pulmonary problem that
                should be apparent or to emotional factors, in which case it could account for non-
                descript episodes of chest pain, faintness, and syncope.
6.   What do dilated veins on the anterior chest wall signify?
       ANS.:   Obstruction to the superior vena cava, impeding flow to the right atrium, will
                cause dilated collateral veins on the chest wall with caudal flow. Obstruction to
                the inferior vena cava will cause the dilated chest veins to flow in a cephalad
                direction.

*7. What is a shield chest, and what does it suggest?

ANS.: It is a broad chest with a greater angle than usual between the manubrium and body of the sternum, as well as widely separated nipples. In a female with neck webbing, wide carrying angle, and short stature (under 5 feet in height) it suggests Turner's syndrome and concomitant coarctation. In a male it is called Noonan's or Ullrich's syndrome and is commonly associated with PS.

REFERENCES

1. Antia, A. U. Familial skeletal cardiovascular syndrome (Holt-Oram) in a polygamous African family. *Br. Heart J.* 32:241, 1970.

2. Beuren, A. J., Schultze, C., Eberle, P., Harmjanz, D., and Aptiz, J. The syndrome of supravalvular aortic stenosis, peripheral pulmonary stenosis, mental retardation and similar facial appearance. *Am. J. Cardiol.* 13:471, 1964.

3. Davies, H., Williams, J., and Wood, P. Lung stiffness in states of abnormal pulmonary blood flow and pressure. *Br. Heart J.* 24:129, 1962.

4. Gorlin, R. J., Anderson, R. C., and Blaw, M. Multiple lentigines syndrome. *Am. J. Dis. Child.* 117:652, 1969.

5. Holt, M., and Oram, S. Familial heart disease with skeletal malformations. *Br. Heart J.* 22:236, 1960.

6. King, S. P., and Franch, R. H. Production of increased right-to-left shunting by rapid heart rates in patients with tetralogy of Fallot. *Circulation* 44:265, 1971.

7. Kozam, R. L., Esguerra, O. E., and Smith, J. J. Cardiovascular beriberi. *Am. J. Cardiol.* 30:418, 1972.

8. Mellins, R. B., and Fishman, A. P. Digital casts for the study of clubbing of the fingers. *Circulation* 33:143, 1966.

9. Myers, A. R., and Willis, P. W., III. Clinical spectrum of supravalvular aortic stenosis. *Arch. Intern. Med.* 118:553, 1966.

10. Noonan, J. A. Hypertelorism with Turner phenotype. *Am. J. Dis. Child.* 116:373, 1968.

11. Phornphutkul, C., Rosenthal, A., and Nadas, A. S. Cardiomyopathy in Noonan's syndrome. *Br. Heart J.* 35:99, 1973.

12. Schrire, V., Beck, W., and Chesler, E. The heart and the eye. *Am. Heart J.* 85:122, 1973.

13. Siggers, D. C., and Polani, P. E. Congenital heart disease in male and female subjects with somatic features of Turner's syndrome and normal sex chromosomes (Ullrich's and related syndromes). *Br. Heart J.* 34:41, 1972.

14. Somerville, J., and Bonham-Carter, R. E. The heart in lentiginosis. *Br. Heart J.* 34:58, 1972.

15. Walker, B. A., and Murdoch, J. L. The wrist sign. *Arch. Intern. Med.* 126:276, 1970.

16. Zvaifler, N. J. Chronic postrheumatic fever (Jaccoud's) arthritis. *N. Engl. J. Med.* 267:10, 1962.

METHOD OF PALPATING THE ARM PULSES

1. Why is it best to palpate both the brachial and radial pulses of one arm at the same time?

   ANS.: a) It speeds up the physical examination, since one must examine both radials anyway.

   Note: A missing radial pulse is very likely due to arterial occlusive disease. If a radial pulse is absent, feel for unilateral absence of the ulnar pulse. An ulnar pulse is not normally unilaterally absent, although it may be bilaterally absent as a normal variant [27].

   b) One may estimate the blood pressure without a sphygmomanometer in this way.

2. How should you hold the arm for easy simultaneous palpation of the brachial and radial arteries?

   ANS.: Since the brachial artery is a medial vessel, it should be approached medially. The radial is a lateral vessel and should therefore be approached laterally.

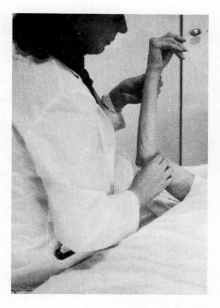

Simultaneous palpation of the radials and brachials speeds up the process and reminds you to palpate the brachials, where you can more easily appreciate rates of rise, the bisferiens pulse, pulse volume, and the hardened vessels of medial sclerosis.

---

* indicates material that is for electives or fellows in cardiology, or concerns rare phenomena, of interest primarily to cardiologists.

Boldface type indicates that the term is explained in the Glossary.

3.   When should you compress the brachial artery with the fingers, and when should you use a thumb?

ANS.:   If the brachial vessel has a good volume, the thumb is preferable because

a) The brachial may roll under the finger; the thumb is better able to fix it.

b) If more than one finger is used, a pulse wave may be felt to pass from the proximal to the distal finger, giving a false impression of a shoulder or even a double beating effect on the pulse.

The fingers, however, are actually more sensitive than the thumb and thus are better for small pulse pressures or volumes.

4.   Where should you look for the brachial artery relative to the biceps muscle?

ANS.:   In a younger patient, it may be hidden just under the biceps. In older patients, tortuosity of the brachials tends to bring these vessels out medially, away from the biceps.

Note: Some degree of arm flexion is often helpful, because extension hides the brachial pulsations in some patients.

5.   What are the questions you must answer as you palpate a peripheral pulse?

ANS.:   a) What is the rate of rise, i.e., is it slow, normal, or fast?

b) What is the contour of the rise, i.e., is there a shoulder on the upstroke or a midsystolic dip, shudder, or thrill?

c) What is the pulse volume or pulse pressure, i.e., is it small, normal, or large?

d) How hard is the vessel, i.e., does it roll too easily under the fingers?

e) What is the blood pressure?

RATES OF RISE

Normal Rates of Rise

1.   What is the significance of a normal rate of rise of an arterial pulse?

ANS.:   It suggests that there is no significant "fixed-orifice" obstruction to left ventricular (LV) outflow into the aorta, i.e., there is no **aortic stenosis.** It also suggests that there is no important obstruction in the arterial tree just proximal to the peripheral artery that is being palpated. (See p. 39 for an exception to this rule.) Therefore you feel only the sharp peak.

In subjects over age 45, however, the straight upward rise often ends in a change of slope to a late peak known as the tidal wave. The change of slope is called the anacrotic shoulder. It is often necessary to vary your finger pressure on the carotid to bring out an anacrotic shoulder. When the correct pressure is applied, you will feel a sharp tap, followed by a more slowly rising pulse.

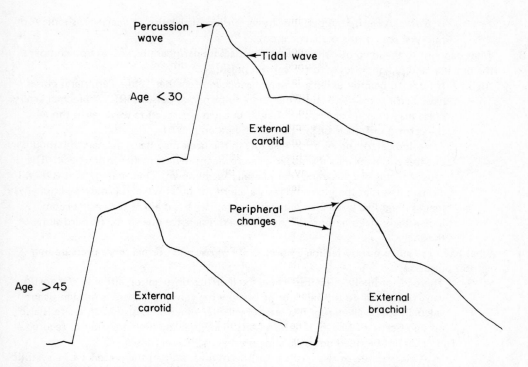

Percussion wave

←Tidal wave

Age < 30

External carotid

Age > 45

External carotid

Peripheral changes

External brachial

The normal percussion wave (first peak) is felt as a sharp tap. In the older age groups an ana-crotic shoulder occurs, resulting in a late tidal wave which is felt as a further outward motion after the initial tap. More peripherally, the shoulder to a high tidal wave disappears.

*2.   Why does the tidal wave increase with aging relative to the percussion wave and so finally develop an anacrotic shoulder?

ANS.:   The percussion wave occurs near the peak of velocity of flow; the tidal wave occurs at peak aortic pressure. The greater the peripheral resistance, the rela-tively higher is the tidal wave. It becomes relatively low after amyl nitrite lowers peripheral resistance and relatively high after administration of a vasopressor agent and with the decreased aortic distensibility of advancing age [24, 25].

After an artificial rise in blood pressure, the tidal wave (T) becomes higher than the percussion wave (P), just as in older age groups and in hypertension.

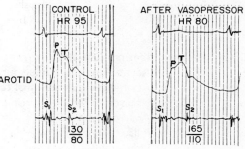

CONTROL   AFTER VASOPRESSOR
HR 95   HR 80

CAROTID

P   T   P   T

S₁   S₂   S₁   S₂

130   165
80   110

Note: A cardiomyopathy or hypertension may cause an anacrotic shoulder of the type seen in the older age group.

3.   What happens to the anacrotic shoulder as you palpate peripherally, i.e., as you compare the brachial and radial pulses with the carotid pulse?

ANS.:   It tends to be attenuated and may disappear altogether [25]. Peripheral pulses have a straighter rise or upstroke than do proximal pulses [59]. A brachial artery pulse may have no anacrotic shoulder but just a percussion wave, even though the carotid may have both. (See the figure on p. 37.)

As indicated, the carotid pulse low in the neck may have an anacrotic shoulder, but this shoulder may disappear just a few centimeters higher in the neck. The cause for this disappearance peripherally is unknown. One analogy that is used to explain it is that the increased resistance to the pulse wave as it moves peripherally makes it act like a wave coming into shore, i.e., the crest of the wave becomes increasingly steep because of the increased resistance due to the upward slope of the shore.

4.   What have you ruled out by feeling a normal rate of rise and normal pulse pressure in a carotid pulse?

ANS.:   There is not likely to be important fixed-orifice obstruction either at the aortic valve, just distal to the valve, or just below the valve, i.e., there is no significant valvular, supravalvular, or discrete subvalvular aortic stenosis (AS). There is also no significant aortic regurgitation (AR). However, mild obstruction or regurgitation cannot be ruled out by feeling normal peripheral pulses.

A normal rate of rise in the elderly is of great help in the presence of a systolic murmur that sounds like the murmur of AS but is really due to **calcific aortic sclerosis**. The murmur in the presence of normal pulses is probably the 50/50 murmur (see p. 273).

Slow Rates of Rise

1.   How can you recognize a slow rate of rise by palpation?

ANS.:   A caressing lift will be felt as a gently undulating, rounded rise and fall. There is no tapping sensation, only a push or nudge.

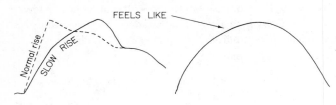

The normal rise is a tap; the slow rise is a caress.

2.   What conditions produce a slowly rising pulse?

ANS.:   a) Aortic stenosis, valvular, supravalvular, or discrete subvalvular.

b) Arterial stenosis proximal to the site of palpation.

3.   List the names given to the slowly rising pulse of AS.

ANS.:   a) Anacrotic pulse.

b) Pulsus parvus.

c) Plateau pulse.

4.   What is meant by an anacrotic pulse?

ANS.:   Anacrotic is derived from the Greek *ana,* meaning "up," and *krotos,* meaning "beat." The literal translation of an "upbeat pulse" has no meaning. By usage, however, the term has come to mean any slowly rising pulse. Since the literal meaning is so far from the usage meaning, the term is best avoided.

Note: The terms *anacrotic shoulder* and *anacrotic notch* are useful terms to retain since they refer to a shoulder or notch on the upstroke.

5.   Why is the term *plateau pulse* often appropriate?

ANS.:   Because with moderate finger pressure, an apparently normal initial rise is followed by a sustained **thrill**, during which the pulse does not seem to rise or rises very little. This kind of pulse is usually only palpable in the carotid.

If an almost normal tap is followed by a sustained thrill, this is the plateau pulse of AS. In the above figure L$_2$ = lead 2, and 2 RIS means that the microphone was in the second right interspace.

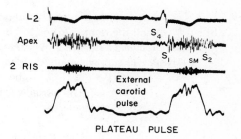

PLATEAU PULSE

Note: A thrill on the upstroke of a carotid is sometimes called a *carotid shudder,* a term that historically was introduced to describe a very short vibration effect that occurs when a patient with combined AS and regurgitation has the double systolic outward movement known now as a bisferiens pulse (see p. 42).

(see p. 42)

6.   What happens to the height of an anacrotic shoulder in a patient with AS as you palpate more and more peripherally?

ANS.:   The anacrotic shoulder tends to move higher and may even disappear if the AS is mild or moderate.

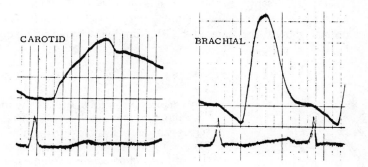

Carotid and brachial pulse contours in a patient with mild AS. By the time the pulse wave reached the brachials, it had become normal.

Note: If the AS is significant or the ventricular contraction weak, an anacrotic shoulder will not disappear at the periphery.

7. What does a slow upstroke of the carotid pulse tell you about the degree of aortic valve **gradient**?

ANS.:   In the presence of a fairly normal myocardium, the gradient is probably over 50 mm Hg.

Note: a) If the patient has a **cardiomyopathy,** then even in mild AS there may be a slowly rising pulse that is transmitted to the periphery. If, however, the aorta is very rigid due to **medial sclerosis,** as in elderly patients, the percussion wave is exaggerated, and no anacrotic pulse is felt. In this situation, only an ejection time (see p. 386) will tell you that AS is the cause of the failure.

*b) If a hypertensive patient with AS has a normal rate of rise, lowering the blood pressure can bring out the anacrotic shoulder.

*8. When will the right carotids and brachials have a normal rate of rise and the left carotids and brachials a slow rise? Why?

ANS.:   In supravalvular AS, in which there is streaming of the jet toward the innominate artery.

Note: The pulses will also be stronger and the blood pressure higher on the right than on the left.

Fast Rates of Rise with Normal Pulse Pressure

1. In which conditions are there very rapid rates of rise but normal pulse pressures?

ANS.:   a) If a large volume in the LV is being ejected through two orifices, i.e., mitral regurgitation (MR) or **ventricular septal defect** (VSD). (See Glossary for explanation of VSD and its hemodynamics.)

b) If there is left ventricular hypertrophy (LVH) due to a delayed obstruction to outflow, as in **hypertrophic subaortic stenosis** (HSS) (see p. 39).

2. Why is there an increased volume in the LV in MR?

ANS.:   During diastole the ventricle receives from the left atrium both the blood it would normally receive from the pulmonary veins plus the blood regurgitated backward into the left atrium during the previous ventricular systole.

Note: The same reasoning explains the large volume in the LV in VSDs; i.e., the LV must receive the blood it shunted into the right ventricle (RV), as well as the normal amounts that entered the RV from the systemic circulation.

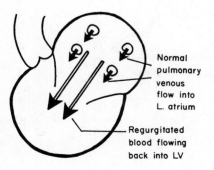

Normal pulmonary venous flow into L. atrium

Regurgitated blood flowing back into LV

This depicts the extra diastolic flow through the mitral valve that takes place when MR occurs during the previous ventricular systole. In MR, the normal pulmonary venous return to the LV is added to the returning regurgitant flow to increase the volume in the LV beyond normal. Thus, in MR, the left atrium is volume-overloaded during ventricular systole and the LV is volume-overloaded during ventricular diastole.

3. Why does the ejection of a large volume in the LV produce a rapid rate of rise in the peripheral arteries if there are two outlets for systole, as in MR or VSD?

ANS.: The stretched myocardium at the end of diastole creates a **Starling effect**. Therefore, during systole the two outlets (mitral and aortic valves or VSD and aortic valves) receive their share of the blood with greater velocity. The fact that the period of ejection into the aorta is no longer than normal in MR or VSD demonstrates that the LV does not take longer than normal to eject its larger volume. Therefore, it must be moving it at a very rapid rate.

Note that the arrows representing ejection into the aorta are equal, i.e., the forward stroke volume in MR is not reduced unless the MR is very severe or there is cardiac damage.

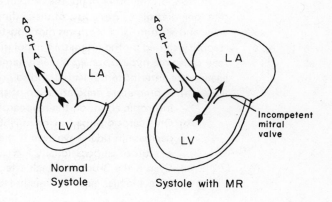

Normal Systole

Systole with MR

Incompetent mitral valve

4. In what kind of AS is there a rapid rate of rise? Why?

ANS.: Hypertrophic subaortic stenosis. In HSS, there is no obstruction until the outflow tract contracts and approximates the septum to the mitral valve. (See figure on p. 277.) When the LV contracts, the **inflow tract** contracts first and the outflow tract (see under **inflow tract**) contracts last. In HSS, early systole is so rapid that as much as 80% of ejection has already occurred during the first third of systole.

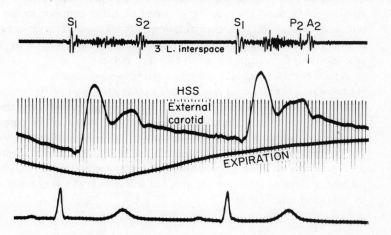

S₁   S₂   S₁   P₂ A₂
3 L. interspace

HSS
External
carotid

EXPIRATION

This is a phonocardiogram and pulse tracing from a 34-year-old woman with HSS. The outflow gradient was 70 mm Hg. Some mitral regurgitation was present. There was an S_3 on auscultation and a large LV on x-ray. Note the rapid rate of rise to a high percussion wave and the midsystolic dip that produce the "pointed-finger" carotid pulse contour.

*5.   How can a pulse pressure following a premature ventricular contraction (PVC) help to
       diagnose HSS?
       ANS.:   In HSS, the pulse pressure of the post-PVC beat often is the same or smaller than
                that of the normal beats [77] . This is known as the Brockenbrough effect, and
                it occurs in only about a third of patients with HSS. In normal subjects or in
                those with AS due to a fixed obstruction, the Starling effect of the long diastole
                on the LV produces a greater stroke volume and a pulse with a larger amplitude
                than the normal pulse.

                In HSS, on the other hand, the drop in aortic pressure that occurs by the end
                of a long diastole causes a loss of distending force for the LV outflow tract (mitral
                valve and septum) and produces more obstruction. Furthermore, increased con-
                tractility caused by the premature depolarization, as well as by the Starling effect,
                may cause the hypertrophied hyperdynamic septum to clamp down more tightly
                against the anterior mitral leaflet and so produce more obstruction.

                Note: a) A premature depolarization of the ventricle produces an increased
                            inotropic effect on the myocardium for unknown reasons.
                         b) On a carotid pulse tracing in HSS the post-PVC beat will show a
                            decrease in tidal wave even if the overall pulse pressure is widened as
                            a result of an occasionally increased percussion wave [19] .
                         c) Even if the Brockenbrough effect is negative, the post-PVC beat will
                            have a longer ejection time in HSS and a shorter ejection time in valvular
                            AS.

6.   What are some names given to the pulse with a rapid rate of rise but with a normal pulse
       volume?
       ANS.:   A brisk or jerky pulse.

Rapid Rates of Rise with Increased Pulse Pressures

1.   What should be thought of if there is a rapid rate of rise and a large pulse volume?
       ANS.:   Although AR causes the most rapid rise of all, other common causes are **patent
                ductus arteriosus** (PDA) and **coarctation**. Thyrotoxicosis, pregnancy, and severe
                anemia may also cause rapidly rising, bounding pulses. More rarely, a large
                arteriovenous fistula may cause this kind of pulse.
                Note: A PDA is actually a kind of arteriovenous fistula.

2.   Why should there be a rapid rate of rise and large pulse pressure in AR?
       ANS.:   When the ventricle expands in diastole in AR, it receives not only the regurgitated
                blood that leaks back from the aorta but also the normal blood coming from the
                lung via the pulmonary veins and left atrium through the mitral valve. Therefore,
                the LV receives blood from two sources and is stretched at end-diastole to produce
                a Starling effect. Since there is only one outlet for systole, it takes longer than
                normal to eject its increased volume, but still does it at a very rapid rate because
                of the end-diastolic stretch.

This illustration represents ventricular diastole in a patient with aortic regurgitation. The reason for the large volume in diastole in AR is obvious, since the LV fills from two sources. As long as the LV is healthy, it will eject the usual 60–75% of its increased end-diastolic volume, i.e., its ejection fraction will remain normal. Thus, the aorta will receive a large stroke volume with each systole.

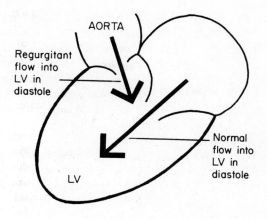

AORTA

Regurgitant flow into LV in diastole

Normal flow into LV in diastole

LV

*3.   How can you exaggerate the rapid rate of rise of AR?

ANS.:   By raising the patient's arm high or by having him stand up [29, 30]. (In subjects *without* AR, standing produces a decrease in the rate of rise.)

   Note: In patients with AR, the increased rate of rise of the pulse on standing does not mean that more AR occurs on standing. Since the tendency to increase the amount of AR caused by the increased peripheral resistance on standing is attenuated by the decreased venous return, there is no change in the quantity of the AR [29].

   The rate of rise of brachial pressure increases on standing in patients with AR and not in normal subjects because the supine AR patient has more peripheral vasodilation than normal (which produces the low diastolic pressure). Therefore, he may have less sympathetic tone than normal in the supine position. When he stands, an exaggerated increase in sympathetic tone occurs because of the need for enough peripheral vasoconstriction to maintain mean pressure. The increased catecholamines or sympathetic outflow causes a more rapid rate of rise of the peripheral pulses [29].

4.   What are some of the names given to the pulse in AR?

ANS.:   *a) **Corrigan's pulse** [14].
   *b) **Water-hammer** pulse.
   *c) Collapsing pulse.
   d) Bounding pulse.

   Note: Since the term *Corrigan's pulse* omits the description of what you feel, *water-hammer pulse* requires that you remember the name of an obsolete toy (see p. 425), and *collapsing pulse* omits the rate of rise, it may be best to call it a *bounding pulse,* or simply to describe it as a rapidly rising or slapping pulse with a large volume.

5.   Why is there a large volume in the LV in PDA, creating a rapid rise and large pulse pressure?

ANS.:   The LV receives both the blood shunted from the aorta to the pulmonary artery and the normal pulmonary venous blood (see **patent ductus arteriosus**).

6.   When may severe AR not produce a large-volume pulse pressure?
     ANS.:   In sudden, severe AR, for the following reasons:
              a) The stroke volume may be low or normal because the high diastolic pressure
                 in the LV may close the mitral valve in mid-diastole (premature closure of
                 mitral valve) and limit filling from the left atrium.
              b) The aortic diastolic pressure may not drop very low because the low output
                 and absence of large pulse pressure may keep the peripheral resistance high.

7.   What traditionally characteristic signs of severe AR can be picked up by auscultation of
     the femoral arteries?
     ANS.:   a) Traube's "pistol-shot femorals," the loud sound heard when the stethoscope
                 is placed over the rapidly rising large-volume pulsations of femoral artery.
              Note: Venous pistol-shot sounds have been described as the loud systolic
              sounds heard over a femoral vein in the presence of severe tricuspid regurgita-
              tion [35].
              b) Duroziez's double murmur; this is
                 1) The systolic murmur produced by placing the stethoscope chest piece on
                    the femoral artery and gradually compressing the artery proximally, plus
                 2) The diastolic murmur produced by gradually compressing the artery distal
                    to the stethoscope. This murmur is due to backflow as the blood in all the
                    large arteries flows backward toward the aorta in diastole [7, 58].
              Note: a) A double sound over the groin can be heard when a strong atrial
                        contraction occurs. The first sound is from the femoral vein and the
                        second, from the femoral artery [1].
                     b) These signs are more of historical than practical interest, since the
                        same information is usually gained by the time the palpation of the
                        pulses and the taking of the blood pressure are completed.

PULSUS BISFERIENS

1.   What is meant by a bisferiens pulse?
     ANS.:   *Bis* means "twice," and *feriens* means "beating," i.e., it is a twice-beating pulse.
             Actually, it is a double-peaked pulse, the two peaks occurring during systole.

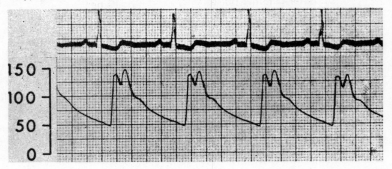

This bisferiens pulse was found in a brachial intra-arterial pressure tracing from a patient with AR.
The midsystolic dip that produces this bisferiens pulse is due to the rapid ejection of the excessive
volume in the LV.

2.   What causes the bisferiens pulse in patients with a good pulse volume?

ANS.:   Since it is associated with a rapid ejection of blood through the aortic valve early in systole, one theory proposes that at the peak of flow there is a **Bernoulli effect** on the walls of the ascending aorta, causing a sudden fall in pressure on the inner aspect of the aortic walls. Support for this theory is found in the correspondence of the dip in pressure with the time of the peak flow rate through the valve.

3.   What causes the most marked bisferiens pulse? Why?

ANS.:   A combination of moderate AS and severe AR [78]. Moderate AS causes an extra high-velocity jet to be shot out, and this is exaggerated by an increased volume flow due to severe AR during the previous diastole. In 1945, *carotid shudder* was suggested as a term for this double pulse movement [17].

   Note: A bisferiens pulse will not be present if myocardial contractility is depressed [36].

The fall in lateral-wall pressure during peak velocity requires a high velocity of ejection. This implies the presence of a relatively healthy myocardium.

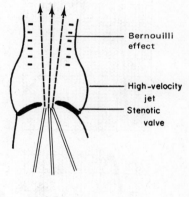

Bernouilli effect

High-velocity jet

Stenotic valve

AS + AR

4.   Can normal subjects have a bisferiens pulse?

ANS.:   Yes, if the term *bisferiens* is used to refer to a very slight double peak at the height of systole. It may merely signify a hyperkinetic circulatory state. This slight bisferiens often feels like a short thrill at the peak of the carotid pulse. If it is subtle, it will often be picked up only with just the right amount of external pressure on the artery.

   Note: A bisferiens pulse can be picked up by an intra-aortic tracing only if it is marked.

*5.   What kind of pure AS can produce a bisferiens pulse?

ANS.:   Hypertrophic subaortic stenosis, because in this condition there is initially no obstruction to outflow, and about 80% of the entire stroke volume is ejected in early systole. The obstruction occurs in midsystole, when the mitral valve approximates the hypertrophied septal area. Then there is a sudden dip in the pulse as flow virtually ceases, followed by a secondary rise as the LV overcomes the obstruction.

   Note: a) The cessation of flow in midsystole can be shown by Doppler techniques.

b) The bisferiens pulse in HSS is often difficult to feel and is a relatively rare palpatory phenomenon; nor is the midsystolic retraction seen in the external carotid tracing of some patients with the ballooned (prolapsed) valve syndrome (see p. 308) usually palpable [3] .

*THE PALPABLE DICROTIC WAVE

*1.   What is the dicrotic wave?
      ANS.:   The small wave that follows the dicrotic notch in an external carotid pressure trac-
              ing. (When the same notch is referred to in an aortic pressure tracing, the word
              incisura is more commonly used.)

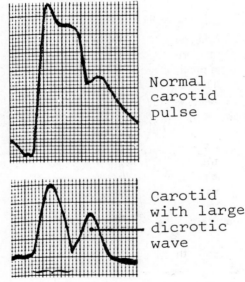

Normal
carotid
pulse

Carotid
with large
dicrotic
wave

Short ejection time

At first glance, a large dicrotic wave gives the appearance of a bisferiens pulse because of the short ejection time seen in all patients with severe heart failure; the large dicrotic wave is usually seen only in such patients.

*2.   When does a dicrotic wave become palpable?
      ANS.:   When there is a very low output and a soft, elastic aorta. The commonest causes
              of a palpable dicrotic wave are:
              a) Severe congestive failure, usually secondary either to an idiopathic or an alcoholic
                 cardiomyopathy.
              b) **Tamponade** [49] .
              c) The low output state following open heart surgery, especially after aortic valve
                 replacement for AR [2] .
              Note: a) A low stroke volume is probably necessary to produce a palpable dicrotic
                     wave, since it is more likely to appear or to become accentuated after a
                     sudden short diastole, after the weaker beats of a pulsus alternans, in the
                     straining phase of a Valsalva maneuver, the inspiratory phase of respira-
                     tion, or when there is a pulse rate of over 90.

b) Soft, elastic blood vessels seem to be necessary to make a dicrotic wave palpable, as shown by the rarity of the palpable dicrotic wave when blood pressure is over 140 and in subjects over 40 [49].

c) Occlusive pressure distal to the site of palpation will tend to bring out the dicrotic wave during inspiration.

*3. What are the quantitative characteristics of the indirect carotid pulse wave in a patient with dicrotism, i.e., with an excessive dicrotic wave?

ANS.: a) The dicrotic notch is abnormally low, i.e., 10% or less of the total pulse pressure [18].

b) From dicrotic notch to peak of the dicrotic wave is about 50% or more of the pulse pressure [18].

PALPATION OF THE PERIPHERAL LEG PULSES

1. What can you learn about the heart from palpating the popliteal arteries?

ANS.: Enough peripheral vascular disease of the lower extremities to produce **intermittent claudication** is highly correlated with the presence of coronary disease.

2. What is the most important aid in palpating the popliteal pulses?

ANS.: You must not try to feel the popliteal blood vessel, but instead must concentrate on trying to feel an area of transmitted pulsation. You may only feel this as a faint, diffuse pulsatile mass in a small segment of popliteal space. It does not feel like a carotid or brachial artery.

3. How do you examine for faint popliteal pulses with the patient in the supine position?

ANS.: a) Place the fingers of both hands in the popliteal space with the palms of your hands in complete contact with the patient's skin. (Air over one part of the palm with skin over another part may prevent the detection of a faint pulsatile kinesthetic sensation in one area.)

b) Relax the muscles around the popliteal area by bouncing his knee up and down a few times.

c) Squeeze with the entire hand (i.e., with the thumbs as well as the fingers), so that the sensation is equal all through the hand.

It will not be necessary to place the patient in the prone position if you remember that the key to popliteal palpation is to feel for an area of transmitted pulsation.

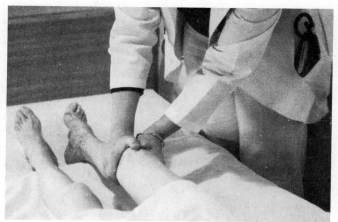

4.   How can you sometimes bring out a faint posterior tibial or dorsalis pedis pulse?

ANS.:   Maximum dorsiflexion. Use two hands and dorsiflex the foot to various degrees
        with one hand as you palpate with the other. A tendon passes diagonally over
        the dorsalis pedis, and the extensor retinaculum of the ankle crosses perpendicu-
        larly over it. Plantar flexion may tighten these overlying structures and obliterate
        the pulse. Dorsiflexion separates them from the artery beneath them.

        Note: There are many normal variations of foot pulses. The dorsalis pedis may
        not be palpable in the usual line between the great and index toe, or may be absent
        in as many as 10% of normal subjects [37]. Normal adult subjects may have a
        palpable posterior tibial or dorsalis pedis only on one side.

        The foot pulses are more important to palpate as a baseline for future follow-up
        when you are looking for the development of peripheral vascular problems.

BLOOD PRESSURE

1.   What controls arterial systolic and diastolic pressure levels?

ANS.:   Systolic blood pressure (the highest pressure reached by the arteries) is controlled
        by the stroke volume of the heart and the stiffness of the arterial systemic vessels
        that receive the stroke volume. Diastolic blood pressure (the lowest pressure found
        in the aorta and its branches after maximal runoff into the periphery) is controlled
        primarily by peripheral resistance.

2.   What is normal blood pressure?

ANS.:   In the adult, the upper limit of normal blood pressure should probably be con-
        sidered to be about 140/90 mm Hg.

        *In infants and children, you may use the rule that by age 1 year the systolic
        pressure is about 90 mm Hg and increases by 5 mm Hg about every three years,
        so that by age 13 or 14, it has reached the adult level of 120 mm Hg.

        A rough rule of thumb then would be that the systolic blood pressure in a child
        would be roughly:

$$90 + \frac{(\text{the age} \times 5)}{3}$$

        The diastolic pressure tends to be about 60 ± 10 mm Hg in infants and children of
        all ages.

3.   What can cause a rise in systolic pressure and leave diastolic pressure normal?

ANS.:   "Pipestem" blood vessels, secondary to medial sclerosis in elderly patients. Their
        sclerotic arteries are relatively nondistensible.

4.   Does AS usually cause a blood pressure that is lower than normal?

ANS.:   No. This is because, first, the stroke volume may be maintained even with severe
        obstruction by such compensatory mechanisms as LVH and an increased left atrial
        contraction, which causes a high **filling pressure** in the LV. Second, as the stroke
        volume falls, peripheral resistance rises and keeps the blood pressure normal. In
        very severe AS, however, a decrease in blood pressure may occur as the patient
        goes into failure.

        Note: The highest blood pressure reported in severe valvular AS is 280/140
        mm Hg.

5. How does AR affect blood pressure?

ANS.: The increased stroke volume causes a higher systolic pressure than normal, while the decreased peripheral resistance causes a lower diastolic pressure than normal. However, in young subjects with soft blood vessels, even severe AR may not raise the blood pressure to more than about 140 mm Hg. In older patients with stiff vessels, even moderate AR may raise the systolic pressure to as high as 180 mm Hg. In hypertensive patients, the increased peripheral resistance can produce a normal or even high diastolic pressure, despite severe AR.

Note: The low diastolic blood pressure in AR is due mostly to the low peripheral resistance that is presumably a reflex response to the large pulse pressure in the carotid and aortic baroreceptors.

BLOOD PRESSURE DIFFERENCES IN THE ARMS

1. What should you suspect if the blood pressure is higher in one arm than in the other?

ANS.: a) If it is higher on the right, it may be due to supravalvular AS, which directs its jet preferentially up the innominate artery. A difference in carotid pulsation, as well as the presence of a murmur of AS, gives you additional helpful information. (See p. 30 for the facies of supravalvular AS.)
b) Arterial obstructive disease may be present.
c) It may be an artifact due to the lack of simultaneous recording.

2. In what percentage of patients is there a difference in systolic blood pressure between the arms of 10 mm Hg or more, if the pressure in both arms is taken (a) separately or (b) simultaneously?

ANS.: If taken separately, 25% of patients will have this difference in systolic blood pressure. If taken simultaneously, only 5% will have such a difference [32].

Note: A difference of over 20 mm Hg between the arms, even when not taken simultaneously, occurs in only 5% of normal arms and therefore should be looked on with suspicion.

3. In what percentage of patients is there a difference of 10 mm Hg or more in *diastolic* pressure between the arms if the pressure in both arms is taken (a) separately or (b) simultaneously?

ANS.: If pressures are taken separately, about 15% will have such a difference in blood pressure. If pressures are taken simultaneously, only 5% will have such a difference [32].

Note: The greatest normal differences between arms tends to occur in hypertensive patients.

*4. Why should you take the blood pressure in both arms if the history suggests vertebral-basilar insufficiency?

ANS.: If the blood pressure is lower in one arm than the other, a **subclavian steal** should be suspected [68]. (See Checklist, p. 14.)

*BLOOD PRESSURE BY PALPATION ALONE

*1. How can you take a systolic blood pressure by palpation alone, i.e., without a blood pressure cuff or stethoscope?

ANS.:   While simultaneously palpating the brachials and radials, apply slight, moderate, and marked pressure on the brachials in an attempt to obliterate pulse transmission to the radial. If slight pressure on the brachial obliterates the radial pulse, the systolic pressure is probably 120 mm Hg or less. If it takes moderate pressure, the pressure is probably between 120 and 160. If it requires marked pressure, the blood pressure is probably over 160 mm Hg.

Note: If too little pressure is applied to the radials, the pulse will appear to be falsely obliterated. If you do not apply a pressure on the brachial artery perpendicular to a tangent to the arm, but instead push the artery to one side, no amount of pressure on the brachial will obliterate the radial pulse. Comparing both arms helps to counteract a false reading.

*2.   How can you take a blood pressure by cuff (sphygmomanometer) and palpation alone, i.e., without auscultation?

ANS.:   With the thumb on the brachial just under the distal edge of the cuff, you can easily palpate the systolic pressure as the cuff is deflated and the pulse returns. As the cuff is further deflated toward diastole, the brachial pulse becomes more slapping and hyperdynamic, until a point is reached when it suddenly changes to a more normal rate of rise. This point correlates well with the diastolic pressure at about the time of muffling [16]. Blood pressure by palpation is closely correlated with that taken by auscultation [55].

Note: a) The diastolic point is difficult to appreciate at the radial pulse.

b) It is useful to obtain the diastolic pressure by palpation alone in subjects in shock and in those without a sharp disappearance or muffling point, as in AR, when the Korotkoff sounds may be heard down to zero [16].

KOROTKOFF SOUNDS

1.   What is meant by Korotkoff sounds?

ANS.:   The sounds produced by the pulsations of the artery under a partially constricting blood pressure cuff (described by the Russian physician Korotkoff in 1905).

Note: Arterial-wall oscillations have been shown to cause the major components of the sounds [69].

2.   Does one hear the heart sounds at the brachial area?

ANS.:   Rarely. If they are very loud, they may be transmitted by bone conduction to that area, e.g., prosthetic aortic valve sounds. Korotkoff sounds, however, are *not* transmitted heart sounds.

3.   What can make the Korotkoff sounds difficult to hear?

ANS.:   a) A slow rate of rise in pressure, as in AS.

b) Poor blood flow to the limbs.

c) A poor myocardial contraction and small pulse pressure, as in shock.

4.   How can inaudible blood pressure sounds in a limb be made audible, or soft ones made louder?

ANS.:   a) Have the subject open and close his fist about 10 times. If the popliteal or foot blood pressure is being taken, have him flex and extend the ankle. This increases flow and dilates the forearm or leg blood vessels. Thus, it may increase the gradient of blood volume and pressure between the proximal and distal cuff blood vessels.

Note: Mildly exercising the hand or foot does not affect blood pressure.

b) Elevate the arm before you inflate the cuff. This empties the vessel beyond the cuff, thus increasing the gradient between the arteries proximal and distal to the cuff [5].

c) Inflate the cuff quickly. This diminishes the venous inflow into the vessels distal to the cuff by the time the arterial flow is cut off. This decreases the tissue pressure distal to the cuff and thus increases the flow gradient for the arterial blood passing under the cuff.

5.   Which is the true diastolic pressure, the point of muffling or the disappearance of the Korotkoff sounds?

ANS.:   Comparative studies have shown that muffling is about 10 mm Hg higher than the diastolic pressure by direct intra-arterial needle [26]. The disappearance point is probably more accurate when compared with the intra-arterial manometer in the brachial artery beyond the cuff [45]. In hyperkinetic states such as AR, however, the disappearance point is often very low and also far from the muffling point. In AR, muffling is probably closer to the true intra-arterial diastolic pressure. When the disappearance point is over 10 mm Hg from the muffling point, muffling is probably the more accurate. Recording both the muffling and the disappearance point aids in communication. Thus, a blood pressure might read: 140/70—40.

6.   What are the other advantages of taking the disappearance point rather than muffling as the diastolic pressure?

ANS.:   a) Among physicians, there has been more agreement as to where the disappearance point is than where muffling is. The muffling point has often been controversial because the sounds sometimes change suddenly from loud tapping to quieter tapping to full muffling. Some take the quieter tapping and others take the full muffling as the diastolic point [63].

b) Since the disappearance point will give a slightly lower diastolic pressure, you are less likely to overtreat on the basis of a questionable blood pressure elevation.

c) Repeatedly clenching the fists can eliminate the muffling phase altogether, suggesting its unreliability [61].

Note: The idea of muffling was introduced as denoting diastolic blood pressure by Erlanger in 1921, in an experiment in which an exposed segment of artery with blood pumped into it from the heart was enclosed within an air compression chamber. As the pressure in the chamber was reduced, the Korotkoff sounds muffled just as the artery first became full and round throughout the pulse cycle. Low-frequency muffled sounds (fourth phase of Korotkoff sounds) continued for a further short period of decompression [23].

7.   Is the systolic blood pressure higher by palpation or by auscultation?

ANS.:   The blood pressure by auscultation is higher because the Korotkoff sounds are heard with the slightest pulse movement at the edge of the cuff (at least 5—10 mm Hg higher than by palpation).

8.   Why should you record blood pressure to the nearest 5 or 10 mm Hg despite the fact that manometer dials are graduated in increments of 2?

ANS.:   Recording a blood pressure as 132 instead of 130 mm Hg gives a false sense of accuracy because

a) The blood pressure changes by at least 2 mm spontaneously from moment to moment.

b) The Korotkoff sounds will occur at different levels of cuff deflation if different observors have differences in hearing acuity, deflate or inflate the cuffs at different rates, have different concepts of the diastolic end point, or place the stethoscope at different sites.

c) It is easier to remember three numbers than six numbers between each 10 mm Hg. For example, between 120 and 130 are only 120, 125, and 130 if you record the blood pressure to the nearest 5 or 10; but to the nearest two there are six possibilities, namely, 120, 122, 124, 126, 128, and 130.

9.   When taking blood pressure, where should you place the stethoscope chest piece in relation to the cuff?

ANS.:   As close to the cuff edge as possible, preferably partly under the edge of the cuff. The farther the stethoscope is from the cuff edge, the softer will be the Korotkoff sounds. A diaphragm placed completely under the cuff produces the loudest Korotkoff sounds of all. Even if no Korotkoff sounds at all are heard at the edge of the cuff (as in shock), they can be heard if the diaphragm is placed under the cuff [80].

10.   Should a bell or a diaphragm be used for Korotkoff sounds?

ANS.:   Since soft Korotkoff sounds consist mostly of low and medium **frequencies**, it seems logical that the bell should be used. But it is difficult to get a good air seal on a rounded arm with a large-diameter bell. Since the edge of the diaphragm can be slipped under the cuff edge (and most diaphragms are not very efficient in attenuating low and medium frequencies), it usually makes little difference whether a bell or diaphragm is used. When the sounds are soft, however, it sometimes helps to apply the bell.

*DOPPLER METHOD OF TAKING A BLOOD PRESSURE

*1.   What is a Doppler instrument?

ANS.:   A Doppler instrument has a probe that generates a beam of high-frequency sound. In accordance with the Doppler principle, motion in the path of the sound beam will alter the frequency of the sound. The sound is reflected back into the probe, which can also receive sound. When the instrument placed over a blood vessel receives reflected sound that differs in frequency from the transmitted sound, an audible signal is heard (via an amplifier) that is due to the motion of blood through the vessel. The motion of a blood vessel pulsating can itself also be made to produce sounds.

*2.   When is it especially useful to take blood pressure by Doppler probe rather than by stethoscope?

ANS.:   a) In infants [34].

b) In legs, especially when there is arterial occlusive disease, coarctation, or low output states [11].

c) In shock states [8].

d) In noisy rooms.

e) During cardiopulmonary resuscitation to test for effectiveness of blood flow [74
   Note: The blood pressure obtained by a Doppler probe can be accepted as the sam
as that obtained with a stethoscope [9, 72].

SOURCES OF ERROR IN TAKING BLOOD PRESSURE

1. What is meant by an accurate zero recording for an aneroid manometer?

   ANS.: The zero recording is accurate if the indicator needle is within the zero circle on the dial. The manometer is more likely to be accurate if an accurate zero recording is present, but it still must be periodically checked against a mercury manometer.

   Note: About 15% of hospital manometers were found to be wrong by about 10 mm Hg or more when tested against a mercury manometer [54]. There appears to be no place for an aneroid manometer in office practice, where bulk is not a significant deterrent to using the more accurate and stable mercury manometer.

2. What precautions must be taken in recording a sitting or standing blood pressure in the arm?

   ANS.: The brachial artery must be at heart level. If it is below heart level, gravity will add its pressure to the brachial artery pressure.

3. What is the advantage of beginning to decrease the inflation pressure slowly?

   ANS.: Spasm of the artery occurs on initial compression. Also, the patient may have anxiety and apprehension on feeling the discomfort of the pressure. This would make the blood pressure too high. Slow deflation will give spasm and anxiety a chance to disappear by the time blood flow occurs under the cuff.

   Note: Deflation of a mercury manometer cuff at the slow rate of 2–3 mm Hg per heartbeat is usually recommended to prevent air pockets from forming above the mercury column.

4. What errors occur if the rubber part of the cuff balloons beyond its covering, or if the cuff is so loose that central ballooning occurs?

   ANS.: Both will require excessive cuff pressure to compress the artery, and the readings will be falsely high.

5. How does the blood pressure with an average cuff on a fat arm compare with intra-arterial pressure?

   ANS.: Since the cuff will be too small, most often the pressure is too high, sometimes by as much as 100 mm Hg [4]. Strangely enough, however, the error may occasionally be the other way. If the cuff is large, there should be no significant difference. It is more important to have increased cuff width than increased wrapping length.

6. In which kind of obese patient is the blood pressure most likely to be significantly overestimated with an ordinary 13 X 20 cm cuff?

   ANS.: In those with a ponderal index of over 4. (Ponderal index is weight divided by height in inches.)

   Note: Most patients with this kind of obesity are actually hypertensive.

7. How can you overcome the small-cuff problem in a fat arm if there is no large cuff available?

   ANS.: Place the cuff on the forearm and auscultate at the radial artery.

8. How can you accurately determine if the cuff is the correct diameter for the limb?

   ANS.: For most adult arms it must be at least 20% wider than the diameter of the arm. An easy way to determine this is to multiply the diameter of the limb by 1.2. Since it is easier to relate cuff width to circumference than to diameter, the cuff width according to the above formula should be at least 40% of the arm circumference.

One study showed that as long as the width of the cuff is at least 12 cm, and the length of the bladder encompasses at least one-half the circumference of the arm, the reading will be reliable even for the fat arm when compared with intra-arterial pressures. This requires that the rubber bladder be placed over the brachial artery. Larger or longer cuffs were found to be no more accurate for the fat arm [9].

Note: a) The ideal cuff width and length of bladder according to the above formula are easy to remember because they should both be roughly one-half the arm circumference.

b) However, several studies have shown that the ideal pneumatic bag bladder pressure is transmitted with the least delay to the underlying artery when the bag completely encircles the arm. Since some studies have also shown that there are no falsely low readings when unusually wide cuffs are used, the width may even be over half the arm circumference in the long, thin arm of the child or the fat, conical obese arm [69].

c) Maximum accuracy in pediatric age groups requires cuffs of several sizes. From birth to age 1, a cuff at least 2.5 cm in width should be available. For ages 1–4, a 5-cm cuff is usually needed. For ages 4–8, a 9-cm cuff may be needed to achieve a width that is almost half the circumference of the arm.

*9. What is the effect of calcified brachial arteries (pipestem brachials) on blood pressure as taken by cuff?

ANS.: Medial sclerosis of the brachial arteries (Mönckeberg's arteriosclerosis) may be severe enough to prevent compression by a blood pressure cuff. This could give a falsely high systolic pressure. One case report showed a cuff pressure of over 300 mm Hg and an intra-arterial needle blood pressure of 130 mm Hg [71].

THE AUSCULTATORY GAP

1. What is meant by an auscultatory gap?

ANS.: It is the silence separating the first appearance of Korotkoff sounds from a second appearance at a lower blood pressure level.

Note: It has been said to occur only when there is venous distention in the arm. This statement, however, appears to reflect a vague understanding of the fact that Korotkoff sounds may be faint when the tissue pressure is high distal to the cuff. These sounds can be made louder by simply raising the arm and inflating the cuff quickly before listening [57].

2. What proof is there that the auscultatory gap is dependent on decreased blood flow to the extremities?

ANS.: a) It can be induced in some elderly subjects with coronary disease by using a tourniquet to decrease flow to the arms [60].

b) It can be eliminated by exercising the hand for about 20 sec before taking the blood pressure [62].

Note: If the Korotkoff sounds are soft, exercise the hand and inflate the cuff quickly with the arm elevated to be sure the patient does not have an auscultatory gap.

3.   What kind of pulse is necessary before a reduced blood flow can produce an auscultatory gap?

ANS.:   An anacrotic shoulder, as in subjects with AS and in elderly subjects with sclerotic aortas.

BLOOD PRESSURE AND PULSES IN THE LEGS

Normal Pressures

1.   How does the blood pressure in the legs compare with that in the arms?

ANS.:   It depends on the cuff size used and on whether the pressure is measured by an intra-arterial needle, by Korotkoff sounds, or by Doppler techniques. With the blood pressure cuff, the leg systolic pressure in adults should be either the same or up to 20 mm Hg higher in the legs than in the arms. In children, the pressure in the legs is usually about 10 mm Hg higher than in the arms [51]. Taken carefully, the systolic pressure in the legs is not normally lower than in the arms [20]. If it is lower, occlusive disease in the vessels of the legs should be suspected [10].

Note: If an intra-arterial manometer is used, the systolic and diastolic pressure in the legs is usually the same as in the arms [6, 51, 52]. By Doppler methods, with the cuff placed above the malleolus, the blood pressure in the foot vessels is normally slightly higher than in the brachials [79].

2.   If the usual arm cuff is used on the thigh, will the blood pressure be too high or too low in the legs in comparison with intra-arterial measurements?

ANS.:   It will be too high, because only a relatively small amount of inflatable rubber cuff is over the limb. Therefore, more compression is required to occlude the artery.

3.   What happens to popliteal blood pressure if the thigh cuff is too short?

ANS.:   If there is not enough length to double the thickness of the edges, the edges will bulge when the cuff is inflated, so that less of the cuff contacts the skin. This will require more pressure to compress the artery, and the blood pressure will appear too high.

4.   How can the blood pressure reading tell you that the cuff is too small for the thigh?

ANS.:   Even though the systolic pressure may normally be higher in the leg, the diastolic pressure tends to remain the same as in the arm. Thus, if the diastolic pressure is higher in the leg, the cuff is probably too small.

5.   Where is the most reliable place to auscultate for blood pressure in the legs?

ANS.:   Over the popliteal artery, with a large cuff on the thigh.

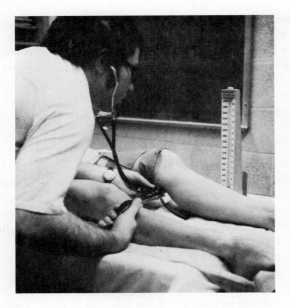

The usual commercial leg cuff, such as that shown here, must be rolled diagonally around the thigh to keep the edges snug against the skin. The systolic blood pressure in the legs should not be over 20 mm Hg higher than in the arms and should not be lower.

Note: a) In severe AS, the slow rate of rise may make it impossible to hear Korotkoff sounds in the popliteals because the audibility of the sounds depends partly on the rate of rise.

b) Compressing the thigh with a blood pressure cuff can cause severe discomfort in some patients. This may cause a false elevation of pressure so that accurate comparisons with the brachials will require simultaneous arm and thigh measurements.

6. How can you fit a cylindrical cuff to the usual conical thigh?

ANS.: It is impossible to make an exact fit.

Note: By making a slightly sickle-shaped leg cuff you achieve an exact fit. A second-best method is to use either an extra-large cuff, so that the edges can be well doubled, or an extra-thick canvaslike material that cannot bulge easily.

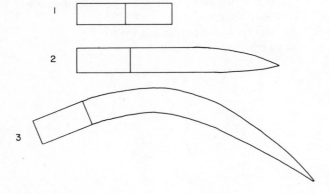

1. Arm cuff. 2. Commercial leg cuff. 3. Curved leg cuff to fit conical thigh and long enough for obese patient.

7.   How can a blood pressure be taken in the lower legs?
      ANS.:   Place an ordinary arm cuff over the lower part of the calf, just above the malleolus,
               i.e., as close as possible to the artery used for asucultation, but without including
               the protuberance of the malleolus. Use a small (pediatric) bell to auscultate the
               posterior tibial artery. If no Korotkoff sounds are audible, auscultate or palpate
               the dorsalis pedis instead. If no Korotkoff sounds are present over any foot artery,
               the Doppler method of taking a blood pressure can be used. (See p. 50.)

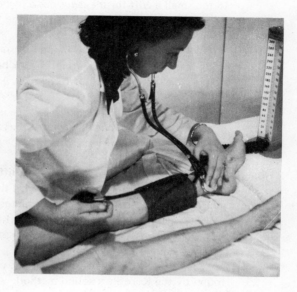

A convenient method of taking a leg
pressure if you do not have a thigh
cuff. A pediatric bell should be used
to achieve an easy air seal behind the
medial malleolus.

8.   What are the advantages of using the foot for taking blood pressure in the lower limbs?
      ANS.:   a) No special size or shape of cuff is necessary.
               b) It is more comfortable for the patient. About 1 in 3 patients complains of
                  pain with the thigh cuff.
9.   What are the disadvantages of using the foot rather than the thigh for blood pressure?
      ANS.:   a) No Korotkoff sounds can be elicited in about 10% of patients.
               b) A marked peripheral constriction, as in a cold room, may cause the blood
                  pressure to be as much as 50 mm Hg lower in the foot than in the arm.
10.   How is blood pressure taken in an infant?
      ANS.:   a) By the flush method: Raise the limb until it is blanched, then inflate the cuff.
                  As you release the cuff rapidly, the first distal flush is read as the *mean* systolic
                  pressure.
               b) By Doppler ultrasound and a cuff about 2.5 cm wide. (See p. 50.)

LEG BLOOD PRESSURE IN AORTIC REGURGITATION

1.   How does AR affect the blood pressure in the legs in comparison with that in the arms?
      ANS.:   It produces a higher cuff pressure in the legs than in the arms.

2.   Why is the cuff blood pressure in AR higher in the legs than in the arms?

ANS.:   The reason is unknown. One theory is that the increased forward initial flinging of blood through the aortic valve causes a percussion wave that builds up as it goes peripherally against resistance, just as an ocean wave often becomes higher and higher as it approaches shore. Another theory is that reflected waves from the periphery summate with forward waves.

Note: Intra-arterial pressure measurements have not always shown this difference in blood pressure, i.e., it may be a cuff artifact [53]. It is not, however, due to too small a cuff for the leg, since a higher pressure in the leg in AR can be elicited with a large sickle-shaped cuff on the thigh or an ordinary arm cuff above the malleolus.

3.   Whose sign is it when there is a higher blood pressure in the legs than in the arms?

ANS.:   Hill's sign [33]. (It is easy to remember because blood pressure goes "uphill" in AR as the examiner goes down the body.)

4.   Is the degree of Hill's sign related to the degree of AR?

ANS.:   Yes, roughly. In mild AR the difference is up to 20 mm Hg; in moderate AR the difference is 20—40 mm Hg; in severe AR the difference is over 60 mm Hg. A difference between 40 and 60 mm Hg may represent either moderate or severe AR [22].

5.   What produces a falsely low Hill's sign, i.e., less difference found between the arms and the legs than would be expected from the severity of the AR?

ANS.:   a) Congestive heart failure or other causes of peripheral constriction. A positive Hill's sign may depend, at least in part, on the low peripheral resistance that occurs with AR and on a strong myocardial contraction.

b) Significant AS.

Note: Mild AS will not eliminate the normal brachial-popliteal gradient usually found by the Korotkoff sound method.

THE LEG PULSES AND BLOOD PRESSURE IN COARCTATION OF THE AORTA

1.   When should you suspect coarctation of the aorta?

ANS.:   In any patient with hypertension.

2.   What are the characteristics of the pulses proximal to and beyond an aortic coarctation?

ANS.:   The proximal pulses; i.e., the carotid and brachial pulses are large, bounding, fast-rising pulses. The parts of the body beyond the left subclavian artery, which is the usual site of the coarctation, receives blood through enlarged collaterals that do not transmit the percussion wave. Therefore, not only do the lower extremity pulses have a low pulse pressure but also their rate of rise is slow and they have a late peak.

3.   Is the delay in femoral pulse peak due to delay in onset of the femoral pulse?

ANS.:   The onset of the femoral pulse is not delayed in the femorals beyond those in the radials.

4.   If the onset of the femoral and radial pulses are simultaneous, what causes the sensation of the delayed peak in the femorals?

ANS.:   Because of the decreased initial flow rate through the femorals, their percussion wave is so low that only the tidal wave is felt in the femorals, i.e., there is an anacrotic shoulder only in the femorals. In the radials, the usual percussion wave is easily felt because there is no obstruction to flow, and the velocity of flow and pulse pressures is increased in the vessels proximal to the obstruction.

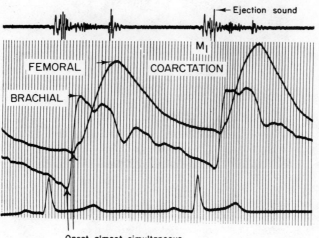

Onset almost simultaneous

This is a simultaneous femoral and brachial intra-arterial pressure tracing in a patient with coarctation. The phonocardiogram was taken at the second left interspace. Any detectable delay in the femoral pulse in coarctation occurs between the percussion wave (initial peak) in the arm and the tidal wave (end-systolic peak) in the femoral. This is because in an artery distal to an obstruction the percussion wave tends to end at an anacrotic shoulder which is imperceptible.

5.   What may make it difficult to compare pulse peaks in the femoral and radial arteries?

ANS.:   They have different pulse pressures, and the finger on the radial may be too far from the finger on the femoral.

6.   How can you overcome the difficulties in comparing the femoral and radial pulses?

ANS.:   a) Place the patient's wrists over your finger, which is on the femoral artery, so that your hands are on top of one another.

b) Vary the compression force until both pulse pressures feel equal.

c) Use the lightest possible pressure, so that you can allow comparison of peaks.

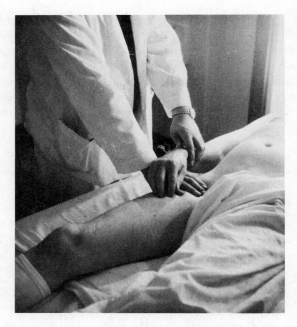

By placing the patient's wrist over his femoral artery as you palpate both, you can best perceive the obvious delay of the femoral pulse peak over that of the arm. In using the radials rather than the brachials to test for differences between the arm and leg, you take advantage of the increased rapidity of pulse rise as you palpate more peripherally down the arm.

7.   When is it especially important to test for femoral pulse peak delay in suspected coarcta-
      tion?
      ANS.:   When AR is present. The femoral pulses may appear normal in volume in the
                presence of AR, because with this condition, all peripheral pulses become more
                bounding, due to reflex peripheral vasodilatation plus strong LV contraction. If
                the AR is severe, the diastolic pressure in the arms may even be normal, despite
                coarctation [10].
          *Note: a) Kinking of the aortic arch without any pressure gradient across the
                        kinked segment (pseudocoarctation) can cause a delay in femoral pulse
                        peak over that of the radials [75]. Experimental progressive constric-
                        tion of the aorta in animals will produce a delayed femoral peak when
                        the aorta is constricted to 40% of its cross-sectional area, whereas a
                        gradient will not develop until the aorta is narrowed to 30% of its
                        original area [75].
                   b) Supravalvular AS [44] can also cause a radial-femoral lag. Only a delay
                        between the *right* radial and femoral will occur. The left radial may also
                        be delayed.
                   c) The blood pressure may not be elevated in the arms in coarctation in
                        patients in whom there is
                        1) Significant AS plus a PDA [40].
                        2) Severe MR [76].

*8.   How can palpation of arteries in a patient with coarctation suggest that the coarctation is abdominal?

ANS.:   If a strong aortic pulsation in the epigastrium suddenly disappears lower down, an abdominal aortic coarctation should be suspected [56].

PULSUS ALTERNANS

1.   What is meant by pulsus alternans?

ANS.:   An alternating fluctuation in pulse pressure, i.e., in every other beat, the blood pressure is lower.

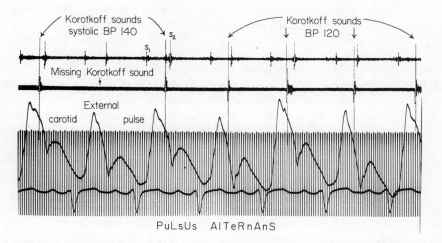

PuLsUs AlTeRnAnS

The heart sounds are shown in the top line. The next line is taken with a microphone over the brachial artery distal to a blood pressure cuff. Note the doubling of the number of Korotkoff sounds when the cuff has been deflated from 140 to 120 mm Hg.

2.   What is the significance of pulsus alternans?

ANS.:   a) It is usually associated with myocardial damage of the type that is either

   1) Severe enough to cause obvious gross failure, or

   2) Mild, but associated with LVH, as in hypertension, AR, or AS.

   Note: Pulsus alternans is rare, even in severe congenital AS under age 35, when a relatively healthy myocardium is assumed to be present. On the other hand, it is common in acquired severe AS in patients over age 35, when a damaged myocardium is more likely.

   b) It may be secondary to tachycardias even in a normal heart [41].

3.   What can start a short run of pulsus alternans in a patient who either had been or is in heart failure?

ANS.:   a) A PVC.

   b) A sudden increase in venous return due to deep inspiration [43].

c) A sudden decrease in venous return due to onset of a tachycardia or sitting up. (Always test for pulsus alternans in the sitting position if it is absent in the supine position.)

d) Exercise [64].

*Note: There is no significance to the disappearance of pulsus alternans at rest in a patient who has been or is in failure, because pulsus alternans may disappear with either improvement or worsening of the failure [64].

4. How much difference in pulse pressure is detectable by finger palpation?

ANS.: At least 20 mm Hg must usually be present between beats [41]. Since in pulsus alternans there is usually less than a 10-mm Hg difference between the beats, a blood pressure cuff is usually required to detect it.

5. What is the cause of pulsus alternans?

ANS.: Three theories are widely held:

*a) It is due to an atrial-carotid reflex started by a sudden strong or weak beat.

*b) It is due to a sudden critical change in diastolic filling period.

c) It is due to an alternation in the number of cardiac fibers contributing to each systole.

*6. What is the atrial-carotid reflex explanation for pulsus alternans?

ANS.: A sudden strong beat (as in a post-PVC beat) reflexly weakens atrial contraction via the carotid sinus, resulting in decreased LV contraction and a small carotid pulse, which in turn reflexly stimulates the carotid sinus to excite the atrium to a stronger contraction. The mechanism for alternation is thereby set up [65].

Note: This theory is weakened by the finding of pulsus alternans in the pulmonary artery or jugulars and not in the aorta or carotid in the same patient [21, 81]. It also is an unlikely theory in view of the fact that when a fourth heart sound (S_4) is present, it is loudest before the weak beats [42].

*7. How has a change in diastolic filling period been postulated to account for pulsus alternans?

ANS.: If a sudden, short diastole is produced (as by a premature beat), a poor contraction and a short systolic ejection period result. The following increased diastole and end-diastolic volume produce a larger stroke volume and longer systolic contraction. The next diastole will be short, and the poor volume results in a poor contraction, and the setup for pulsus alternans is produced [50].

Note: Although total electromechanical systole (Q to A_2) is unchanged in the weak and strong beats, most subjects show prolongation of isovolumic relaxation time in the strong beats, thus encroaching on the next diastolic filling period [66]. The longer isovolumic relaxation time of the LV is presumably due to the strong beats having a higher systolic pressure and therefore a higher aortic valve closing pressure. Thus, it takes longer for LV pressure to drop down to left atrial pressure to open the mitral valve [67]. This theory is weakened by the finding of alternating pulmonary artery pulse in the presence of atrial fibrillation [28].

8. Is electrical alternans (alternating differences in QRS configuration) associated with pulsus alternans?

ANS.: Pulsus alternans occurs in about 10% of patients with electrical alternans.

PULSUS PARADOXUS

1.   What is meant by pulsus paradoxus?
     ANS.:   It is a marked drop in systolic blood pressure on inspiration, usually due to **tamponade** but sometimes seen in **constrictive pericarditis.**

Normal Effect of Respiration on Blood Pressure

1.   Does the systolic blood pressure normally increase or decrease with inspiration? Why?
     ANS.:   It decreases because
        a) Lung capacity increases with inspiration; therefore, less blood comes from the lung into the left heart.
        b) Intrathoracic pressure decreases with inspiration. Since the aorta is an intrathoracic organ, its pressure will also drop.
2.   If the systolic pressure normally decreases with inspiration, what is paradoxical about a pulsus paradoxus?
     ANS.:   Nothing. It is just an exaggeration of a normal phenomenon.
3.   Why did the term *paradoxus* come into use?
     ANS.:   Kussmaul, in the late 1800s, originally described a marked drop in, or even loss of, blood pressure on inspiration in patients with constrictive pericarditis [38]. He decided to call it a "pulsus paradoxus" because he noticed that the apex beat did not change in any way, despite a loss of pulse with inspiration. He also thought it was paradoxical that although the peripheral pulse appears at first to be irregular, it actually comes and goes regularly [73].
4.   What might be a more descriptive term than *pulsus paradoxus?*
     ANS.:   A marked inspiratory fall in blood pressure of X number of millimeters of mercury.
5.   How much systolic pressure is normally lost with (a) normal, (b) deep, and (c) very deep inspiration?
     ANS.:   a) 2–6 mm Hg.
        b) Up to 10 mm Hg.
        c) Up to 15 mm Hg.

How to Elicit an Abnormal Inspiratory Fall in Blood Pressure

1.   With what kind of respiration is the test done?
     ANS.:   With not more than moderate respiration. If the patient is breathing too shallowly, tell him to breathe "just a little more deeply, but not too deeply," just enough to see the chest movements easily out of the corner of your eye.
           Note: If respirations are rapid or irregular, raise your arm for inspiration and lower it for expiration, and ask the patient to follow the movements of your hand.
2.   On moderate inspiration and expiration what is a positive paradoxus, i.e., how much BP fall on inspiration is definitely abnormal?
     ANS.:   10 mm Hg or more is generally agreed on in the literature. With practice, however, experience shows that about 6 mm Hg inspiratory fall is the upper limit of normal. Some of the probable reasons for believing that 10 mm Hg could be normal are errors such as the following:
        a) The subject is asked to breathe too deeply or even to hold his breath on inspiration and expiration.

      b) The physician may fail to realize that as he is lowering the cuff pressure slowly below the level of the first Korotkoff sound on expiration, the blood pressure itself is often falling. Therefore, after he hears the Korotkoff sounds both on inspiration and expiration for the first time, he fails to reinflate the cuff to see if the systolic pressure has actually dropped while he was performing the test. One need not reinflate the cuff from a zero point, but merely up from where the sounds were heard on both inspiration and expiration.

3.   Why should you always test for pulsus paradoxus when taking a patient's blood pressure for the first time?

    ANS.:   a) It takes practice to do it well. Therefore, when it becomes part of the differential diagnosis, practice will make your results more reliable.

           b) You automatically pick up pulsus alternans or pulsus bisferiens this way.

The Mechanism of Inspiratory Fall in Tamponade or Constriction

1.   Why does the cardiac output drop markedly on inspiration in constriction or tamponade?

    ANS.:   Because much less blood enters the left atrium on inspiration than in normal subjects.

2.   Why does much less blood enter the left atrium on inspiration in constriction or tamponade?

    ANS.:   Because on inspiration the left ventricular and left atrial pressures do not drop as much as intrathoracic pressure drops. Thus, the pressure in the left atrium may even exceed the pressure in the pulmonary veins. Blood may even flow backward into the lungs on inspiration.

3.   Why does left atrial and left ventricular pressure not drop proportionately to intrathoracic pressure in the presence of constriction or tamponade?

    ANS.:   The following is one plausible explanation: Tamponade or constriction almost always affects both sides of the heart. The venae cavae are largely extrathoracic, so that their pressure does not drop with inspiration, but actually may rise. Thus, the filling pressure of the right ventricle is increased with inspiration. The right pericardium is stretched, and its intrapericardial pressure is increased. This increased intrapericardial pressure is transmitted to the left ventricle and atrium, and their pressure is raised during inspiration [15].

Cause of False-Positive and False-Negative Tests for Inspiratory Fall in Blood Pressure

1.   What is meant by (a) a Valsalva maneuver and (b) a Müller maneuver?

    ANS.:   a) A Valsalva maneuver is an expiratory straining against the closed glottis. This raises intrathoracic pressure.

           b) A Müller maneuver is an inspiratory effort against a closed glottis. This lowers intrathoracic pressure.

2.   Why may some asthmatic patients seem to have a marked inspiratory fall in blood pressure?

    ANS.:   If expiration raises intrathoracic pressure too high as a result of bronchospasm (Valsalva maneuver), inspiration will by contrast seem to lower the systolic pressure excessively. Actually, it is an expiratory rise in blood pressure, not an inspiratory fall. There are, however, patients with emphysema who also have some inspiratory obstruction that causes an exaggerated inspiratory fall of intrathoracic pressure as well (Müller maneuver). In short, the blood pressure is merely reflecting changes in intrathoracic pressure.

It is surprising how severe chronic emphysema can be with only a slight expiratory rise in blood pressure.

Note: The pulse of tamponade may differ from the pulse of a patient with bronchospasm and a marked expiratory rise in blood pressure because in bronchospasm, the pulse pressure remains about the same on inspiration and expiration because the cardiac output is not affected by the phasic changes in intrathoracic pressure. In tamponade, on the other hand, the pulse pressure (as well as the systolic pressure) decreases on inspiration because the cardiac output drops markedly on inspiration. Consequently, although the tamponade pulsus paradoxus may occasionally be palpable, that due to bronchospasm alone never is.

The diastolic pressure in tamponade changes very little, while in bronchospasm, it varies as much as does systolic pressure.

3.   Which patients have the greatest inspiratory fall in systolic pressure, those with constriction or those with tamponade?

ANS.:   Only with tamponade are inspiratory drops of 20 mm Hg or more found during quiet breathing [39].

In chronic constrictive pericarditis, a pulsus paradoxus is actually uncommon unless it is subacute, with some fluid still present.

Note: In the effusive-constrictive type of pericarditis, a tense effusion adds pressure to a constricting visceral pericardium, which still causes constriction even after complete pericardiocentesis. While the relatively small effusion is present, there is likely to be a marked pulsus paradoxus, just as in pure tamponade [31].

*4.   Why may congestive heart failure by itself sometimes cause a falsely exaggerated inspiratory fall in blood pressure?

ANS.:   This is unknown. It is always associated with marked cardiomegaly when it does occur. It may be partly due to the cardiomegaly's being so great that it stretches even the normal pericardium to its maximum, thus making it behave like a noncompliant restrictive pericardium.

*5.   What conditions that are neither cardiac nor bronchospastic can cause a marked inspiratory fall in blood pressure? Why?

ANS.:   a) Extreme obesity, which possibly causes excessive compression of the inferior vena cava at the thoracic inlet on inspiration.

b) Pregnancy, presumably because the large uterus obstructs the free forward flow of blood in the inferior vena cava during expiration. (Blood flows forward in the abdomen mainly during expiration, when intraabdominal pressure is lowest.)

c) Compression, on inspiration, of one subclavian artery by a fibrous band or anterior scalenus muscle due to an unexplained anatomical anomaly may account for the occasional unilateral paradoxus effect [13, 70].

d) Acute pulmonary embolism, usually found in the presence of a cardiomyopathy [12, 48].

e) Shock.

Note: Shock can cause a marked inspiratory fall in blood pressure only if it is associated with hypovolemia. This is presumably because the depletion of the venous reservoir will cause less blood than normal to be ejected into the lungs on inspiration. The pulmonary reservoir is therefore underfilled, so that with inspiration an excess amount of pulmonary blood is withheld from the LV, thus markedly decreasing the left ventricular output and blood pressure during inspiration.

*6.   What is the cause of the marked inspiratory fall in blood pressure seen in some patients with a large acute pulmonary embolism?

    ANS.:   The reason is unknown, but since it is associated with a decrease in pulse pressure during inspiration, there are several possibilities.

        a) An acutely dilated RV on inspiration may encroach on the LV in diastole and reduce the LV stroke volume. This is a reversed **Bernheim effect**.

        b) The lungs are so empty that there may be excessive pooling in the lungs on inspiration.

*7.   When will there be no significant inspiratory fall in blood pressure despite marked tamponade?

    ANS.:   If AR is present, the LV can fill from the aorta during inspiration. Therefore, if dissection of the aortic root causes both AR and tamponade, do not expect a pulsus paradoxus.

        Note: Hypertrophic subaortic stenosis has been reported to cause a reversed pulsus paradoxus [47]. The reason for this is unknown.

SUMMARY OF HOW TO TAKE ARM BLOOD PRESSURE BY AUSCULTATION AND LISTENING FOR KOROTKOFF SOUNDS

1.   Ask the patient to extend his arm with the palm upward. This exposes the brachial artery position clearly.

2.   Be sure that the cuff bladder is over the brachial artery, and that the indicator needle is in the zero area on the dial of an aneroid manometer. (A mercury manometer should be used in the office to avoid having to calibrate your aneroid manometer repeatedly.)

3.   Place the diaphragm chest piece partly under the cuff.

4.   Raise the cuff pressure to a reasonable level, such as 140 mm Hg, and drop the arm to the heart level and listen for Korotkoff sounds. If they are present at 140 mm Hg, pump the cuff up another 10 mm Hg. Repeat the listening and pumping until no Korotkoff sounds are heard. (This avoids applying unnecessarily excessive painful pressure.)

5.   If the Korotkoff sounds are very soft, have the patient open and close his hand about ten times, raise the arm up at 45 degrees, and pump up the bladder quickly to eliminate any auscultatory gap. (This is rarely necessary in the young patient without significant cardiac failure or AS, and in whom the Korotkoff sounds are not very soft.)

6.   Deflate the cuff at a rate of about 2 mm Hg per heartbeat only during expiration until the first Korotkoff sounds are heard during expiration. This is approximately the systolic blood pressure. Read it to the nearest 5 or 10 mm Hg.

7.   If this is the first time that you are taking a blood pressure in this patient, deflate the cuff very slowly until the pressure returns on inspiration. If the difference between the inspiration and expiration blood pressure is over 6 mm Hg, reinflate the cuff and repeat (5) and (6) above to see if systolic pressure was dropping while you were testing for inspiratory fall.

8.   Listen for pulsus alternans while testing for inspiratory fall.

9.   Deflate the cuff further until muffling is heard. Then deflate further until the sound disappears. If the difference between pressures at the muffling point and disappearance point is less than 10 mm Hg, report the disappearance point as the diastolic pressure. If, however, the difference is greater than 10 mm Hg, report both numbers (to the nearest 5 or 10).

10.   If the arm is so fat that the cuff width or bladder length is less than half the arm circumference, use a thigh cuff. If no thigh cuff is available, use an arm cuff above the radial artery.

CAPILLARY PULSATION

1.   How do you elicit capillary pulsation (Quincke's sign)?
       ANS.:   Compress the skin of the face or hands with a glass slide, or exert slight pressure on the nail beds and watch for intermittent flushing. You can also transilluminate the nail bed with a flashlight against the pad of the patient's finger while shading the finger with your other hand.
2.   What causes capillary pulsation? What noncardiac conditions can cause it?
       ANS.:   The transmission of the arterial pulse through the open capillaries to the subpapillary venous plexus. It is found in any condition that causes capillary dilatation, such as hot weather, a hot bath, fever, anemia, pregnancy, or hyperthyroidism.
3.   Which cardiac conditions cause capillary pulsation?
       ANS.:   Any cardiac condition that causes a large pulse pressure, such as AR, systemic hypertension, or marked bradycardia, as in complete atrioventricular block.
               Note: All the preceding cardiac conditions can cause such marked capillary pulsation that it may be seen by mere inspection of the palms, cheeks, or forehead, without compressing the skin [46].

REFERENCES

1. Alzamora-Castro, V., and Battilana, G. The double femoral sound. *Am. J. Cardiol.* 5:764, 1960.
2. Barner, H. B., Willman, V. L., and Kaiser, G. C. Dicrotic pulse after open heart operation. *Circulation* 42:993, 1970.
3. Benchimol, A., Harris, C. L., and Desser, K. B. Graphic techniques in cardiology. Midsystolic carotid pulse wave retraction in subjects with prolapsed mitral valve leaflets. *Chest* 62:614, 1972.
4. Berliner, K., Fujiy, H., Lee, D. H., Yildiz, M., and Garnier, B. Blood pressure measurements in obese persons. *Am. J. Cardiol.* 8:10, 1961.
5. Berry, M. R. The mechanism and prevention of impairment of auscultatory sounds during determination of blood pressure of standing patients. *Staff Meet. Mayo Clin.* 15:699, 1940.
6. Bertrand, C. A. Arm and leg blood pressures. *J. A. M. A.* 227:942, 1974.
7. Braunwald, E., and Morrow, A. G. A method for the detection and estimation of aortic regurgitant flow in man. *Circulation* 17:505, 1958.
8. Buggs, H., Johnson, P. E., Gordon, L. S., Balguma, F. B., and Wettach, G. E. Comparison of systolic arterial blood pressure by transcutaneous Doppler probe and conventional methods in hypotensive patients. *Anesth. Analg.* 52:776, 1973.
9. Burch, G. E., and Shewey, L. Sphygmomanometric cuff size and blood pressure recordings. *J. A. M. A.* 225:1215, 1973.
10. Campbell, M., and Baylis, J. H. The course and prognosis of coarctation of the aorta. *Br. Heart J.* 18:475, 1956.

11. Carter, S. A. Clinical measurement of systolic pressures in limbs with arterial occlusive disease. *J. A. M. A.* 207:1869, 1969.

12. Cohen, S. I., Jupersmith, J., Aroesty, J., and Rowe, J. W. Pulsus paradoxus and Kussmaul's sign in acute pulmonary embolism. *Am. J. Cardiol.* 32:271, 1973.

13. Cohn, J. N., Tristani, F. E., and Pinkerson, A. L. Mechanism of parodoxical pulse in clinical shock. *J. Clin. Invest.* 46:1744, 1967.

14. Corrigan, D. J. Permanent patency of the mouth of the aortic valves. *Edinb. Med. Surg. J.* 37:225, 1832.

15. Dornhorst, A. C., Howard, P., and Leathart, G. L. Pulsus paradoxus. *Lancet* 1:746, 1952.

16. Enselberg, C. D. Measurement of diastolic blood pressure by palpation. *N. Engl. J. Med.* 265:272, 1961.

17. Evans, W., and Lewes, D. The carotid shudder. *Br. Heart J.* 7:171, 1945.

18. Ewy, G. A., Rios, J. A., and Marcus, F. I. The dicrotic arterial pulse. *Circulation* 39:655, 1969.

19. Falicov, R. E., and Wang, T. Analysis of postextrasystolic beats in the diagnosis of idiopathic hypertrophic subaortic stenosis. *Am. J. Cardiol.* 33:931, 1974.

20. Felix, R., Jr., Hochberg, H. M., George, M. E. D., Schmalzbach, E. L., and Vaserberg, R. Ultra-sound measurement of arm and leg blood pressures. *J. A. M. A.* 226:1096, 1973.

21. Ferrer, M. E., Harvey, R. M., Cournand, A., and Richards, D. W. Cardiocirculatory studies in pulsus alternans of the systemic and pulmonary circulations. *Circulation* 14:163, 1956.

22. Frank, M. J., Casanegra, P., Migliori, A., and Levinson, G. The clinical evaluation of aortic regurgitation. *Arch. Intern. Med.* 116:357, 1965.

23. Freis, E. D. Auscultatory indication of diastolic blood pressure. *Cardiol. Digest* 3:13, 1968.

24. Freis, E. D., Heath, W. C., Luchsinger, P. C., and Snell, R. E. Changes in the carotid pulse which occur with age and hypertension. *Am. Heart J.* 71:757, 1966.

25. Freis, E. D., and Kyle, M. C. Computer analysis of carotid and brachial pulse waves. *Am. J. Cardiol.* 22:691, 1968.

26. Freis, E. D., and Sappington, R. F., Jr. Dynamic reactions produced by deflating a blood pressure cuff. *Circulation* 38:1085, 1968.

27. Friedman, S. A. Prevalence of palpable wrist pulses. *Br. Heart J.* 32:316, 1970.

28. Gould, L. Pulmonary artery alternation with atrial fibrillation. *J. A. M. A.* 207:1515, 1969.

29. Gould, L., and Lyon, A. F. Postural changes in the brachial artery first derivative in the normal and pathologic state. *Dis. Chest* 53:476, 1968.

30. Gould, L., and Shariff, M. Comparisons of the left ventricular, aortic, and brachial artery first derivative. *Vasc. Surg.* 3:34, 1969.

31. Hancock, E. W. Subacute effusive-constrictive pericarditis. *Circulation* 43:183, 1971.

32. Harrison, E. G., Jr., Roth, G. M., and Hines, E. A., Jr. Bilateral indirect and direct arterial pressures. *Circulation* 22:419, 1960.

33. Hill, L., and Rowlands, R. A. Systolic blood pressure: (1) in change of posture, (2) in cases of aortic regurgitation. *Heart* 3:219, 1911–1912.

34. Hochberg, H. M., and Saltzman, M. B. Accuracy of an ultrasound blood pressure instrument in neonates, infants, and children. *Ther. Res.* 13:482, 1971.

35. Hultgren, H. N. Venous pistol shot sounds. *Am. J. Cardiol.* 10:667, 1962.

36. Ikram, H., Nixon, P. G. F., and Fox, J. A. The haemodynamic implications of the bisferiens pulse. *Br. Heart J.* 26:452, 1964.

37. Ison, J. W. Palpation of dorsalis pedis pulse. *J. A. M. A.* 206:2745, 1968.

38. Kussmaul, A. Ueber schweilige Mediastinopericarditis und den paradoxen Pulse. *Klin. Wochenschr.* 10:443, 1873.

39. Lange, R. L., Botticelli, J. T., Tsagaris, T. J., Walker, J. A., Gani, M., and Bustamante, R. A. Diagnostic signs in compressive cardiac disorders, constrictive pericarditis, pericardial effusion, and tamponade. *Circulation* 33:763, 1966.

40. Little, J. A., Leight, L., Davis, L. A., and Haller, J. A., Jr. Coarctation of the aorta associated with aortic stenosis and a patent ductus arteriosus. *Am. J. Cardiol.* 12:570, 1963.

41. Littmann, D. Alternation of the heart. *Circulation* 27:280, 1963.

42. Littmann, D. Cardiac alternation. Alternation of heart sounds and murmurs. *Am. J. Cardiol.* 14:420, 1964.

43. Liu, C. K., and Luisada, A. A. Halving of the pulse due to severe alternans (pulsus bisectus). *Am. Heart J.* 50:927, 1955.

44. Logan, W. F. W. E., Jones, E. W., Walker, E., Coulshed, N., and Epstein, E. J. Familial supravalvar aortic stenosis. *Br. Heart J.* 27:547, 1965.

45. London, S. B., and London, R. E. Critique of indirect diastolic end point. *Arch. Intern. Med.* 119:39, 1967.

46. MacGregor, G. A. Spontaneous capillary pulsation in complete heart block. *Br. Heart J.* 21:225, 1959.

47. Massumi, R. A., Mason, D. T., Zakauddin, V., Zelis, R., Otero, J., and Amsterdam, E. A. Reversed pulsus paradoxus. *N. Engl. J. Med.* 289:1272, 1973.

48. McDonald, I. G., Hirsh, J., Jelinek, V. M., and Hale, G. S. Acute major pulmonary embolism as a cause of exaggerated respiratory blood pressure variation and pulsus paradoxus. *Br. Heart J.* 34:1137, 1972.

49. Meadows, W. R., Draur, R. A., and Osadjan, C. E. Dicrotism in heart disease. *Am. Heart J.* 82:596, 1971.

50. Mitchell, J. H., Sarnoff, S. J., and Sonnenblick, E. H. The dynamics of pulsus alternans: Alternating end-diastolic fiber length as a causative factor. *J. Clin. Invest.* 42:55, 1963.

51. Park, M. K., and Guntheroth, W. G. Direct blood pressure measurements in brachial and femoral arteries in children. *Circulation* 40:231, 1970.

52. Pascarelli, E. F., and Bertrand, C. A. Comparison of blood pressures in the arms and legs. *N. Engl. J. Med.* 270:693, 1964.

53. Pascarelli, E. F., and Bertrand, C. A. Comparison of arm and leg blood-pressures in aortic insufficiency: An appraisal of Hill's sign. *Br. Med. J.* 2:73, 1965.

54. Perlman, L. V., Chiang, B. N., and Keller, J. Accuracy of sphygmomanometers in hospital practice. *Arch. Intern. Med.* 125:1000, 1970.

55. Putt, A. M. A comparison of blood pressure readings by auscultation and palpation. *Nurs. Res.* 15:311, 1966.

56. Pyorala, K., Heinonen, O., Koskelo, P., and Heikel, P. E. Coarctation of the abdominal aorta, review of twenty-seven cases. *Am. J. Cardiol.* 6:650, 1960.

57. Ragan, C., and Bordley, J. The accuracy of clinical measurements of arterial blood pressure. *Bull. Johns Hopkins Hosp.* 69:504, 1941.

58. Rittenhouse, E. A., and Strandness, D. E., Jr. Oscillatory flow patterns in patients with aortic valve disease. *Am. J. Cardiol.* 29:568, 1971.

59. Robinson, B. The carotid pulse. II. Relation of external recordings to carotid, aortic, and brachial pulses. *Br. Heart J.* 25:61, 1963.

60. Rodbard, S., and Ciesielski, J. A relation between auscultatory gap and the pulse upstroke. *Am. Heart J.* 58:221, 1959.

61. Rodbard, S., and Ciesielski, J. Duration of arterial sounds. *Am. J. Cardiol.* 8:18, 1961.
62. Rodbard, S., and Margolis, J. The auscultatory gap in arteriosclerotic heart disease. *Circulation* 15:850, 1957.
63. Rose, G. Standardization of observers in blood-pressure measurement. *Lancet* 1:673, 1965.
64. Ryan, J. M., Schieve, J. F., Hull, H. B., and Oser, B. M. Experiences with pulsus alternans, ventricular alternation and the stage of heart failure. *Circulation* 14:1099, 1956.
65. Sarnoff, S. J., Gilmore, J. P., Brockman, S. K., Mitchell, J. H., and Linden, R. J. Regulation of ventricular contraction by the carotid sinus; its effect on atrial and ventricular dynamics. *Circ. Res.* 8:1123, 1960.
66. Spodick, D. H., Khan, A. H., and Quarry, V. M. Systolic and diastolic time intervals in pulsus alternans. *Am. Heart J.* 87:5, 1974.
67. Spodick, D. H., and St. Pierre, J. R. Pulsus alternans: Physiologic study by noninvasive techniques. *Am. Heart J.* 80:766, 1970.
68. Sproul, G. Basilar artery insufficiency secondary to obstruction of left subclavian artery. *Circulation* 28:259, 1963.
69. Steinfeld, L., Alexander, H., and Cohen, M. L. Updating sphygmomanometry. *Am. J. Cardiol.* 33:107, 1974.
70. Swinton, N. W., Jr., Nelson, W. P., Hall, R. J., and Harrell, J. E. Paradoxical pulse. *Arch. Intern. Med.* 124:492, 1969.
71. Taguchi, J. T., and Suwangool, P. "Pipe-stem" brachial arteries. *J. A. M. A.* 228:733, 1974.
72. Tahir, A. H., and Adriani, J. Usefulness of ultrasonic technique of blood pressure determination. *Anesth. Analg.* 52:699, 1973.
73. Wagner, H. R. Paradoxical pulse: 100 years later. *Am. J. Cardiol.* 32:91, 1973.
74. Waltemath, C. L., and Preuss, D. D. Determination of blood pressure in low-flow states by the Doppler technique. *Anesthesiology* 34:77, 1971.
75. Wang, K., Harrington, D., and Gobel, F. L. Delayed systolic peak of the femoral pulse from kinking of the aortic arch. *Am. J. Cardiol.* 33:286, 1974.
76. Wigle, E. D., and Auger, P. Coarctation of the aorta associated with severe mitral insufficiency. *Am. J. Cardiol.* 21:190, 1968.
77. Wigle, E. D., Heimbecker, R. O., and Gunton, R. W. Idiopathic ventricular septal hypertrophy causing muscular subaortic stenosis. *Circulation* 26:325, 1962.
78. Wood, P. Aortic stenosis. *Am. J. Cardiol.* 1:553, 1958. Classic article.
79. Yao, S. T., Hobbs, J. T., and Irvine, W. T. Ankle systolic pressure measurements in arterial disease affecting the lower extremities. *Br. J. Surg.* 56:676, 1969.
80. Zahir, M., and Gould, L. A new method for measurement of blood pressure in clinical shock. *Am. Heart J.* 79:572, 1970.
81. Zoneraich, S., and Zoneraich, O. Alternation in jugular pulse. *Ann. Intern. Med.* 78:610, 1973.

4
The Jugular Pulse

VENOUS PRESSURE BY JUGULAR INSPECTION

1. With which chambers of the heart are the jugulars in continuity in systole and in diastole?
    ANS.: In systole, the jugular is in continuity only with the right atrium, because the tricuspid valve is closed. In diastole, when the tricuspid valve is open, the jugulars are in continuity with both the right atrium and the right ventricle (RV). Therefore, examination of the jugulars reveals to you the contour and pressures in the right atrium and ventricle without the need for intubation.

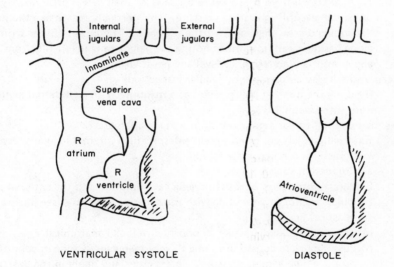

VENTRICULAR SYSTOLE   DIASTOLE

In diastole, the atrium and ventricle are in continuity and become an "atrioventricle." Note also that the internal jugulars are in a more direct line with the superior vena cava than are the external jugulars.

---

* indicates material that is for electives or fellows in cardiology, or concerns rare phenomena, of interest primarily to cardiologists.

Boldface type indicates that the term is explained in the Glossary.

2.   Where are there working valves between the jugulars and the superior vena cava?

ANS.:   In the external jugulars. (These may often be demonstrated in the supine position by preventing flow from above by finger occlusion.)

3.   Do these valves interfere with the use of the jugulars as a manometer for measuring venous pressure, i.e., as reflectors of right atrial events?

ANS.:   The valves in the external jugulars could interfere with pressure measurements that depend on filling from below. This should interest you in learning to look for information from pulsations of the internal jugulars, which do not have effective valves separating them from the superior vena cava and right atrium.

Note: If the venous valves of the arm are destroyed by phlebitis, as in chronic heroin users, the normal jugular pulsations will be transmitted to the arm veins [1]. Any vein in the body may transmit jugular pulsations if there is marked elevation of venous pressure or volume of pulsations, as in severe tricuspid regurgitation. Varicose veins of the leg are especially likely to pulsate with severe tricuspid regurgitation because their valves are incompetent.

4.   What besides the presence of valves makes the use of "filling from below" a poor criterion for elevated jugular pressure?

ANS.:   All jugulars fill from below up to the level of their valves or, if no valves are present, up to the level of right atrial pressure. This normally may make the jugulars visible, depending on the angle of the patient's chest. Therefore, "filling from below" alone has no meaning without noting the height to which it fills from below, i.e., above some stated reference level and chest angle.

5.   How can you tell venous pressure by jugular inspection?

ANS.:   By using the internal jugular veins as a manometer. The external jugulars make a poor manometer [7].

6.   Why is the external jugular a poor vein to use as a manometer?

ANS.:   External jugulars are often invisible despite high internal jugular pressures. False low pressures can occur because of

a) Competent valves.

b) Poor transmission of superior vena cava pulsations to the external jugulars, which are not in direct line with the superior vena cava (see illustration for question 1).

c) The external jugulars may be poorly developed anatomically.

d) Possible severe constriction due to very high venous tone in conditions that produce high venous pressure. This is especially likely in shock states.

7.   Can you see an internal jugular vein?

ANS.:   Only in the presence of severe tricuspid regurgitation is it visible as a discrete structure.

8.   If you cannot ordinarily see internal jugular veins, how can they be used as a manometer?

ANS.:   The *pulsations* of the internal jugulars are transmitted to the skin of the neck. The top level of neck pulsations is taken as the venous pressure. Thus, the jugulars are used as a "pulsation manometer."

9.   Why should the right rather than the left jugulars be used?

ANS.:   Normally, the pressure in the right jugulars is either slightly greater than or the same as that of the left. Upper levels of normal have been established for the right side. In some arteriosclerotic patients, the left jugular pressure may be falsely elevated due to compression of the innominate vein between the sternum anteriorly and large tortuous arteries arising from a high aortic arch below and posteriorly. (An aortic **aneurysm** can occasionally be the cause of innominate vein compression, but this is rare in comparison with arteriosclerotic compression.)

Note: a) Giving diuretics or lowering the blood pressure can reduce the compression of the innominate vein by a hypertensive tortuous aorta and normalize the left jugular pressure [10].

   b) A persistent left superior vena cava draining into the coronary sinus will make the pressure in the left jugulars slightly higher than the right, possibly due to their having a relatively greater emptying resistance [19]. A persistent left superior vena cava is especially likely in the presence of an atrial septal defect (ASD) [13].

10.   How can you bring out jugular pulsations that are difficult to perceive?

   ANS.:   a) Shine a light tangentially either behind the neck to throw a jugular shadow anteriorly, or in front of the neck to throw the jugular shadow posteriorly.

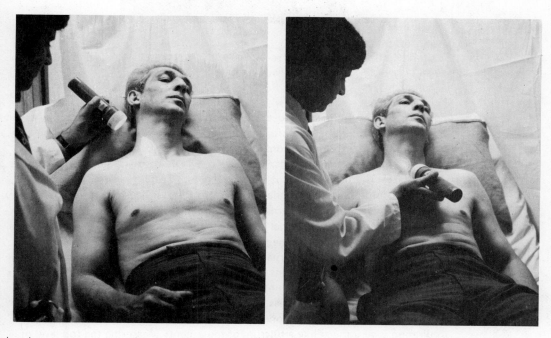

Jugular movements may be very subtle. Any slight movement of the hand holding the light can produce as much artifactual movement as movement from the jugulars themselves. Therefore, you must support your hand on either the pillow behind or the chest in front.

   b) Examine the silhouette of the neck for pulsations. This is the most accurate way of finding the top level of pulsations. When you are using the right side of the neck, you must lean over to the left side of the patient or stand on the left side of the bed temporarily to judge the silhouette of the right neck.

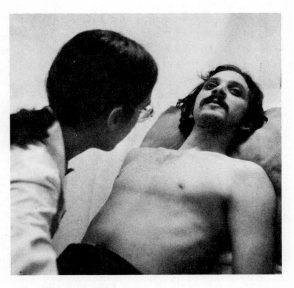

Leaning over to the left side of the patient to view an outline of the neck against the pillow will show you more subtle motion than could be seen even with an oblique light. Therefore, the true upper level of motion is best seen from this viewpoint.

       c) Check for slight earlobe movement. If the internal jugular pressure is high, the earlobes often pulsate. Unfortunately, strong carotid pulse pressures can also cause slight earlobe pulsations.

11.   Why is the phrase "distended neck veins," which is so widely used as a sign of high venous pressure, a poor expression?

    ANS.:   This expression suggests that the observer probably is accustomed to looking only at external jugulars, since internal jugulars are rarely visibly distended. A high level of pulsation in the internal jugulars may be associated with invisible external jugulars. If you wish to use the jugulars as a manometer, you should state the height of the top level of internal jugular pulsations in centimeters above a certain reference point with the patient in a certain position. You should be interested in the top level of pulsations, not in distention.

        Note: One of the difficulties in judging the top level of jugular pulsations is that they tend to diminish as one reaches the upper level, i.e., the top level of pulsation is very much like a fulcrum of movement. Measuring the top level of venous pressure really means looking for the fulcrum of internal jugular movement.

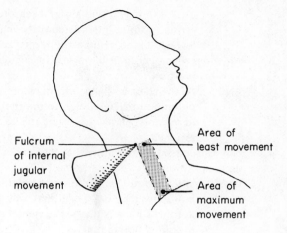

The top level of pulsations is really an area of subtle disappearance. The accuracy is probably within about 0.5 cm.

Fulcrum of internal jugular movement

Area of least movement

Area of maximum movement

HOW TO READ THE JUGULAR MANOMETER

1. What reference level may be used as zero? Why?

    ANS.:   The **sternal angle.** This landmark was once thought to bear a constant relationship to the right atrium with the body in either the recumbent or sitting position. Although this is doubtful, an arbitrary zero level is practical, provided normal standards for venous pulsations above this zero are established.

2. What upper limits of normal have been suggested for jugular pulsations in (a) the supine and (b) the 45-degree position?

    ANS.:   a) The upper limit is 2 cm.

    b) The upper limit is 4.5 cm. (It is easy to remember 4.5 cm at 45 degrees.)

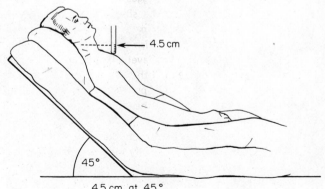

The upper normal above an arbitrary zero level of the sternal angle is 4.5 cm. Some cardiologists insist on adding an assumed distance of 5 cm between the bottom of the right atrium and the sternal angle to make the upper normal 9.5 cm of blood. This seems to be an unnecessary additional step, since the distance between the right atrium and sternal angle is really an unknown factor.

4.5 cm

45°

4.5 cm at 45°

Note: If you find a normal absolute venous pressure when you suspect a low cardiac output, inquire about the ingestion of diuretics and you may find that a lowered blood volume has normalized the venous pressure.

3.   Why does the upper limit of normal for jugular pulsations above the sternal angle depend on chest position?

ANS.:   As the chest is changed from recumbent to upright in bed, the top level of jugular pulsation rises in relation to the sternal angle. This may be due to an actual change in relation between the right atrium and the sternal angle as the upright position is assumed.

4.   Why is it important to know what the venous pressure is at 45 degrees rather than in the supine position?

ANS.:   When the subject is supine, the jugulars may be normal, and yet the top level of pulsations may be so high that they are above the angle of the jaw. This is because in some supine patients, the sternal angle may even be above the level of the jaw if measured horizontally.

Note: Normal subjects have been shown to have about the same absolute venous pressure in the supine as in the 45-degree chest position relative to the right atrium. Those with peripheral edema and high venous pressure have a venous pressure level slightly lower (by less than 1 cm) at 45 degrees than in the supine position.

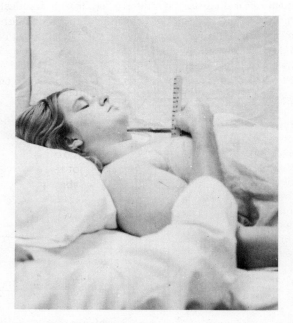

The 2-cm level is above the angle of the jaw in this patient. Therefore, only if her top level of pulsations were lower down at sternal-angle level would the upper level be measurable. At 45 degrees, her top level of jugular pulsations was below jaw level and was measurable.

5. What does inspiration do to the absolute height or top level of jugular pulsations in the normal subject?

  ANS.: The height on the neck may be lowered because the drop in intrathoracic pressure on inspiration may be reflected in the jugulars. Inspiration may, however, make jugular pulsations easier to see, because the right atrium has more vigorous pulsations on inspiration.

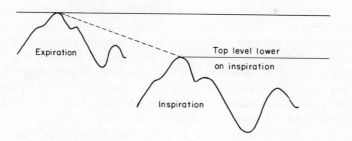

Note the higher absolute level but smaller amplitude of pulsations on expiration. With bronchospasm, jugular pulsations with normal pressures may only be visible above the clavicle during expiration due to the effect of straining, which elevates intrathoracic pressure with each expiration.

THE ABDOMINAL COMPRESSION TEST (HEPATOJUGULAR REFLUX)

1. How can you tell that a venous pressure that is below the upper limit of normal is actually abnormally high for a particular person?

  ANS.: Abdominal compression will cause and maintain a rise of at least 1 cm in the top level of pulsations only if the venous pressure is high. The higher the rise with abdominal compression, the higher is the venous pressure. This is called the *hepatojugular reflux* (not *reflex*).

    Note: The effect of abdominal compression is more important than the absolute jugular pressure in determining whether or not the venous pressure is normal.

2. What happens to the top level of jugular pulsations if abdominal compression is applied to a patient without heart failure?

  ANS.: In the normal patient, the jugular pulsation level will either remain the same or fall.

3. In the normal subject, what causes the drop in jugular pressure if abdominal compression is maintained?

  ANS.: a) Pressure on the abdomen obstructs femoral venous return almost as effectively as venous tourniquets on the thighs. Thus, less blood reaches the right atrium.

    b) The response of many patients to interference with diaphragmatic descent by abdominal compression is to breathe in a more inspiratory position. This causes a decreased intrathoracic pressure, which is reflected in the jugulars as a decrease in jugular pressure.

Note: One bonus derived from testing for jugular pressure with abdominal compression is the possible discovery of a low vital capacity. If abdominal compression causes an increase in dyspnea or the use of accessory muscles of respiration, this implies that the patient cannot tolerate any decrease in vital capacity produced by pushing up on the diaphragm. Therefore, a markedly reduced vital capacity must already be present.

4.   What is wrong with the term *hepatojugular reflux*?

ANS.:   It is a historical term, first applied in 1885, when it was thought that pressure on the liver was an essential part of the abdominal compression test. Actually, the effect can be achieved with a normal-sized liver and with compression on any part of the abdomen. However, it is true that right upper quadrant pressure gives the greatest response. This may be either because it is easier to compress the inferior cava here, or because pressure upward on a large RV, causing a decrease in its ability to expand, may produce part of the effect. But if the right upper quadrant is tender, do not hesitate to compress other areas instead.

Note: The term *hepatojugular reflux* must be retained because it is so widely known that it is useful for indexing, referencing, and communication among physicians.

5.   What is different about a congestive failure patient that makes his venous pressure rise on abdominal compression?

ANS.:   a) In peripheral congestive failure, there is an increased venous tone, which counteracts the thigh tourniquet effect and decreases the ability of the veins of the head and arms to dilate and absorb the displaced visceral blood.

b) In congestive failure blood volume may also be increased, and there may even be a disproportionate increase in splanchnic over total blood volume [31]. This causes more blood to be displaced from the splanchnic area with abdominal compression.

c) The congestive failure patient also commonly has a large RV, and right upper quadrant compression of the RV could interfere with its filling [15]. This may account for the fact that in patients with failure, right upper quadrant pressure very often causes a decrease in cardiac output despite the apparently higher **filling pressure.**

6.   What causes the increased venous tone in congestive heart failure?

ANS.:   Inadequate cardiac output eventually causes

a) Sympathetic outflow along the autonomic nerves.

b) Increased catecholamines in the blood.

Note: The increased sympathetic outflow and catecholamines are reflected in the sinus tachycardia seen in patients with heart failure. Their increased venous tone, or tension, has been proved by plethysmography, in which volume and pressure in an encased limb are used to solve for tension by using Laplace's law: pressure is proportional to $\dfrac{\text{tension}}{\text{volume}}$.

Increased venous tone has been found in all patients with so-called **rightventricular failure**, i.e., peripheral congestive failure (increased venous pressure and peripheral edema due to inadequate cardiac output) [34]. If the cardiac output is nearly normal at rest, even though it is inadequate for exertion, an equivocal abdominal compression test result is usually obtained. If diuretics have normalized the absolute height of venous pressure, abdominal compression may still demonstrate the increased tone.

7.   What can cause a false rise in the height of jugular pulsations with abdominal compression?
ANS.:   a) Inability to tolerate the resistance of downward movement of the diaphragm caused by pressure on the abdomen, as in patients with severe obstructive pulmonary disease or in any other condition that causes severe loss of vital capacity [24].
b) Increased blood volume [18].
c) Increased sympathetic stimulation due to such causes as nervousness, pain, intravenous catecholamines, or an acute infarct [6].
d) An obstruction to the superior vena cava below the azygos vein.

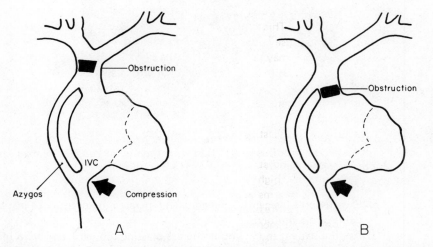

(A) Partial obstruction of the superior vena cava above its junction with the azygos will elevate jugular venous pressure. Abdominal compression will not elevate it further because the displaced abdominal blood can reach the area below the obstruction. (B) Obstruction, partial or complete, below the junction of the azygos with the superior vena cava will also elevate venous pressure, and abdominal compression will prevent the jugular blood from emptying freely into the azygos, thus further elevating the jugular pressure.

8.   How does a patient with marked chronic obstructive pulmonary disease (emphysema) respond to abdominal compression?
ANS.:   During inspiration he resists with his abdominal musculature, thus raising both his intra-abdominal and intrathoracic pressures on inspiration. Since bronchospasm may be present and bronchospasm causes intrathoracic pressure to be high also on expiration, a reason exists for high intrathoracic pressures on both inspiration and expiration. Since the jugulars reflect intrathoracic pressures, their pressures will rise in response to abdominal compression. This applies only to severe chronic obstructive pulmonary disease.

9.   How should you compress the abdomen in order to prevent false elevations due to sympathetic outflow?
ANS.:   a) Compress with warm hands or with a garment or sheet between your hand and the abdomen.
b) Spread the fingers apart, so that there is as little local pressure as possible.

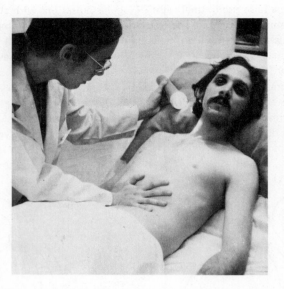

Spreading the fingers allows you to distribute pressure over a large area, so that more pressure can be applied without producing discomfort. Sometimes, only marked abdominal pressure will raise jugular pulsations enough to show that they are abnormal.

      c) Start by pressing gently, and gradually increase the pressure to just below the point of discomfort.

      d) Ask the patient to tell you if you are pressing too hard, and warn him that it spoils the test if you produce discomfort.

*10.   What is Kussmaul's sign?

ANS.:   The rise in the height of jugular pulsations during inspiration in patients with chronic constrictive pericarditis. It is found in only a minority of patients with constrictive pericarditis, and rarely ever found in tamponade [21].

Note: In any patient with high venous pressure, it may be raised further on inspiration because inspiration raises intra-abdominal pressure and can act like abdominal compression [39]. Also, any patient with a strong right atrial contraction can have a stronger one on inspiration, because that is when more blood is drawn into the right atrium; the increased stretch of the atrium makes it contract harder, and the jugular pressure will appear higher.

11.   Besides an abdominal compression effect, what may be the cause of a positive Kussmaul's sign in **tamponade** or **constrictive pericarditis**?

ANS.:   It may be that the inspiratory downward pull on the diaphragm pulls in turn on the pericardium to make the latter more constricting. (The diaphragm is firmly attached to the pericardium.)

ANTECUBITAL MANOMETRY

1.   Are the effects of abdominal compression transmitted as reliably to a manometer at the antecubital veins as they are to the jugulars?

ANS.:   Jugular effects are usually more marked. Thus, with a very mild increase in venous tone, only the jugulars may show a rise with abdominal compression.

2.   What are the causes of poor antecubital manometry, and how are they prevented?

ANS.:   a) Obstruction to the thoracic inlet. This can be prevented by placing the arm at a 45-degree angle from the body.

b) Venospasm. This can be overcome by waiting about 5 minutes after the needle is in the arm to allow the initial spasm to disappear, so that the venous pressure returns to its lowest level.

3.   When a manometer is used at the elbow, what is the top limit of normal for venous pressure?

ANS.:   It depends on where the zero level is arbitrarily placed. With a zero level 5 cm below the sternal angle, the top limit of normal is 120 mm H_2O. With the zero level at 10 cm from the back, the top limit of normal is 150 mm H_2O; this is more commonly used because it has been shown to be closer to actual right atrial level with the greatest variation of chest shapes, especially with chronic obstructive pulmonary disease.

Note: As with the jugulars, abdominal compression is more important than an absolute upper level in determining the presence of increased venous tone.

JUGULAR PULSE CONTOURS

The Normal Jugular Pulse Contours

1.   What is the difference between jugular and right atrial pulse contours?

ANS.:   None, for all practical purposes, except when jugular pulse tracings pick up carotid artifacts. Therefore, the right atrial contours will be explained first, since it is right atrial changes that produce the jugular contours.

Note: The delay between right atrial and jugular events used to record the jugular pulsations depends on the recording system used. The narrow external jugulars show a much more delayed response than that of the larger internal jugulars. Thus, among various investigators, the delay has been found to vary from an insignificant 10 msec (0.01 sec) at the jugular bulb to as much as 100 msec (0.10 sec) at the external jugulars.

2.   What is the normal right atrial contour, and what are the letters given to the important crests and descents?

ANS.:   The normal right atrial contour consists of the waves A, C, and V, and the descents X, X prime, and Y.

The atrial and jugular waves are very similar. The crests are A, C, and V; the descents are X, X', and Y.

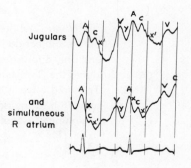

Jugulars

and simultaneous R atrium

3.   What produces the A wave? Relate the right atrial A wave to the ECG.

ANS.:   The A wave is produced by right atrial contraction, which begins at about the peak of the P wave.

Note: The right atrial pressure rise begins at about 90 msec after the onset of the P wave. (Left atrial pressure begins to rise about 30 msec later.)

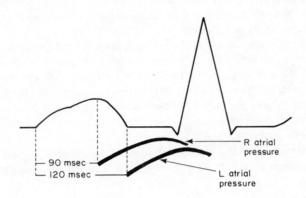

The A wave of the atrium and jugular pulse is produced by right atrial contraction, which in turn is produced by depolarization of the right atrium, as represented by the first third of the P wave. (The last two-thirds of the P wave represents left atrial depolarization.)

4.   What produces the X descent?

ANS.:   Atrial diastole or atrial relaxation. It occurs just before the ventricle contracts.

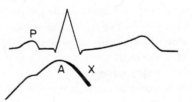

Atrial relaxation produces the drop in pressure known as the X descent.

Note: The literature on jugular contours shows that about half the writers on the subject do not actually name the atrial diastolic descent as a separate entity, and only about half call it the X descent [5].

5.   What produces the C wave in the right atrial pressure pulse?

ANS.:   Tricuspid valve closure due to RV contraction, which causes the valves to bulge upward into the right atrium, raising its pressure slightly. This occurs at the beginning of **isovolumic contraction**.

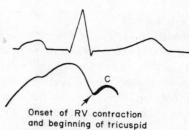

Onset of RV contraction
and beginning of tricuspid
valve upward movement

The right atrial C wave is probably due to tricuspid valve bulging, but in the jugulars only the first part of the C wave is due to such bulging. The huge jugular C waves seen in some tracings are certainly not all due to tricuspid valve movement.

6. What produces the C wave in the jugular tracings taken with a cone or other pickup device applied to the neck?

ANS.:   It is a fusion of the tricuspid bulging effect plus carotid artifact. It is usually (although not always) due to carotid artifact on the pulse tracing; i.e., when iso-volumic contraction finishes, and the aortic valve opens, the aortic pressure rises and expands the carotid arteries. The expansion of the carotid pulse is picked up by the pulse unit on the neck, in an attempt, usually unsuccessfully, to isolate the jugular pulse.

*Note: Mackenzie [22], in 1902, in his book on the pulse, was the first to call this the C wave to symbolize the word carotid, because he believed that it was always entirely carotid artifact. He described an experiment in which pure jugular tracings were taken before and after the jugulars were dissected away from the carotid. The carotid C wave, which had been present before, disappeared after the dissection. He also described the various amplitudes of C waves that could be obtained merely by varying the pressure or site of the pickup. The theory attributing the C wave to upward bulging of the tricuspid valve was tested and also found wanting by Wiggers [38], who described right atrial pressure and jugular pulses taken at various levels. When he recorded volume changes at successively higher levels, from the right atrium to low in the neck, the changes in contour that were due to tricuspid valve closure completely disappeared, and only the carotid arti-fact C wave remained.

In complete atrioventricular (AV) block, simultaneous jugular and right atrial pulse tracings have shown a persistent C wave in the jugulars following the onset of each ventricular contraction even when absent in the atrial tracing [9].

If the carotid arterial component is electronically subtracted from the jugular tracing, the C wave becomes diminutive or disappears [26].

*7. When will a tricuspid closure C wave bulge be seen in a jugular pulse tracing?

ANS.: a) In AV block or left bundle branch block, because left ventricular events may be so delayed that a bifid C wave may be seen, the first part of which is due to tricuspid bulging [32].

b) If there is right atrial and RV overload, as in ASDs, mitral stenosis (MS) with atrial fibrillation, and congestive heart failure [2].

8.   What causes the X prime (X′) descent?

ANS.:   Right ventricular contraction. If you watch carefully the next time you see a cineangiogram of a ventricle contracting, you will note that the base of the ventricle (floor of the atrium) descends toward the apex with ventricular contraction. Physiologists have called this the systolic "descent of the base," meaning the descent of the AV ring. Since the atria are firmly attached by their tributary veins to surrounding structures, pulling down of the atrial floor results in a decline in atrial pressure.

Note: The anatomy of the left ventricle (LV) lends itself well to a downward pull on the atrial floor, because its syncytium has two prominent columns parallel with the long axis of the ventricle, each inserting into the trigones of the AV ring [14].

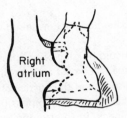

The broken lines represent systole. The apex does not rise significantly during ventricular contraction. The drawing down of the AV valve ring (*see arrows*) is the major method of contraction of a ventricle.

This fall in atrial pressure during systole produces a descent in the atrial and jugular pulses. Physiologists have called this venous collapse during systole "the systolic collapse of the venous pulse."

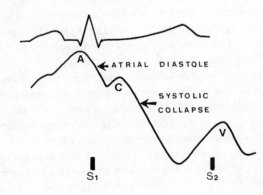

The systolic depression seen in the jugulars is the deepest, fastest collapsing movement that the eye can see in the neck.

Note: a) The other explanations for the systolic jugular descent do not stand up well against criticism. Atrial relaxation has been said to be partly responsible. Since this requires that the atria continue to expand during ventricular systole, this explanation should be abandoned except under abnormal circumstances, such as in reference to the left atrium in the presence of MS. Studies have indeed shown that contraction of the left atrium in MS may be prolonged, so that atrial relaxation can occur during ventricular systole and therefore can produce most of the systolic descent following the C wave [4, 41]. However, this has been shown only in the left atrium and only in the presence of MS [30]. Also, in MS, the A wave reaches high levels and produces a large prolonged X descent. Because the left atrium in MS is stiff, the X' may be eliminated by the rapid rise in pressure due to filling from the pulmonary veins; i.e., the filling wave (V wave) begins too early to allow a fall in pressure due to the descent of the base. In a subject without MS, however, the atrium has completed its expansion or relaxation by the time the ventricle starts to contract, and an X' descent should be seen. Furthermore, the LV in MS often shows an alteration in contraction that may decrease the descent of the base [40].

If venous return is reduced by limb tourniquets plus tilting, a jugular tracing will show a progressively smaller A wave and larger C, until the A wave is eliminated. The systolic descent, although smaller, remains [25].

Another explanation given for the systolic descent is that it is caused by the pressure drop in the thorax, secondary to the loss of blood from the chest due to LV ejection. This ignores the increase in thoracic blood volume that occurs during RV systole. Flowmeters and angiograms have shown that forward flow into the heart occurs chiefly during RV systole, which produces a "suction effect" as it draws the floor of the atrium down [11, 37].

b) In going over the nomenclature used by 36 authors who have described jugular contours, it was noted that almost half of these authors left the systolic venous collapse unnamed [5]. It was called "X" by seven authors; it was combined with atrial relaxation under the letter X by an equal number; and it was called "X prime (X')" by nine authors [5].

9. What are the advantages of the term *X prime* (X') for the systolic jugular descent?

ANS.: a) It compromises with those who have always used an X to represent the descent of the base.

b) There has been no other name given to it by anyone who wanted to distinguish it from the X of atrial diastole ever since it was first used by Mackenzie [23], in 1907, in what was apparently the first attempt to distinguish the atrial diastolic descent from a systolic collapse. He shows a tracing with a delay in ventricular contraction due to a first-degree AV block (long P–R interval). The systolic jugular descent was so obviously not due to atrial diastole, which showed its descent long before, that he felt obliged to give a different name to and origin for the descent during systole, calling it "X'."

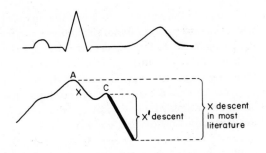

The X′ descent is due to a different phenomenon than the X and so requires a different name.

10.   What causes the ascending limb of the V wave?
       ANS.:   During systole, the tricuspid valve is closed, and atrial filling from the venae cavae
                finally overcomes the "descent of the base" and causes the atrial pressure to rise.
                Since the V wave is built up during systole, it is crucial to remember that the V
                wave is mainly a systolic event, resulting entirely from blood pouring into the
                right atrium while the tricuspid valve is closed.
                    Note: The X′ descent ends at a nadir called the X′ trough, from which the
                V wave begins its rise.

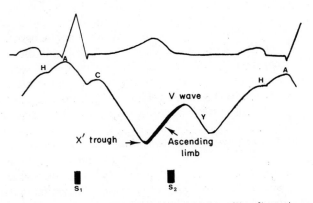

The jugular V wave is built up during systole, and its height will reflect the rate of filling and the
elasticity of the right atrium. Between the bottom of the Y descent (Y trough) and beginning of
the A wave is the period of relatively slow filling of the "atrioventricle" or diastasis period. The
wave built up during diastasis is the H wave. The H wave height also reflects the stiffness of the
right atrium.

11.   What causes the Y descent, or descending limb, of the V wave?
       ANS.:   When ventricular systole ends and the ventricle expands with the fall in pressure,
                the ventricular pressure will quickly fall to below right atrial pressure, which is at
                about 5 mm Hg. At this point the tricuspid valve opens, and there is rapid inflow
                into the expanding RV. This causes a rapid drop in right atrial pressure because
                the right atrium empties more rapidly than it can fill. This fall in right atrial pulse
                is known universally as the *Y descent,* and the bottom of the descent is known as
                the *Y trough.*

Note: a) You can best explain that the right atrium empties faster than it fills if you assume that RV expansion is not a passive but an active process, which can create a "suction effect" on the right atrium.

b) The common chamber produced by the opening of the tricuspid valves might be called an "atrioventricle."

*12. What is the wave called that is produced by the passive pressure rise in the atrioventricle as it fills in diastole after the Y trough?

ANS.:   The diastasis wave, or H wave. (See figure on p. 84.)

CONTOUR RECOGNITION BY INSPECTION

Normal Jugular Movement

1. Can you see an A, C, and V wave by inspection of the normal jugulars?

ANS.:   No. The C wave is not normally visible, since it is mostly carotid artifact.

2. Can you tell the X from the X' descent by eye?

ANS.:   Not easily, since the C wave that separates them is almost invisible.

Note: After much experience, a subtle double descent can be seen in some subjects during systole, denoting a separate X and X'.

3. Is the V wave visible in the normal jugular pulse?

ANS.:   The V wave in the normal adult is often so small that it may be invisible to the eye even though it is usually seen on a jugular pulse tracing. This is because on the right side, i.e., in the right atrium, the V wave and subsequent Y descents are very small. The reason for this is probably because in the right atrium the V wave reflects the building up of pressure in a very compliant or distensible chamber, i.e., the right atrium is too distensible to allow its pressure to rise much when the tricuspid valve is closed.* (The left atrium is a thicker chamber and has a much better V wave and Y descent.)

4. Why is it easier to decipher jugular movements by observing the descents, or downward-collapsing movements, rather than ascents, or upward movements?

ANS.:   a) The jugular descents or collapsing movements are larger than the ascents. The eye perceives and times the fastest, deep descents more easily than it does the shallow ascents.

b) The normal carotids have fast rises but slow falls. By noting the rate of descent you can easily distinguish the jugular from the carotid impulse at a glance.

5. How can knowing that the normal jugular is mainly a systolic descent (X + X') help you to recognize easily whether or not a jugular contour is normal?

ANS.:   Since the descent of the base effect, or the X' descent, is a systolic event, it must end before the second heart sound (S_2), which is due to aortic and pulmonary valve closure at the end of systole. With your stethoscope on the chest, you can time the dominant jugular descent or collapse and see if it appears to fall onto the S_2. If it does, it is an X + X', and the wave preceding it is an A wave. If, on the other hand, the dominant descent does not fall onto the S_2, it must be a Y descent, and the preceding dominant wave is a V wave.

Note: If there is only a V wave and Y descent, the peak of the jugular pulse will coincide with the S_2.

6.   If the X′ actually ends *before* the S₂, why does it appear to end *at* the S₂?
   ANS.:   The eye sees movement later than the ear hears sound; i.e., a movement that ends
        just *before* a sound appears to end *at* the sound. (Visual perception has been
        shown to be delayed by about 60 msec over auditory perception.)

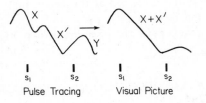

Although the X′ trough actually ends *before* the S₂, to the eye and ear it seems to end *at* the S₂;
i.e., the jugular descent seems to fall onto the S₂.

    Note: With this technique, the type of wave present can be inferred from the
    recognition of descents. If, for example, in sinus rhythm, an X′ descent is present
    and very little Y, there is a dominant A wave present. If, on the other hand, there
    is a large Y and very little X′, the presence of a dominant V wave can be inferred.
    If we see an equal X′ and Y descent, we can infer that the A and V wave are nearly
    equal in amplitude.

*7.   What relation should the X′ and Y descents have to the carotid pulse as felt with the finger?
   ANS.:   The X′ should seem to be immediately initiated by the peak of the carotid pulse.

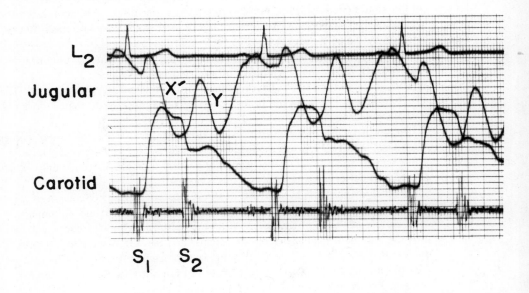

Note that the peak of the carotid pulse occurs at the beginning of the X′ descent.

Note: If you say "C" for carotid and "down" for the jugular descent, the rhythm will be "C-down" as quickly as you can say it. The Y descent should seem to come about the same distance from the carotid that the two heart sounds are from one another, so that if you say "C-down" slowly enough to equal the lub-dup of a first and second heart sound rhythm, you will have it about right.

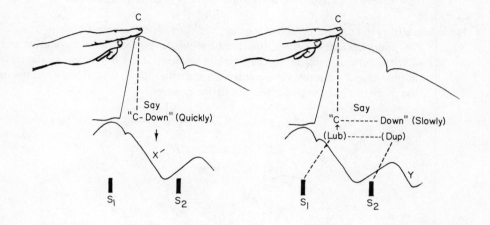

With a quick "C-down," the "down" will time with the X′ descent. With a slow "C − − − down," the "down" will time with the Y descent.

8.   When is it normal to have a moderately easily visible Y descent, i.e., a fair V wave? Why?
      ANS.:   In young people. This is because a V wave is an atrial filling wave during ventricular systole, when the tricuspid valve is closed. If the circulation time is slightly fast, as in most young people, the atrial filling wave or V wave will be slightly exaggerated. But the X′ descent will still be dominant.

Making Jugular Movements More Visible

1.   Which jugulars should you examine for contours, the internal or the external jugulars?
      ANS.:   Because they have the freest communication with the right atrium, the internal jugulars are best, not only for measuring pressures but also for seeing all the contours. Occasionally, however, the external jugulars show the only easily analyzable movement, and then they must be used.

2.   In what position do you place the patient to examine for jugular contours?
      ANS.:   In the supine position, because in this position more blood returns to the right atrium. Further, when the chest is raised, the jugulars may disappear below the clavicles.

3.   How can you exaggerate jugular movement that is too small for easy timing?
      ANS.:   Try to increase the venous return by the following maneuvers:
      a) Elevate the subject's legs.
      b) Have the subject take deeper breaths. Deep inspiration can draw more blood into the right atrium and make movements of larger amplitude.

Note: Holding the breath is sometimes necessary when the use of accessory muscles of respiration interferes with jugular visibility. This, however, often produces a Valsalva maneuver, which may eliminate all venous movement.

DIFFERENTIATING THE JUGULAR FROM A CAROTID PULSE

1.   How does sitting the patient up affect jugulars and carotids differently?

ANS.:   The more upright the chest, the lower the jugular pulsations are in relation to the clavicle. This is because the right atrium becomes lower in relation to the clavicle in the upright position. The carotid, on the other hand, is seen higher in the neck the more upright the patient in the sitting position.

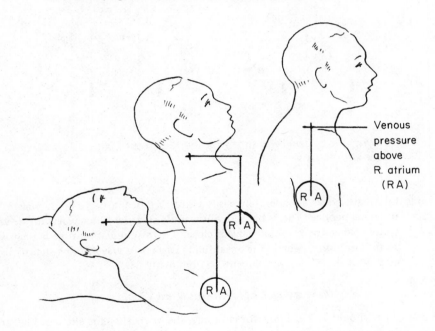

The horizontal line represents the top level of jugular pulsations. Note that jugular pulsations fall relative to the clavicle with a subject in the upright position. Visible carotid pulsations remain the same distance superior to the clavicle in all chest positions.

2.   How can you tell a jugular from a carotid by palpation?

ANS.:   Normal jugulars are not palpable. If venous pressure is high, you may occasionally feel a very compressible, gentle undulation. The carotids produce a strong, almost incompressible impulse.

3.   How does abdominal compression differ in its effect on jugular and carotid pulsations?

   ANS.:   In normal subjects, sudden abdominal compression momentarily displaces some blood into the RV, which therefore has a greater output for a few beats. This produces a greater descent of the base effect and so a more marked X' descent; and because of the momentary increase of venous return, the V wave may also become higher for a few beats. In patients with congestive failure, the jugulars can be made more visible for as long as abdominal compression is maintained. Abdominal compression has no effect on carotid pulsations.

4.   What is the effect of inspiration on the jugular and carotid pulsations?

   ANS.:   It increases the amplitude of jugular pulsations, but has little visible effect on carotid pulsations.

5.   Why will inspiration increase the amplitude of jugular pulsations?

   ANS.:   Inspiration decreases intrathoracic pressure, which in turn acts as an expanding bellows or suction pump to bring more blood into the RV during systole. The greater RV contraction in response to this increased volume will cause a greater "descent of the base" (the X' descent). A greater filling wave (V wave) and Y descent should also be produced.

6.   How can pressure on the neck reveal whether one is dealing with a jugular or a carotid pulsation?

   ANS.:   Moderate pressure on the neck below the level of pulsations can obliterate jugular but not carotid pulsations. Pressure low in the neck can also cause distention of the external jugulars, which will collapse on release of pressure.

   Note: When jugular pressure is high, obliteration of its pulsation may only occur with compression at least one-third or even one-half of the way up the neck.

A very strong jugular pulsation with a high venous pressure will not be eliminated by pressure just above the clavicle, probably because the sternomastoid tendons prevent adequate pressure against the vein.

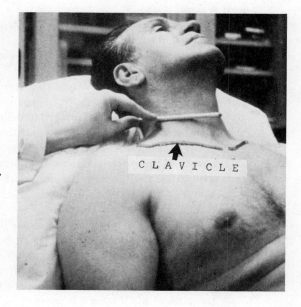

CLAVICLE

Summary of Jugular Versus Carotid Recognition

1. The carotid pulse has only one descent, or collapse; the jugular often has two, the X' and the Y.

2. The carotid descent is slow; the jugular X' descent is rapid. If the fastest and greatest movement is a collapse, or descent, it is a jugular pulse.

3. A pencil pressed firmly 1—5 cm above the clavicle will obliterate all jugular pulsations, but will not affect carotid pulsations.

4. Inspiration may exaggerate jugular pulsations (although it may lower their vertical level) and will, if anything, diminish carotid pulsations.

5. Sitting up makes the carotids appear higher in the neck, but the jugulars will appear lower in the neck.

6. The carotid, if visible, is always easily palpable with firm pressure. The normal jugular is rarely palpable, except as a slight fluttering sensation with light pressure. The jugular with high pressure is relatively easily compressible.

7. The X' descent appears to end at the S_2, while the carotid descent appears to begin with the S_2.

8. Sudden abdominal compression makes the jugular momentarily more visible, but has no effect on the carotids.

ABNORMAL JUGULAR CONTOURS

Abnormalities of the A Wave

1. What can cause a stronger-than-normal atrial contraction and so produce an exaggerated or giant A wave?

    ANS.:   a) Obstruction to outflow from the atrium, as in tricuspid stenosis (TS) or right **atrial myxoma** [29].

    b) A poorly compliant (stiffer) RV, as in pulmonary stenosis (PS) or pulmonary hypertension.

2. Why does RV systolic (pressure) overloads as in PS or pulmonary hypertension, cause a stronger right atrial contraction?

    ANS.:   When the RV has a **pressure load** to overcome, it becomes thicker and less compliant than normal. Since in diastole the atrium and ventricle are in continuity, the pressure in this "atrioventricle" rises very rapidly as it fills with blood. The stretch of the atrium produces a **Starling effect** and a powerful atrial contraction, which stretches the ventricle just before it contracts. This in turn produces a Starling effect on the ventricle, which can result in a ventricular contraction that is 30% more powerful than usual.

    Note: There may seem to be only one wave in the jugular pulse in PS because RV systole may be so prolonged that the V wave is also prolonged. (Remember that the V wave is built up during ventricular systole when the AV valves are closed.) By the time the V wave finishes and the AV valve opens, the atrium is ready to contract. Therefore, the giant A wave may begin to rise almost as the late peak of the V wave is reached.

3.   What besides a stronger atrial contraction increases the amplitude of the A wave?
     ANS.:   a) A stronger ventricular contraction can lower the depth of the X' descent, so
               that to the eye the amplitude of the A wave appears to be greater, even though
               its absolute height is unchanged.
             b) A higher-than-normal venous pressure, as in heart failure, because the stretched
               atrium is stimulated by the Starling effect.
             c) An atrial contraction during ventricular systole will occur when the tricuspid
               valve is closed. This large A wave is called a "cannon wave." A cannon wave
               occurs in the presence of either **atrioventricular dissociation** or an early P wave,
               such as that in a premature atrial contraction.
             Note: Cannon waves are very difficult to see unless the atrial contraction is
             extra-strong, due to loss of **compliance** (increased stiffness) of the RV, as in
             pulmonary hypertension. They are easily recorded and probably were given
             the name "cannon waves" from the appearance of recordings rather than
             from the appearance of the slight variation of jugular pulsation amplitude
             seen in the neck.

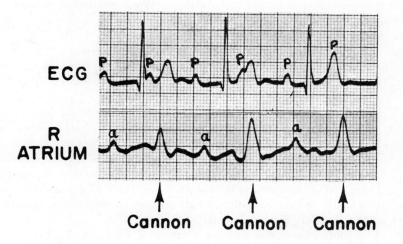

Note that in this patient with complete **Atrioventricular block**, every other P wave happens to
fall on a T wave, i.e., it occurs during ventricular systole when the tricuspid valve is closed. Thus
there is a cannon A wave with every other P wave.

*4.   How can the jugular A wave suggest **hypertrophic subaortic stenosis** in a patient with an
      aortic ejection murmur?
      ANS.:   If on inspiration the jugulars rise in height due to a larger A wave, RV outflow
              obstruction due to an excessively thick septum is suggested. Inspiration can cause
              a strong right atrial contraction by bringing more blood into the noncompliant
              "atrioventricle" in diastole.
*5.   What can you hear by auscultation over a jugular with a giant A wave?
      ANS.:   The large A wave can produce a presystolic sound [8].

Abnormalities of the X' Descent

1. What can produce a stronger right ventricular contraction so that a deeper X' descent results?
   ANS.:   a) Increased volume in the RV, such as in **atrial septal defect** (ASD) and **ventricular septal defect** (VSD).
   b) Increased pressure in the RV, such as in pulmonary hypertension or PS.

2. What can cause a smaller-than-normal or even absent X' descent?
   ANS.:   a) Tricuspid regurgitation (TR). The X' descent is encroached on, proportionally to the degree of regurgitation.
   b) A poor RV contraction, as in heart failure or absence of atrial presystolic Starling effect stretch, as in atrial fibrillation.
   c) A loss of compliance of the right atrium, as when filled by a tumor (right atrial myxoma or thickened by hypertrophy, as in TS [29].
   Note: Increased stiffness of the atrium causes the venous filling to overcome the descent of the base effect earlier than normal and will tend to exaggerate the V wave.

*3. What condition besides increased volume in the RV can produce an increased X' descent?
   ANS.:   **Pericardial tamponade.**

*4. Why may the X' descent in tamponade be very deep?
   ANS.:   In tamponade, the major restriction in movement is in diastole. Cardiac output can only be maintained either by tachycardia, more complete systolic emptying, or both. If more emptying occurs, the base may be drawn further down and a deep X' descent produced.
   Note: In constrictive pericarditis, systole is also often restricted, as shown by the below-normal or low-normal cardiac output and stroke volume at rest. This is not a mechanical effect, as demonstrated by the fact that an inotropic agent such as isoproterenol can increase the stroke volume in constrictive pericarditis by about 60% [28]. The pressure-volume loop, velocity of myocardial fiber shortening, and tension-velocity relationships are all abnormal in constrictive pericarditis [36].

*5. How can a jugular contour help differentiate constrictive pericarditis, effusive-constrictive pericarditis (see p. 63), and tamponade?
   ANS.:   In constrictive pericarditis, the Y descent is dominant. In effusive-constrictive pericarditis, the X' descent is either dominant or equal to the Y, even in atrial fibrillation. In tamponade, there is almost always a dominant X' descent and occasionally no Y at all.
   Note: When the X' descent is dominant, an S_3, or pericardial knock (p. 238), is usually absent [20].

*6. How may the X' descent help you diagnose the presence of tamponade or effusive-constrictive pericarditis?
   ANS.:   In the presence of atrial fibrillation and a high venous pressure, a deep X' (as well as a deep Y) is rarely seen in the absence of tamponade or effusive-constrictive pericarditis. In the presence of a high venous pressure, even in sinus rhythm, a deep X' together with a deep Y is also rare in the absence of tamponade or effusive-constrictive pericarditis.
   Note: In severe, chronic mitral regurgitation (MR) and aortic regurgitation (AR) (and perhaps in other conditions causing LV dilatation), a **Bernheim effect** may occur that may have the same effect as tamponade [33, 35]. This may produce a deep X' descent (as well as a Y) in the presence of a high venous pressure.

Abnormalities of the V Wave

1.   What can cause a high jugular V wave?
     ANS.:   a) Rapid right atrial filling. This is because the tricuspid valve is closed during
             the production of the V wave.
             b) Poor descent of the base of the RV, as in poor RV stroke volume.
             c) Tricuspid regurgitation, if one calls the regurgitant wave a V wave.
             d) A high venous pressure, as in congestive heart failure.
             e) Loss of compliance of the right atrium, as in constrictive pericarditis, in an
             atrial tumor, or after cardiopulmonary bypass surgery in which sutures are
             placed in the right atrium [17].

2.   What can cause a rapid atrial filling and so produce a relatively high V wave?
     ANS.:   a) Rapid **circulation times**, such as occur in exercise, anemia, anxiety states, and
             hyperthyroidism.
             b) Filling of the right atrium from extra sources, as in ASD, **anomalous pulmonary
             venous drainage** into the right atrium, or TR.
     Note: *a) A patent foramen ovale may be stretched by severe MR or a large left-
             to-right shunt such as patent ductus arteriosus or VSD, thus producing
             an atrial septal shunt that can enlarge the right atrial V wave [27].
             b) In ASDs, the overloaded right atrium contracts strongly, due to the
             Starling effect, and the large volume ejected by the RV causes a deep
             X' descent. The large V wave, as well as the deep X + X', produces a
             characteristic jugular pulse with both deep X + X' and deep Y descents,
             i.e., a high A and a high V wave. (See figure on p. 359.)

3.   Why will double filling of the right atrium by TR not produce a deep X' and Y descent as
     with ASDs?
     ANS.:   Because in TR the tendency to increase the descent of the base is counteracted by
             the regurgitant stream with the pressure of the RV behind it; i.e., in TR, the right
             atrium fills from another source, not only with increased volume but also with an
             increased pressure. Therefore, with increasing amounts of TR, the X' becomes
             more and more shallow and the Y increasingly deep.

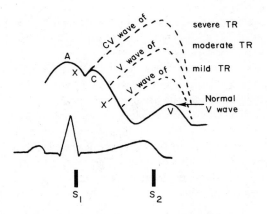

As the degree of TR increases, the X' descent is increasingly encroached upon With severe TR, no
X' descent is seen, and the jugular pulse wave is said to be "ventricularized."

*4.   With which lesion is severe TR confused on inspection of the jugulars alone? Why?
       ANS.:   With severe AR. The large single regurgitant CV wave looks like the large carotid
                pulse wave of AR.
*5.   Why will a poor descent of the base, as with a poor RV contraction, cause a high V wave?
       ANS.:   Both the X′ descent and the V wave are produced during systole, while the tricuspid
                valve is closed. The V wave can appear only when atrial filling can overcome the
                drop in pressure produced by the descent of the base. A poor descent of the base
                can be overcome much earlier by atrial filling from the venae cavae, and so a larger
                V wave will result.
*6.   What is the jugular H wave?
       ANS.:   It is the diastolic wave between the Y trough and the next A wave that results from
                filling of the "atrioventricle." During most of this period, known as "diastasis,"
                the ventricle is filling relatively slowly. (See figure on p. 84.)
*7.   Besides in tachycardias, when will the diastasis, or H wave, be absent?
       ANS.:   In TS, because of a too slow Y descent (unless there is a bradycardia with very
                long diastoles).
*8.   How can a jugular tracing help suggest constrictive pericarditis?
       ANS.:   It will reflect the right atrial pressure curve, which usually shows a dominant
                V wave and steep Y descent with a rapid rise to a diastolic plateau type of H wave
                [16]. The diastolic part of this curve reflects RV pressure events known as the
                "early diastolic dip and plateau," commonly seen at cardiac catheterization in
                constrictive pericarditis. One theory attributes this phenomenon to work performed
                during contraction on tissue that is fixed to the ventricular wall; i.e., it is deformed
                in the manner of a "loaded" spring [3]. The sudden release of the "loaded spring"
                in diastole causes the ventricular wall to recoil excessively, resulting in a rapid fall
                in ventricular pressure (which is reflected in the rapid jugular Y descent). The
                limited expansion due to the encasement causes the ventricular pressure to rise
                steeply after the early dip. The same mechanism may be operating in some
                patients with endocardial or myocardial fibrosis or infiltrate, causing a restrictive
                cardiomyopathy.
*9.   How can we account for the large X′ and small V in tamponade, and the large V and small
       X′ in constrictive pericarditis?
       ANS.:   Presumably tamponade via fluid does not have as much effect on atrial compliance
                as does the stiff encasement of an atrium with fibrous tissue and calcium, as in
                constrictive pericarditis.
10.   Why is it logical to call the atrial wave that is caused by TR a V wave, even though it is the
       result of a different mechanism than the usual V wave?
       ANS.:   Other sources besides the usual venae cavae blood often contribute to the V wave;
                e.g., in ASDs, blood from the left atrium is added to it, and an anomalous pul-
                monary vein draining into the right atrium can also contribute to it. Regurgitant
                flow from the RV contributing to the V wave in TR should not force us to use a
                different term for this large wave. However, if the entire X′ is replaced, the systolic
                wave may justifiably be called a CV wave.
                    *Note: a high, sharp CV wave can produce a clicking sound over the jugulars in
                systole.

THE JUGULAR PULSE IN ARRHYTHMIAS

1.   How does atrial fibrillation affect the jugular pulse contour?
      ANS.:   a) No A wave is present.
              b) There is a decreased X', usually with a dominant Y descent.

The dominant descent in atrial fibrillation is almost always the Y descent, i.e., it has the superficial appearance of the pulse wave of TR.

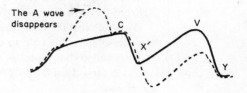

2.   Why is there a diminished X' descent if atrial fibrillation is present?
      ANS.:   The absent "kick" at the end of diastole causes a poor RV contraction because the RV is not stretched at the end of diastole, and so loses some of the Starling effect. By the loss of atrial contraction, the otherwise normal heart can decrease its stroke work by about 10%, but the heart with RV overload may decrease its stroke work by as much as 30%.

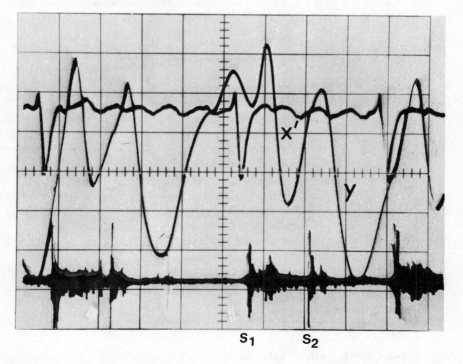

The wave before the X' cannot be an A wave since it is not due to atrial contraction. It is really a prolonged H wave. Note the good X' descent, despite the dominant Y descent, in this patient with moderate rheumatic MR.

3.   What other reasons are there for a poor X′ descent in atrial fibrillation if there is also high venous pressure?
ANS.:   a) A high venous pressure due to heart failure implies poor RV contraction and therefore a poor descent of the base.
 b) A right atrium in a patient in heart failure is under increased tension from excess sympathetic stimulation. Thus the atrium is less compliant than normal and there will be a steeper rise of pressure than normal as it receives its blood from the venae cavae to build up a V wave during ventricular systole.
 Note: Some TR tends to occur when there is atrial fibrillation and high venous pressures. This may help to obliterate the X′ descent.
4.   What is the wave called that precedes the descent of the base in a patient with no atrial contraction (as in atrial fibrillation)?
ANS.:   An H wave.
*5.   How are the jugular pulsations affected by atrial flutter?
ANS.:   Multiple small A waves may result, one for each F wave, with higher ones occurring during systole when the AV valves are closed. These are difficult to see unless the venous pressure is elevated. (Even coarse atrial fibrillation has produced irregular small A waves in jugular tracings.)
*6.   Which arrhythmias will produce irregularly occurring cannon waves?
ANS.:   Any arrhythmia in which a P wave may occur intermittently between the QRS and the end of the T; e.g., in premature atrial or ventricular contractions or in AV dissociation, as in complete AV block.

*HOW TO RECORD A JUGULAR PULSE

*1.   Where must one place a pulse pickup on the neck for best recording of an internal jugular pulsation?
ANS.:   Over the right jugular bulb [17]. This is just above the clavicle, between the insertions of the sternocleidomastoid muscle.
 Note: It is often helpful to remove the pillow from beneath the patient's head and raise his chin slightly and push it to the left in order to expose the right supraclavicular fossa.
*2.   Which is preferable, a photoelectric cell method of recording the silhouette of a jugular as it interrupts a light source, a cone that picks up volume changes, or a pressure-sensitive device that is placed on the jugulars?
ANS.:   The photoelectric method exaggerates carotid artifacts. Thus, either a cone or a pressure sensitive transducer is preferable.
 Note: If the silhouette of the external jugulars is recorded by means of a beam of light passing over them to a photoelectric cell, marked time delays can occur.

*SPECIAL INFORMATION FROM JUGULAR TRACINGS

*1.   What is meant by the P_2 to V peak interval, and what hemodynamic event does this represent?
ANS.:   The distance between the pulmonary component of the S_2 and the peak of the V wave of a jugular pulse tracing represents the isovolumic relaxation time of the right ventricle.

*2.   What controls the P_2 to V peak interval?

     ANS.:   a) Heart rate. Bradycardia makes it longer.

              b) Rapidity of intrinsic ventricular expansion time. In uncomplicated ASDs, the rate of expansion is inordinately rapid.

              c) Height of the pulmonary artery pressure and right atrial V wave pressure. Pulmonary hypertension prolongs isovolumic expansion time and therefore prolongs the P_2 to V peak interval, provided the venous pressure is normal and the V wave height is not thereby increased.

*3.   In what congenital lesion is the P_2 to V peak interval (a) well correlated with mean pulmonary artery pressure or (b) poorly correlated with mean pulmonary artery (PA) pressure?

     ANS.:   a) In isolated VSD. The regression equation for mean PA pressure is $812 \times (P_2$ to V$) - 37$, with a standard error of 12 mm. Roughly, a P_2 to V peak interval of 80 msec (0.08 sec) separates normal from elevated pulmonary artery pressure [12]. It is probable that the kind of pulse unit necessary to make use of these figures is one that utilizes volume displacement by a funnel or cup.

              b) In ASD or in PS the correlation is poor.

REFERENCES

1. Ali, N. Pulsations of arm veins in the absence of tricuspid insufficiency. *Chest* 63:41, 1973.
2. Bonner, A. J., Jr., and Tavel, M. E. The relationship of the jugular "C" wave to changing diastolic intervals. *Am. Heart J.* 84:441, 1972.
3. Burch, G. E., and Giles, T. D. Theoretic considerations of the post-systolic "dip" of constrictive pericarditis. *Am. Heart J.* 86:569, 1973.
4. Cheng, T. O. Mechanism of X descent in atrial pressure pulse. *Arch. Intern. Med.* 132:114, 1973.
5. Constant, J. The X prime descent in jugular contour nomenclature and recognition. *Am. Heart J.* 88:372, 1974.
6. Constant, J., and Lippschutz, E. J. The one-minute abdominal compression test or "the hepatojugular reflux," a useful bedside test. *Am. Heart J.* 67:701, 1964.
7. Davison, R., and Cannon, R. Estimation of central venous pressure by examination of jugular veins. *Am. Heart J.* 87:279, 1974.
8. Dock, W. Loud presystolic sounds over the jugular veins associated with high venous pressure. *Am. J. Med.* 20:853, 1956.
9. Feder, W., and Cherry, R. External jugular phlebogram as reflecting venous and right atrial hemodynamics. *Am. J. Cardiol.* 12:383, 1963.
10. Fred, H. L., Wukasch, D. C., and Petrany, Z. Transient compression of the left innominate vein. *Circulation* 29:758, 1964.
11. Gabe, I. T., Gault, J. H., Ross, J., Jr., Mason, D. T., Mills, C. J., Schillingford, J. P., and Braunwald, E. Measurement of instantaneous blood flow velocity and pressure in conscious man with a catheter-tip velocity probe. *Circulation* 40:603, 1969.
12. Gamboa, R., Gersony, W. M., Hugenholtz, P. G., and Nadas, A. S. External measurement of the isovolumic relaxation phase as an indicator of pulmonary artery pressure in ventricular septal defects. *Am. J. Cardiol.* 16:665, 1965.

13. Gensini, G. G., Caldini, P., Casaccio, F., and Blount, S. G., Jr. Persistent left superior vena cava. *Am. J. Cardiol.* 4:677, 1959.

14. Grant, R. P. Notes on the muscular architecture of the left ventricle. *Circulation* 32:301, 1965.

15. Hamosh, P., and Cohn, J. N. Mechanism of the hepatojugular reflux test. *Am. J. Cardiol.* 25:100, 1970.

16. Hansen, A. T., Eskildsen, P., and Gotzsche, H. Pressure curves from the right auricle and the right ventricle in chronic constrictive pericarditis. *Circulation* 3:881, 1951.

17. Hartman, H. The jugular venous tracing. *Am. Heart J.* 59:698, 1960.

18. Hitzig, W. M. On the mechanism of inspiratory filling of the cervical veins and pulsus paradoxus in venous hypertension. *J. Mt. Sinai Hosp.* 8:625, 1941.

19. Horwitz, S., Esquivel, J., Attie, F., Lupi, E., and Espino-Vela, J. Clinical diagnosis of persistent left superior vena cava by observation of jugular pulses. *Am. Heart J.* 86:759, 1973.

20. Kesteloot, H., and Denef, B. Value of reference tracings in diagnosis and assessment of constrictive epi- and pericarditis. *Br. Heart J.* 32:675, 1970.

21. Lange, R. L., Botticelli, J. T., Tsagaris, T. J., Walker, J. A., Gani, M., and Bustamente, R. A. Diagnostic signs in compressive cardiac disorders: Constrictive pericarditis, pericardial effusion and tamponade. *Circulation* 33:763, 1966.

22. Mackenzie, J. *The Study of the Pulse.* London: Pentland, 1902.

23. Mackenzie, J. The interpretation of the pulsations in the jugular veins. *Am. J. Med. Sci.* 134:12, 1907.

24. Matthews, M. D., and Hampson, J. Hepatojugular reflux. *Lancet* 1:873, 1958.

25. McKay, I. F. S. An experimental analysis of the jugular pulse in man. *J. Physiol.* 106:113, 1947.

26. McKay, I. F. S., and Walker, R. L. True venous pulse wave. *Nature* 205:1220, 1965.

27. Nagel, M. R., Ronan, J. A., Jr., and Roberts, W. C. Left-to-right shunt at atrial level after rupture of papillary muscle from acute myocardial infarction. *Am. Heart J.* 86:112, 1973.

28. Nakhjavan, F. K., and Goldberg, H. Hemodynamic effects of catecholamine stimulation in constrictive pericarditis. *Circulation* 52:487, 1970.

29. Nasser, W. K., Davis, R. H., Dillon, J. C., Tavel, M. E., Helmen, C. H., Feigenbaum, H., and Fisch, C. Atrial myxoma. *Am. Heart J.* 83:810, 1972.

30. Nixon, P. G. F., and Polis, O. The left atrial X descent. *Br. Heart J.* 24:173, 1962.

31. Rapaport, E., Weisbart, M. H., and Levine, M. The splanchnic blood volume in congestive heart failure. *Circulation* 18:581, 1958.

32. Rich, L. L., and Tavel, M. E. The origin of the jugular C wave. *N. Engl. J. Med.* 284:1309, 1971.

33. Russek, H. I., and Zohman, B. L. The syndrome of Bernheim. *Am. Heart J.* 30:427, 1945.

34. Sharpey-Schafer, E. P. Venous tone. *Br. Med. J.* 2:1589, 1961.

35. Spring, D. A., Folts, J. D., Young, W. P., and Rowe, G. G. Premature closure of the mitral and tricuspid valves. *Circulation* 45:663, 1972.

36. Vogel, J. H. K., Horgan, J. A., and Strahl, C. L. Left ventricular dysfunction in chronic constrictive pericarditis. *Chest* 59:484, 1971.

37. Wexler, L., Bergel, D. H., Gabe, G. S. M., and Mills, C. J. Pressure and velocity patterns in the venae cavae of normal human subjects. *Circulation* 36 (Suppl. II):269, 1967.

38. Wiggers, C. J. *Modern Aspects of the Circulation in Health and Disease* (2nd ed.). Philadelphia: Lea & Febiger, 1923.

39. Wood, P. Chronic constrictive pericarditis. *Am. J. Cardiol.* 7:48, 1961.

40. Wooley, C. F., Goodwin, R. S., and Ryan, J. M. Mitral stenosis. *Arch. Intern. Med.* 127:727, 1971.
41. Wooley, C. F., Klassen, K. P., Leighton, R. F., Goodwin, R. S., White, R. P., and Ryan, J. M. The left atrial pressure pulse of mitral stenosis in sinus rhythm. *Am. J. Cardiol.* 25:395, 1970.

5

Inspection and Palpation of the Chest

THE NORMAL APEX BEAT OR APEX IMPULSE

1. What is meant by the term *apex beat* or *impulse*?

    ANS.:   The term was originally meant to refer to the palpable apex of the left ventricle
    (LV). During **isovolumic contraction**, the heart rotates counterclockwise (as
    viewed from below), and some part of the heart, usually the lower part of the
    anterior LV, strikes the anterior chest wall.

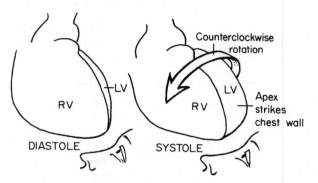

This counterclockwise rotation occurs during isovolumic contraction, i.e., before blood is ejected
from the ventricles.

    Unfortunately, the part of the heart that strikes the chest wall is not necessarily
    the apex as seen on an x-ray or by examination of the heart directly. In patients
    with a large enough right ventricle (RV), the "apex beat" may be due to movement
    of the RV. Therefore, the "apex beat" really means the *most lateral palpable ven-
    tricular movement or most lateral cardiac impulse.*

2. What is the disadvantage of using the term *point of maximum impulse* (PMI) as synonymous
    with the apex beat?

    ANS.:   Maximum precordial pulsations may be due to such abnormalities as a dilated pul-
    monary artery, a ventricular **aneurysm**, or an aortic aneurysm.

---

* indicates material that is for electives or fellows in cardiology, or concerns rare phenomena, of interest
primarily to cardiologists.

Boldface type indicates that the term is explained in the Glossary.

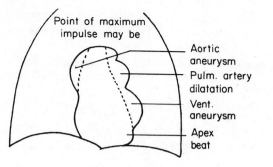

The point of maximum impulse (PMI) should not be equated with the apical impulse.

Palpability of the "Apex Beat" or Most Lateral Ventricular Impulse

1. How often is the normal "apex" beat palpable in the sitting position?
    ANS.:   In about 1 out of 5 subjects over age 40. However, in most children or young adults, even if slightly obese, an "apex" beat is palpable in the sitting position.
    Note: A cardiac impulse is more likely to be palpable in the sitting than in the supine position because in the latter, the heart falls away from the anterior chest wall.
2. How often is a normal LV impulse palpable in the **left lateral decubitus position**?
    ANS.:   In about 4 out of 5 older adults and in almost all children or young adults.
3. Why is it not generally known that a normal LV impulse is not usually palpable in the supine or sitting position in the older adult?
    ANS.:   Perhaps because it is not generally recognized that heart sound vibrations are palpable. One of the heart sounds at the site of the usual lateral cardiac impulse may be palpable and be mistaken for an outward movement of the chest wall. Also, position and age may not have been considered.
4. Why does a thick chest in an obese, normal young person not necessarily make the LV impulse impalpable?
    ANS.:   Possibly because obese people have physiological enlargement, which may make their LV impulse palpable.
5. What kind of chest shape will usually make a normal LV impulse impalpable?
    ANS.:   One with an increase in anteroposterior diameter. The mere palpability of the LV impulse in such a chest suggests cardiomegaly.
6. What is the best phase of respiration to bring the heart closest to the chest wall so that you can best feel the LV impulse?
    ANS.:   Whatever phase of respiration brings an impulse between the ribs. This may therefore be fully held expiration, inspiration, or even halfway between inspiration and expiration.
7. With which part of the hand is a slight localized impulse best felt?
    ANS.:   The fingertips or the area just proximal are best for slight localized movements (see figure on p. 146).
    Note: a) All chest palpation is best done from the right side of the bed, with the patient's bed as comfortably high as possible — ideally, at the level of the examiner's waist.

b) Some cardiologists find that removing the stethoscope from the ears
helps sharpen the kinesthetic sense, so that faint impulses are more
easily appreciated.

c) Try each hand separately. Some examiners find the fingers of one hand
more sensitive than the other in detecting fine movements.

Site of the Most Lateral Cardiac Impulse and Its Normal Limits

1.   Besides the greater likelihood of finding it palpable, what are the advantages of examining
for the site of a lateral cardiac impulse with the patient in the sitting rather than in the
supine position?

ANS.:   The site of a cardiac impulse is best measured in the sitting position with the feet
up on the bed, because

a) The most lateral impulse often moves slightly more to the left and against the
chest wall in this position, so that the most lateral extent is better ascertained.
Note: This lateral shift in the sitting position with the legs up is probably due
to the upward push by the compressed abdominal contents and diaphragm. In
the standing position, for example, the most lateral cardiac movement does not
shift leftward [28].

b) It allows routine palpation from behind, which has several advantages. Occasionally, a very subtle lateral impulse can only be felt when the hand palpates
from a quiet, immobile area like the back. A hand on the anterior chest often
is disturbed by left parasternal movements and heart sound vibrations that mask
any slight motion at the tips of the fingers. Second, a frontal approach may mis-
lead you into thinking that the movement on the front of the chest is the most
lateral LV impulse when in fact it may only be the RV movement or an aneurysm,
and the true most lateral LV movement may be near the posterior axillary line.

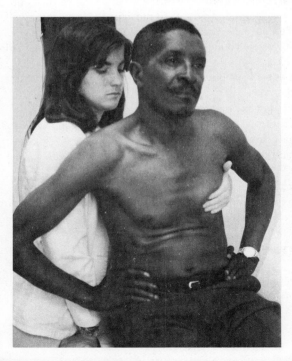

A posterior in addition to an anterior
approach may allow you to feel more
subtle movements, especially if your
left hand is more sensitive than your
right.

c) The sitting position is more like an x-ray position than is the supine position, and we are more familiar with the site of the normal apex on x-ray in each individual type of chest in the upright position.

*d) It allows you to relate the most lateral impulse site to the circumference of the chest and so offers the use of another method of establishing the normalcy of the impulse's position. This method requires that you imagine the chest as a circular structure, with the heart lying exactly in its center. If you draw an imaginary line from the center of the chest to the midsternum, and another to the most lateral impulse, the angle thus produced is the heart angle, whose upper normal is about 50 degrees [19].

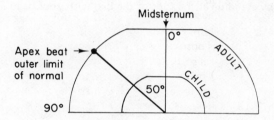

The outer normal limit for a heart angle in adults (with their legs up on a bed) is about 50 degrees.

This angle can be calculated from the formula:

$$\text{Heart angle} = \frac{\text{distance from midsternum} \times 360}{\text{chest circumference}}$$

The following nomogram, taken from the original study in 1941, will expedite matters [19].

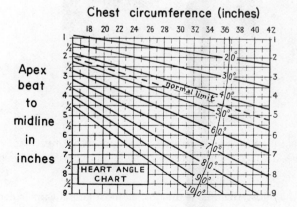

By encircling the chest with a tape measure with the zero mark at the midsternal line, you can measure in one step the circumference of the chest and the distance in inches of the apex impulse from the midsternal line.

2.   With the patient in the sitting position, how can you most quickly judge whether or not
       the most lateral ventricular impulse is in the normal site?
       ANS.:   The normal most lateral ventricular impulse is at about the mid-left thorax, at the
                horizontal level of the fourth or fifth interspace. If it is over 2 cm to the left of
                the mid-left thorax, cardiomegaly should be suspected.
                  Note: The midclavicular line is the more popular site of the normal most lateral
                ventricular impulse. Unfortunately, medical dictionaries equate the midclavicular
                line with the nipple line, to which it may bear no relation. The term also has a
                false aura of accuracy about it, as if the site of the most lateral impulse were not
                a rough measurement. Instead of trying to find the exact lateral end of the clavicle,
                which is often difficult to ascertain, it is quicker and easier simply to view the left
                thorax by standing at the foot of the bed with your head in line with the mid-left
                thorax.

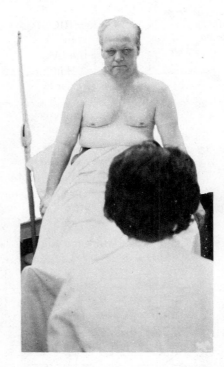

The mid-left thorax as viewed from the front is a good measure of cardiac impulse displacement.
An impulse that is over 2 cm to the left of the mid-left thorax is probably abnormally displaced.

3.   How far from the midsternal line is the normal most lateral ventricular impulse?
       ANS.:   The upper limit of normal is 10 cm from the midsternal line. This is surprisingly
                useful, because over 10 cm has a good correlation with cardiomegaly, even in a large
                chest. This may be due to the fact that when the chest is so large that, say, 11 cm
                is normal for that chest, a ventricular impulse should not be palpable in that chest;
                i.e., if it is palpable at all in a huge chest, cardiomegaly is probably present.

Note: In the left lateral decubitus position, the normal ventricular impulse site is unknown because it then depends on mediastinal mobility.

4. What is the present status of chest percussion in determining heart size?
    ANS.:   It is not used by many cardiologists because
    a) A palpable ventricular impulse tells the heart size quickly and easily.
    b) When a ventricular impulse is not palpable because of a thick chest or over-aeration due to pulmonary disease, percussion becomes unreliable.
    c) Dressler [10], who devoted 20 pages of his clinical cardiology book to percussion of the chest for cardiac abnormalities, begins by stating that he finds it impossible to percuss cardiac borders.
    Note: Dressler worked out a system for defining "areas of cardiac dullness," which gave him much information. However, it requires great skill, as well as a study of his findings, in order to make use of percussion to detect abnormalities.

CAUSES OF A DISPLACED LEFT VENTRICULAR IMPULSE

1. Does left ventricular hypertrophy (LVH) displace the LV impulse to the left?
    ANS.:   No. There must be dilatation as well as LVH in order to displace an LV impulse. Pure LVH tends to encroach on the ventricular cavity by growing inward as much as outward.
    Note: Dilatation without some hypertrophy of a ventricle is very rare. If a ventricle is dilated for a long enough time, it will nearly always hypertrophy in obedience to Laplace's law, which states that pressure is proportional to tension and inversely proportional to radius or volume. This means that the larger the volume, the greater must be the wall tension in order to maintain pressure. The need for tension seems to stimulate the hypertrophy, which in turn supplies the necessary tension. Exceptions are the acute dilatation that may occur with a ruptured aortic cusp, or the chronic dilatation associated with the diffuse fibrosis of some severe idiopathic **cardiomyopathies.**

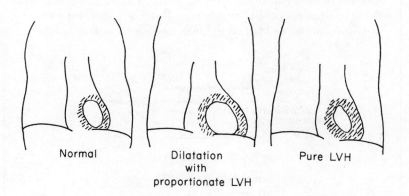

Normal   Dilatation   Pure LVH
                with
          proportionate LVH

Pure LVH causes an encroachment inward on the cavity and has been called "concentric" hypertrophy. Dilatation with proportionate hypertrophy has been called "eccentric" hypertrophy.

A primarily hypertrophied heart, as in aortic stenosis (AS) or hypertension, can become a dilated heart when cardiac decompensation occurs. Therefore, although AS or hypertension will not displace an LV impulse while there is only pure hypertrophy, it may be displaced when the patient goes into failure.

2.   What is meant by concentric and eccentric hypertrophy?

ANS.:   Left ventricular hypertrophy without dilatation is called concentric hypertrophy. The term *concentric* implies the existence of an "eccentric" hypertrophy. Since, however, the latter term suggests that the ventricle is eccentrically hypertrophied, and it does not mean this at all, it is a poor term. Eccentric hypertrophy means that the chamber dilatation (usually with proportionate hypertrophy) has forced the geometric center of the heart to be shifted eccentrically to the left.

*3.   What kind of cardiac **malposition** besides dextrocardia will cause a ventricular impulse to be palpable on the right chest?

ANS.:   Dextroversion (see types of **malpositions of the heart**).

Note: To confirm the presence of dextrocardia by physical examination, percuss for the stomach bubble in order to reveal tympany on the right.

To confirm dextroversion by physical examination, aortic pulsations may be palpable in the second right interspace because of the anterior position of the aorta caused by the rotation of the LV anteriorly.

*4.   What can displace an LV impulse to the left in the absence of cardiomegaly?

ANS.:   a) **Pectus excavatum.**

b) Congenital complete absence of the pericardium.

CHARACTER OF THE LEFT VENTRICULAR IMPULSE

The Normal Left Ventricular Impulse

1.   What is the character of the normal LV impulse?

ANS.:   This is most thoroughly understood by observing it with the patient in the supine position, either flat or with his chest up at 45 degrees. The normal LV impulse rises and retracts quickly by the first half of systole. Listen with your stethoscope to the heart sounds while watching one finger or your chest piece on the impulse. A normal impulse will fall on to the second sound or even before it.

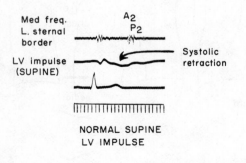

NORMAL SUPINE
LV IMPULSE

In the supine position, the normal LV impulse falls away during systole and appears to end on or before the S_2.

2. What causes the initial outward movement that results in the heart's striking the chest wall?

    ANS.: During isovolumic contraction the heart rotates counterclockwise (as seen from below) and flings the apical area of the heart against the anterior chest wall. (See figure on p. 100.)

3. How can you explain the midsystolic retraction of the normal LV impulse?

    ANS.: The retraction is probably due to the inferolateral LV wall's contracting and pulling away from the anterior chest wall. This retraction occurs after the initial counterclockwise rotation of the heart during isovolumic contraction has flung this part of the heart briefly against the chest wall.

    *One theory has it that when ejection occurs, the circular muscle, which does not extend to the apex, pulls on the oblique muscle of the apex to cause precordial retraction [8]. This theory has two weaknesses: (a) The part of the heart that strikes the chest wall, especially in the supine position, is probably not the apex, but a segment anterior and superior to the actual apex. (b) The outer surface of the apex probably does not really retract, i.e., the angiographic picture of retraction is really an illusion caused by closing in of the sides of the LV wall during systole.

The apparent upward movement of the apex on cineangiograms is an illusion caused by the drawing together of the side walls, closing off the apex from below upward.

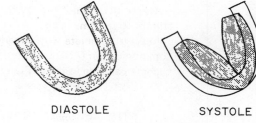

DIASTOLE   SYSTOLE

4. How can you tell that the most lateral impulse is caused by the LV and not by a large RV usurping that area?

    ANS.: a) Only the LV impulse feels like a localized thrust, i.e., as though a golf ball inside the chest were being pushed against your fingers. The RV usually has a more diffuse, poorly circumscribed movement.

    b) The LV impulse almost always will manifest medial retraction. This means that as the heart rotates to thrust the LV outward, the medial aspect of the heart moves posteriorly and pulls the chest-wall muscle and skin with it.

Note the retraction medial to the apex which shows a sustained impulse due to the effect of LVH. Although these tracings were taken in the supine position, medial retraction is best seen in the left lateral decubitus position.

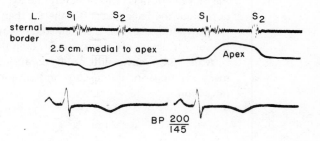

Note: When both the outward and medial movements are large, this is sometimes called a left ventricular rock.

5.   How can you best elicit medial retraction?

ANS.:   First, place one finger on the most lateral impulse and explore with another finger
directly medially, supramedially, and infermedially, noting whether or not the
medial finger retracts while the finger on the lateral impulse rises. If you do not
observe medial retraction, remove the medial finger and examine the skin instead.
Often, the skin will show obvious medial retraction that the finger on the skin did
not; i.e., the skin often amplifies medial retraction.

6.   What cardiac diagnoses are ruled out by the presence of a palpable LV impulse?

ANS.:   a) Any abnormality that causes a dilated RV without concomitant dilatation of
the LV, e.g., secundum-type **atrial septal defects** (ASDs) and **primary pulmonary
hypertension** should not be readily diagnosed if the LV apex beat is found.
Note: In **endocardial cushion defects**, there may be severe mitral regurgitation
(MR) that enlarges the LV. Therefore, this type of ASD can be suggested by identi-
fying the LV impulse.

b) Any abnormality that causes pure right ventricular hypertrophy (RVH), such
as pure pulmonary stenosis (PS). This is because a hypertrophied RV tends to
rotate the heart clockwise (looked at from below). This places the LV posteriorly, so that even if the RV is only hypertrophied and not dilated, the LV is
still usually not palpable.
Note: In severe PS with a marked right-to-left shunt through an intra-atrial
communication (ASD or patent foramen ovale), the LV may enlarge enough to
become palpable in the left lateral decubitus position.

THE LEFT VENTRICULAR IMPULSE IN
LEFT VENTRICULAR HYPERTROPHY

1.   How does the character of the LV impulse in LVH differ from the normal LV impulse?

ANS.:   a) It is sustained.

b) It may have extra humps or dips.

2.   What is meant by a sustained LV impulse?

ANS.:   The sustained impulse continues its outward movement longer than normally
throughout systole.
Note: In order to tell whether or not the impulse is sustained, you must time
the bottom of the fall of the impulse and relate it to the second sound (S$_2$). If
the movement falls onto or before the S$_2$, it is not sustained. If, however, the
bottom of the fall occurs after the S$_2$, then it is sustained. In order to tell whether
the outward movement is sustained, say a word such as *down* at the bottom of
the fall. If the word follows the S$_2$, then the impulse is sustained.
Note: Skin movements can be confusing. It is preferable to watch the movement of a finger or stethoscope on the ventricular impulse in timing the fall or
retraction.

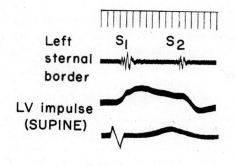

Sustained apex host

If you imagine a sound shortly after the S_2, the sustained apex beat will seem to fall onto it rather than onto the S_2.

3. Sustaining is a normal phenomenon in which position?
    ANS.:   In the left lateral decubitus position.
        Note: In the 45-degree position, the normal LV impulse is not usually sustained, even in the left lateral position [30].

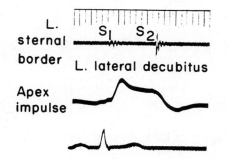

Note the sustained apex impulse in the left lateral decubitus position. In this position the true apex probably recoils against the chest wall and is an opposite and equal reaction to the force of ejection. Since ejection is a sustained activity, the apex reaction against the chest wall should also be sustained.

*4.   In which kind of LVH is there no sustaining?
    ANS.:   When the LVH is proportional to a mild or moderate amount of volume overload, as in moderate aortic regurgitation (AR), patent ductus arteriosus, ventricular septal defect (VSD), or severe anemia, the LV impulse may be overactive but not sustained.
        Note: The degree of AR can be roughly judged by the presence of sustaining. In mild to moderate AR, there is an overactive (larger amplitude of movement) but a nonsustained impulse. Only if AR is at least moderately severe is there a sustained impulse.

*5.   What can cause a sustained LV impulse in the absence of LVH?
      ANS.:   Congenital complete absence of the pericardium. The LV impulse here is generally
              displaced into the midaxillary line.

The Atrial Hump in Left Ventricular Hypertrophy

1.   How does a cineangiogram show the effect of a contracting atrium on the ventricle?
      ANS.:   When contrast material is injected into the LV, a cineangiogram can show that the
              LV suddenly expands at the end of diastole in response to atrial contraction.
2.   When is this end-diastolic or presystolic expansion of the LV palpable on the chest wall?
      ANS.:   It is normally not palpable. Only a very strong left atrial contraction can expand
              the LV with enough force to cause a palpable presystolic hump at the LV impulse.
                 *Note: If the atrial hump effect is too close to the outward movement of the
              ventricular contraction, it may be impalpable even if very high. This can be caused
              by a short P—R interval.

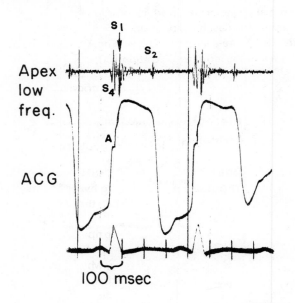

A short P—R of about 80 msec due to a preexcitation abnormality has caused the atrial hump
(A) to be too close to the major ventricular movement to be palpable.

3.   What is the cause of a left atrial contraction strong enough to make a palpable left ventricu-
      lar hump at the LV impulse?
      ANS.:   Severe loss of LV **compliance**, i.e., loss of distensibility of the LV.
                 Note: The strong atrial contraction effect on the LV is often called the "atrial
              kick" or "booster-pump" effect. This is because the expansion of the LV just
              before its contraction produces an increased energy of ventricular contraction or
              Starling effect.

4.   How does the left atrium "get the message" to contract harder when the LV is stiffer?
  ANS.:   In diastole, the mitral valve is open and the atrium and ventricle are in continuity,
       i.e., it is, in effect, an "atrioventricle." When the ventricle is stiff, the atrioven-
       tricle is also stiff, and when blood pours into a stiff chamber, the pressure rises
       steeply. If the atrium is under high pressure at the end of diastole, then, via the
       Starling effect, it will contract more strongly.
         Note: Eventually the atrium itself will hypertrophy in response to its continued
       strong contractions and will then contribute to the stiffness of the "atrioventricle."

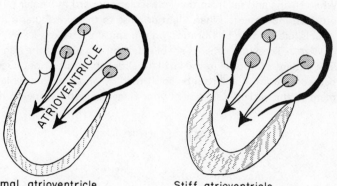

Normal atrioventricle   Stiff atrioventricle

A stiff ventricle must be transmitting its loss of compliance to the atrium during diastole when
the AV valves open.

5.   What is the commonest cause of chronic increased stiffness of the LV?
  ANS.:   Left ventricular hypertrophy secondary to hypertension. The next most common
       is LVH secondary to coronary disease; i.e., the confluent patchy areas of fibrosis
       or infarction can cause a stiff LV.
6.   Which cause of LVH most commonly results in a palpable presystolic atrial hump?
  ANS.:   Coronary disease with residual infarction or fibrosis. This may be because coronary
       disease produces patchy areas of scarring, which leave the ventricle nondistensible
       but only moderately hypertrophied, so that a strong atrial contraction can still
       easily expand the nonscarred myocardium.
*7.   Which type of AS is most likely to produce a palpable atrial presystolic hump at the site of
   the LV impulse?
  ANS.:   Hypertrophic subaortic stenosis (HSS). Perhaps this is because the extremely thick
       septum causes a marked loss of compliance, but the resulting strong atrial contrac-
       tion can easily expand the rest of the LV, which, although thick, is not nearly so
       thick as the septum that caused the strong atrial contraction in the first place. In
       valvular AS, the entire LV is equally hypertrophied, so that it resists the expansion
       of a left atrial contraction.
         Note: A palpable atrial hump in the presence of valvular AS is strongly corre-
       lated with a gradient of at least 75 mm Hg. In HSS, no such correlation can be
       made.

8. Why is it especially important to palpate for an A wave in AS?

ANS.: a) The S_4 may be inaudible because the louder murmur may obscure the soft, low-frequency S_4 (see **frequency**), or the S_4 is mistaken for an S_1 and the murmur that follows is thought to be "midsystolic."

b) A palpable A wave is highly correlated with a systolic gradient of at least 75 mm Hg [18].

c) It tells you that there is no concomitant mitral stenosis (MS), because MS will not permit a large enough atrial hump to be palpable.

9. What does an atrial kick feel like?

ANS.: When strong and far from the ventricular outward movement, it feels like a double outward movement. When slight or close to the ventricular outward movement, it feels like a notch or vibration on the apical upstroke.

Note: These movements are best felt by the part of the hand near the fingertips. The patient should be in the left lateral decubitus position. Occasionally, a suspected faint atrial kick can be confirmed by observing a double outward movement of the patient's skin or of your finger or stethoscope on the LV impulse.

ATRIAL KICK

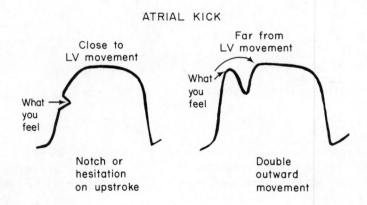

If only a notch or slight hesitation is present on the upstroke, the tips of the fingers must be used to perceive it. If a large double movement is felt, it must be distinguished from a midsystolic dip.

THE LEFT VENTRICULAR IMPULSE IN LEFT VENTRICULAR DILATATION

1. When can you suspect that the LV is enlarged when displacement of the LV impulse is questionable?

ANS.: When the LV impulse is enlarged in area.

2. What is the normal vertical or Y axis extent of the LV impulse area?

ANS.: If we consider interspace distance as the Y axis or vertical spread, then a normal LV impulse should not be felt well in more than one interspace in the Y axis.

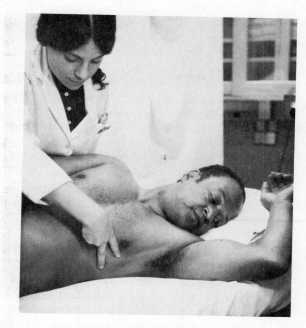

The normal apex beat is not felt through two interspaces during the same phase of respiration.

Note: This does not refer to the normal downward movement of the LV impulse with inspiration that may cause it to be felt one interspace lower on inspiration than on expiration. An impulse is enlarged if it can be easily felt in two interspaces in the *same phase of respiration.*

3.   What is the normal side-to-side, or X axis, extent of the LV impulse?

ANS.:   A normal LV impulse is usually not more than 1½ fingertips wide in the X axis; i.e., if it is felt equally well with two fingers placed side by side perpendicular to the ribs, cardiomegaly should be suspected.

Note: These measurements refer to examination in the left lateral decubitus position.

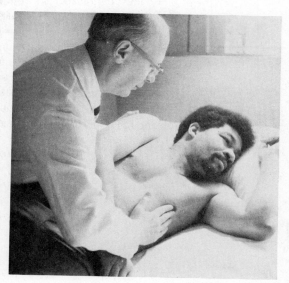

A normal apical impulse is no larger than about 1½ fingertip widths.

4.   What is meant by a "heave" or "lift"?

ANS.:   Any large area of sustained outward movement may be referred to as a heave or lift.

*5.   Why is the LV often palpable as a dilated chamber in the presence of pure, severe MS?

ANS.:   The reason is unknown, because about a third of subjects with the largest hearts and pure MS have the LV larger than the RV without any heart failure to suggest a significant cardiomyopathy [38].

*6.   When can the LV impulse of a nonenlarged heart be palpable in the left axilla in the presence of normal chest anatomy?

ANS.:   In congenital absence of the left pericardium [31].

Note: An inferior or right axis deviation on ECG, and an x-ray showing a prominent main pulmonary artery with marked displacement of the heart to the left of the vertebral column, suggest this cause of a displaced LV impulse.

THE EARLY RAPID FILLING HUMP IN DILATED HEARTS

1.   When does a ventricle expand rapidly, in early, middle, or end-diastole?

ANS.:   In early diastole there is a rapid expansion. This early diastolic rapid expansion suddenly halts and gives way to slow expansion. At the end of the slow expansion phase, the atrium contracts and produces a short period of rapid expansion again at the end of diastole.

Note: The cause of the sudden changeover from early rapid to slow expansion of the LV is unknown. These phases of diastole are also known as "rapid filling" and "slow filling" phases.

2.   What can exaggerate the changeover from early rapid to slow filling phases?

ANS.:   The more rapid the early filling phase, the greater is the difference between early rapid and slow filling phases. Anything that increases the rate of expansion of the LV will increase the rapid filling of the LV, and this will exaggerate the abruptness of the changeover to the slow filling phase. This is most marked when an increased volume of blood must be transported from the left atrium to the LV, as in MR.

*Note: a) The point of changeover from early rapid to slow filling can become palpable in severe MR. Here, the torrential flow into the LV can cause it to expand so rapidly in early diastole that it is pulled up very sharply. The momentum of rapid expansion carries the ventricular movement out so far that when it is pulled up, it can cause the entire ventricle to be pulled in. This causes a palpable hump at the end of the early rapid filling phase. This palpable hump or bump after the main LV impulse rise and fall is always associated with a third heart sound (S_3).

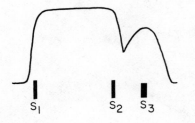

S_1 S_2 S_3

A slight outward movement following the major out-and-back movement suggests a palpable early rapid filling of the LV and is most commonly felt together with an S_3 in severe MR.

b) This extra early diastolic hump is also felt when the end of early rapid expansion is augmented by atrial contraction. This can occur only with an abnormally early P wave, as in first-degree atrioventricular (AV) block plus a short diastolic interval caused by a tachycardia. This effect of an abnormally early P wave is also associated with a very loud sound known as a summation sound. (This will be discussed in Chap. 11.)

*3.   What besides an atrial hump or rapid early filling hump can cause a double outward movement?

ANS.:   A midsystolic dip. This is most often felt in patients with severe HSS. It can, however, occasionally be palpable in patients with the ballooned valve syndrome or with acute myocardial infarction [40].

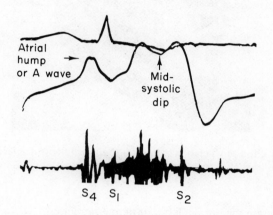

This apex impulse tracing (apex cardiogram) is from a 45-year-old man with HSS. The atrial hump and the midsystolic dip give an impression of a triple outward movement.

Note: A double *diastolic* outward movement is seen in some patients with sudden, severe AR [44]. The second movement occurs after the mitral valve has closed in mid-diastole, and further filling from the aortic valve occurs.

RIGHT VENTRICULAR OVERLOAD PARASTERNAL MOVEMENT

Normal Left Parasternal Movement

1.   What is the normal movement at the lower left parasternal area?

ANS.:   The major movement is a very small retraction. The retraction may be preceded by a short, small-amplitude outward movement in young people or in those with thin chests [7, 12, 22].

Note: Large areas of chest motion, as with usual left parasternal movements, are best palpated with the proximal part of the palm (thenar and hypothenar areas). This method transmits the movement to the entire arm, which may amplify the perception of palmar motion.

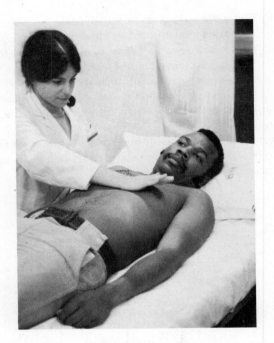

In this patient with MS, the physician is palpating the movement of a large RV, which was producing a right ventricular rock, i.e., a sustained left parasternal impulse and lateral retraction.

2.   What can exaggerate the normal left parasternal retraction?
        ANS.:   a) Any cause of a large LV stroke volume, such as a high output state (anemia or
                   hyperthyroidism) or AR. This is really a large area of apical medial retraction
                   which has extended as far medially as the sternum.
                b) A cardiomyopathy with a large LV can also exaggerate left parasternal retrac-
                   tion, despite the poor stroke volume.
3.   How can you tell that the left parasternal movement is due to RV overload?
        ANS.:   a) The presence of a RV rock, i.e., lateral retraction in the mid- or lateral thorax,
                   occurring simultaneously with outward parasternal movement, suggests a large
                   RV.

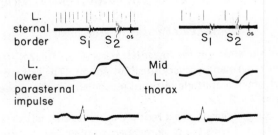

A sustained left parasternal impulse with lateral retraction is a sign of a volume overload of the
RV (and probably also of a pressure overload).

b) The presence of a second left interspace outward systolic movement due to a dilated pulmonary artery suggests a large RV.
Note: This degree of pulmonary artery dilatation is usually only seen either with severe pulmonary hypertension or a large volume RV overload, as in ASD.
c) The presence of an epigastric downward impulse suggests a large RV.
Note: A hand with the fingers pointing upward into the epigastrium during inspiration may feel an impulse coming down and striking the tips of the fingers (a large RV) [20]. If, on the other hand, the impulse strikes the pads of the fingers, it is due to an aortic pulsation. This is an especially useful maneuver if an increased chest diameter hides left parasternal movements.

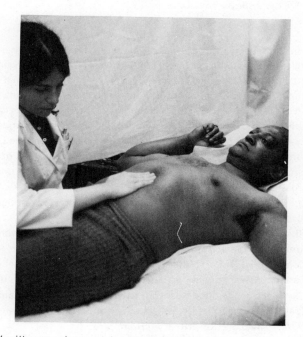

A large RV will come down and strike the tips (not the pads) of your fingers.

*d) The presence of an outward movement that is more marked to the right of the sternum than to the left is usually due to a huge right atrium and implies not only RV overload but severe tricuspid regurgitation (TR) [20].

*4.   How may a biventricular overload, as in VSDs, manifest itself on the chest wall?
ANS.:   A biventricular rock may be present; i.e., both the left parasternal and apical areas may rise with systole, with an area of systolic retraction between them.

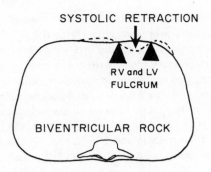

Retraction in the mid-left thorax, with sustained outward movements on either side, tells you that there is a biventricular volume overload.

5.   What conditions may produce large RV stroke volumes without either tricuspid or pulmonary regurgitation? What kind of chest pulsations would this engender?

ANS.:   Shunt flows such as occur in an ASD and a **ventricular septal defect** (VSD) and **anomalous pulmonary venous drainage** into the right atrium.

Note: The LV is often smaller than normal in patients with ASD [23]. The large RV of a moderate ASD may push back the slightly underfilled LV and prevent palpation of the LV impulse and also hide or prevent the LV physiological S_3; a shunt produced by partial anomalous pulmonary venous drainage may not do so. Anomalous pulmonary veins usually must drain an entire lung before the RV enlarges enough to hide LV events.

6.   List some causes of primary tricuspid regurgitation (TR) severe enough to create telltale precordial pulsations.

ANS.:   a) Rheumatic heart disease (almost never without both severe mitral disease and some tricuspid stenosis [TS] as well).

*b) Congenital TR, i.e., either idiopathic or with endocardial cushion defects.

*c) **Carcinoid heart disease** (due to carcinoid plaques on the undersurface, fixing the valves in the open position). (See Glossary for explanation and illustration.)

*d) Traumatic heart disease, i.e., due to ruptured chordae tendineae.

Note: All causes of primary TR are rare.

*7.   List some causes of enough primary pulmonary regurgitation to engender left parasternal pulsations.

ANS.:   a) Congenital absence of the pulmonary valve.

b) The unfortunate result of surgery for PS.

c) Infective endocarditis.

*8.   How may severe TR affect the precordial movements in an unexpected fashion?

ANS.:   a) The left parasternal area may retract instead of expand during systole. This is presumably because the RV, which is like an overdistended balloon in diastole, empties during systole and may cause the entire left parasternal area to retract.

b) The entire right precordium may expand during systole, while the entire left precordium retracts. This is because the right atrium may be so enlarged to the right, and the liver so expanded by the regurgitant volume, that systole may expand the entire right chest.

The Sustained Left Parasternal Impulse

1. How can you tell RVH from RV dilatation by palpation?

    ANS.:   Pure RVH may produce a sustained impulse at the mid- to lower left parasternal area. It will not be very marked in amplitude or very extensive in area. On the other hand, RV dilatation, such as that in uncomplicated ASDs, can produce a large area movement that may have a large amplitude and may not be sustained, but instead may be overactive [22].

      *Note: Eventration of the right diaphragm has been known to produce large and sustained left parasternal systolic movement by displacing the heart anteriorly and to the right.

2. List the commonest causes of a sustained RV heave.

    ANS.:   a) Pulmonary stenosis.

      *Note: The maximum impulse in PS is often a few centimeters away from the parasternal area or even in the mid-left thorax, especially as subjects grow older [24].

      b) Pulmonary hypertension.

      *Note: Although a sustained parasternal movement in a patient with an ASD suggests pulmonary hypertension, some patients with ASDs have sustained RV heaves even without pulmonary hypertension [32]. Since there is no significant RVH in most patients with ASD unless there is pulmonary hypertension, the cause for the occasional sustaining is unexplained [14, 24]. There is, however, trabecular hypertrophy in ASDs, which perhaps could change the pattern of RV contraction [27].

3. Why is there usually a sustained and often marked left parasternal movement in significant, pure MS, despite only a slightly elevated pulmonary arterial pressure?

    ANS.:   This may be due to a combination of the RVH and dilatation produced by the rise in pulmonary artery pressure with exercise, plus the effect of a large left atrium that could hold the RV hard against the left parasternal area [11].

*4. How can palpation of RV pulsation tell you whether PS is valvular or infundibular?

    ANS.:   Since the transmitted systolic movement originates in the high pressure zone *below* the stenosis, in valvular PS a parasternal impulse may be detected as high as the third left interspace; in infundibular stenosis the impulse may be confined to the fourth and fifth left interspaces. The impulse in subinfundibular stenosis (rare) may be detected only in the fifth interspace.

      Note: The dilated pulmonary artery of the poststenotically dilated pulmonary artery in pulmonary valve stenosis is not usually palpable, probably because the pulmonary artery above the valve tends to angulate sharply backward, away from the chest wall.

*Left Parasternal Impulse in the Uncommon Congenital Heart Abnormalities

*1. What left parasternal movement should make you doubt the presence of an Ebstein's anomaly?

    ANS.:   A systolic movement in the fourth or fifth interspace, i.e., over the body of the RV.

      Note: A movement in the third left interspace is not unusual. Apparently, a slight dilatation of the remaining RV due to the TR that is commonly present can cause left parasternal movement, but it will not be low, as in the usual dilated RV of TR or ASD. An impulse below the third left interspace is strong evidence against an Ebstein's anomaly.

*2.   What should you suspect if the murmur and LV impulse of a VSD are identified, but despite the absence of a low RV parasternal impulse there is a pulmonary artery pulsation in the second left interspace?

ANS.:   A VSD with a large shunt that is ejecting its blood mostly into the pulmonary artery without creating much pulmonary hypertension.

Note: If, on the other hand, you think that the patient has a VSD and a disproportionately hyperdynamic parasternal impulse of a marked RV volume overload, it suggests that the VSD is shunting directly into the right atrium. This is because a VSD usually causes only a mild RV volume overload since

a) The LV usually ejects its blood high into the infundibular area and not into the body of the RV.

b) A VSD shunt occurs mainly during systole, when the RV is contracting.

*3.   What precordial movements are expected in truncus arteriosus?

ANS.:   Biventricular volume overload pulsations, unless the pulmonary arteries are small or absent, in which case only the RV impulse is palpable. If a short main pulmonary artery is given off, that vessel may dilate and produce an impulse in the second left interspace.

*4.   What should you suspect in a cyanotic child with a palpable LV and no RV impulse?

ANS.:   Either pulmonary atresia (with intact ventricular septum and small RV), tricuspid atresia, Ebstein's anomaly, or vena cava to left atrial communication.

Note: In one type of pulmonary atresia, however, there is a large right atrium and RV due to TR. This can cause a palpable RV impulse. There is also a rare type of tricuspid atresia with a palpable RV and RV impulse. This is due to the presence of a large VSD, which can cause an increase in RV and pulmonary blood flow.

*5.   What precordial movements are felt in transposition of the great vessels?

ANS.:   A biventricular overload impulse is expected. This is because the pulmonary and systemic circuits operate in parallel and relatively independently of one another. Further, each circuit has an excessive volume of blood, so that even without communications, each circuit is volume-overloaded. Clinically, when pulmonary flow is reduced by severe pulmonary hypertension or stenosis, only the RV impulse will be palpable. The RV is, of course, a systemic ventricle in patients with transposition.

LEFT-SIDED CAUSES OF LEFT PARASTERNAL MOVEMENT

1.   When will mid- to lower left parasternal movement be due to the LV?

ANS.:   a) In young subjects with long, thin chests, the LV impulse may be very medial, i.e., at the left parasternal area.

b) In some subjects in whom the LV is markedly enlarged, it may extend medially to the left parasternal area (as well as laterally).

*c) In congenitally corrected transposition of the great vessels. This is because the septum may be rotated to a position more perpendicular to the chest wall than normal, thus swinging the left-sided ventricle (an anatomical RV) more medially than normal.

2. When will the left parasternal outward movement be due to a left atrium? Why?

    ANS.:   In severe, chronic MR. The left atrium is a mid-chest structure, i.e., it is not really
    a left atrium but a posterior atrium.

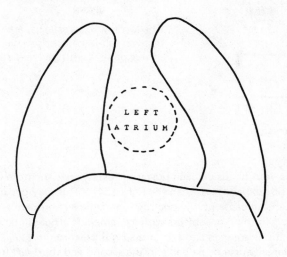

The "left" atrium is really a posterosuperior atrium, since it is behind and above the right atrium.
Although it is slightly to the left of the right atrium, it is a midline structure.

    If the posterior atrium expands markedly, it can push the RV (which is an
    anterior structure) against the chest wall [29]. If MR is severe enough, the left
    atrium will expand greatly during ventricular systole as it receives the regurgitant
    blood from the LV. The expanding left atrium can then push the RV forward
    against the chest wall.

*3. How can you tell whether or not an expanding left atrium is the cause of a marked left
    parasternal movement?

    ANS.:   a) You should suspect it only in the presence of severe *chronic* MR. It is not
    expected in acute MR because the healthy left atrium does not usually
    enlarge enough to push the RV forward significantly [35]. However, an acute
    event such as ruptured chordae occurring as a complication of chronic MR is
    very likely to cause marked left parasternal movement.

    b) Compare the LV impulse movement with the left parasternal movement by
    placing a finger on each. A left atrial lift will begin and end slightly later than
    the LV thrust. Right ventricular movement will begin and end at the same
    time or even before the LV thrust.

    c) There is a more precipitous parasternal collapse when MR is the cause of the
    left parasternal lift.

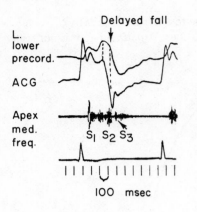

The left lower parasternal area movement shows a delayed fall in comparison with the apical impulse in this patient with severe chronic rheumatic MR.

d) Place your hands on each posterior hemithorax and note whether or not the left side expands less than the right [34]. This may occur because a large left atrium can cause partial obstruction of the left bronchus.

Note: In the rare subjects with extreme left atrial dilatation, the sustained pulsations are seen and felt in the right precordium [17].

*4.   When will an enlarged aorta be palpable in the second and third *left* interspace? Why?

ANS.:   In corrected transposition of the great vessels, because the aorta is excessively anterior and to the left, due to the rotation of the septum, which lies more perpendicular than parallel to the frontal plane of the chest. Thus, the left-sided RV (which ejects into the aorta) is more rightward and anterior than normal and carries the aortic root anteriorly against the chest wall.

MISCELLANEOUS CHEST PULSATIONS

Ventricular Aneurysms

1.   What is felt on the chest wall with a ventricular **aneurysm**?

ANS.:   Surprisingly, the commonest sign of a ventricular aneurysm is a larger-than-normal area of LV apical movement. This is completely indistinguishable from the impulse of a dilated and hypertrophied LV. In others, an aneurysm is felt as a sustained systolic bulge, separate from an LV impulse but too low for a pulmonary artery and too lateral for the RV.

Note: The term *paradoxical pulsation* is often used to describe the precordial movement that is palpable with a ventricular aneurysm. This is a poor term for any precordial systolic bulge. The term refers to what is seen in an open-chested dog or by fluoroscopy during an acute infarction: the infarct area bulges outward with systole while the rest of the heart contracts [13]. On the chest wall, an outward movement during systole separate from the LV impulse may not be due to an aneurysm. A large pulmonary artery, RV, or left atrium can cause an ectopic systolic expansion on the chest wall that we do not call paradoxical. Also, an aneurysm at the apex of the LV, on palpation of the chest wall, will cause the same movement as an enlarged LV [13].

2.   What is meant by a physiological aneurysm?

ANS.:   During acute anterior infarction, the lower left sternal border area may bulge with systole; but when healing occurs, this bulging may cease. Such a bulge, when felt during life but not seen at autopsy, is sometimes called a physiological aneurysm.

*3.   When will the most lateral ventricular impulse retract deeply in systole without the initial outward movement that is seen in RV overload?

ANS.:   In constrictive pericarditis [3]. Here, the left parasternal area retracts slightly also, but the right parasternal area may rise in systole. It is usually followed by a diastolic outthrust [15].

Aortic and Arterial Pulsations on the Chest Wall

*1.   How do you look for an aortic aneurysm by palpating the chest wall?

ANS.:   Look for right or left sternoclavicular joint area pulsations.

Note: a) An aortic aneurysm can occasionally be suspected if it depresses the left bronchus with each pulsation. Depression of a left bronchus will in turn pull down the trachea. Stand behind the seated patient and apply steady, upward pressure on the cricoid cartilage with the tip of one forefinger, and you will readily detect the downward pull on the trachea with each expansion. This phenomenon is known as the tracheal tug.

b) A dilated right aortic arch can also cause a right sternoclavicular pulsation. This, however, usually occurs only in the presence of cyanotic congenital heart disease, because only then is the aortic arch likely to be both on the right and dilated. In the presence of cyanosis, a right aortic arch suggests tetralogy, especially with pulmonary atresia, because only severe tetralogy, i.e., with severe PS or atresia, will cause a right aortic arch to be dilated enough to produce a palpable impulse. The more severe the PS, the larger the shunt into and diameter of the aorta. This pulsation should be sought specifically just below the right sternoclavicular junction.

2.   How may **coarctation** produce pulsations on the chest wall?

ANS.:   The posterior intercostal arteries (enlarged collaterals) may be both visible and palpable. You can best make their pulsations visible by having the patient bend forward and let his arms hang, to stretch the skin of the back. Project a light from above, to create a shadow below the posterior ribs.

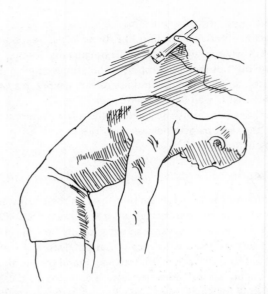

In the proper light, the dilated subcostal collateral arteries can be seen to pulsate.

3.   What should you suspect if a patient with coarctation has no posterior chest-wall collateral
      vessel pulsations?
      ANS.:   Coarctation of the abdominal aorta [37].
                  Note: In the usual thoracic coarctation, there may also be no visible or palpable
                  intercostal pulsations, no matter how severe the coarctation.
*4.   What noncardiac condition can cause the entire left anterior chest wall to heave with systole?
      ANS.:   A large aneurysm of the descending aorta directly behind the heart.

GRAPHIC DISPLAYS OF CHEST MOVEMENTS

Methods

*1.   What methods are most commonly used to show a visual record of chest movements on an
      oscilloscope or paper?
      ANS.:   The apex cardiogram, the kinetocardiogram, and the impulse cardiogram.
2.   What is meant by an apex cardiogram (ACG)?
      ANS.:   It is a tracing of the movements of the chest wall taken in the left lateral decubitus
                  position by applying a chest piece (held on the chest by a hand or strap) that can
                  transmit the movement to a transducer.
                  Note: A transducer is an instrument that can convert a mechanical signal into
                  an electrical one, or vice versa. The mechanical signal often comes from a funnel,
                  cone, or small cup placed over the skin of the chest (chest piece) in which the air
                  is displaced by movements of the chest wall. The air pressure change is the
                  mechanical signal that affects the transducer. Also common is a pressure-sensitive
                  pin or disk whose movement affects a diaphragm that undergoes pressure changes
                  that are transmitted to a transducer.

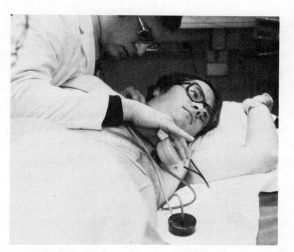

The pulse transducer is the black cylinder that is connected by a rubber tube to a side hole in a funnel held against the apical movement. The funnel is attached to a microphone, which the physician holds between his fingers. In this way, a simultaneous pulse tracing and phonocardiogram can be taken over the exact same area of the apex.

*3.   What part of the ventricle does a tracing of the movement of the cardiac "apex" represent?

      ANS.:   Apex cardiograms done on the exposed human heart during open heart surgery, or on dogs on different layers from skin to pericardium, show that the ACG represents the entire ventricular pulsation and not only movement of the apex itself. During ejection, you are recording the recoil of the ventricle against the chest wall as blood is ejected from the aorta. During ejection, it is thus not surprising that the ACG follows Newton's second law and reflects the exact opposite of the forces of ejection. Only with the patient in the left lateral decubitus position are you close enough to the actual apex to record the opposing ballistic force of ejection. With the patient in the supine position you are probably including the free-wall contraction in the tracing. Thus, in the supine position, the tracing is better called something other than an apex cardiogram. An *apex precordiogram* has been suggested as a suitable compromise. Perhaps we should use the term *impulse cardiogram* for supine recordings of ventricular motion, but even the latter term has already been given a specific meaning.

*4.   What is the specific meaning of *impulse cardiogram*?

      ANS.:   It is a tracing of movements of the chest wall in the supine or 45-degree chest position taken by applying to the impulse a pin whose movement is transmitted in such a way that it can obstruct a photoelectric cell beam proportionate to the pin's displacement. The entire unit is fixed to a clamp on a bedside stand.

*5.   What is meant by a kinetocardiogram?

      ANS.:   It is a tracing of movements of the chest wall, taken by the application to the chest wall of a pin that is *not* held by hand or strap to the chest. Instead, it is held in place by a rod that is fixed to the floor or bedstand; i.e., the chest movement is related to a fixed point in space. The chest movement is transmitted via the pin to a metal air-filled bellows and thence to a transducer.

*6.   Why is the ACG the most popular of the preceding methods?

ANS.:   a) It is more easily and quickly applied to the cardiac impulse in all chest positions.

b) The same chest piece and transducer can be used for carotid or jugular tracings.

c) There is a greater literature on the information from an ACG.

Note: By exaggerating peaks and troughs, the kinetocardiogram gives fine details of chest-wall movements, which are recorded routinely from all the areas in which a chest electrode of an ECG are taken. This kind of information is easy for a technician to obtain and has a growing literature that can be very useful.

*The photoelectric technique gives you the best representation of what the hand feels. However, there is very little in the literature on its use, and what is felt by the hand is often of limited value for purposes to which apical movements have been applied. For example, although the other methods exaggerate peaks and troughs, this is often an advantage when they are used as reference tracings for timing sounds and murmurs and when analyzing relative heights and rates and shapes of movements.

*7.   What is necessary before an ACG or impulse cardiogram pulse unit can show a sustained cardiac impulse?

ANS.:   The time constant should be at least three times the length of systole, i.e., at least 1.2 sec. Some investigators have recommended that it should be at least 2 sec, and others think that it is preferable to have it at 3 sec.

Note: a) The *time constant* is the rate at which a constant signal will drop down to the baseline or, to be more precise, the time taken for the signal to drop 36.6% of its original height. An adequate time constant for an ECG machine, for example, is 3.2 sec, i.e., after holding the standardization button down for 3.2 sec, the stylus should drop from 10 mm to not less than 3 mm above the baseline. An ACG or an ECG taken with too short a time constant will overshoot all peaks and troughs and be incapable of showing any sustained movements. It will act like a differential transducer, i.e., it will begin to measure change of rate or velocity with time. Air leaks in crystal transducers can cause a short time constant [26]. It is also thought that too much air in a large funnel can shorten the time constant.

b) As long as the low-frequency cutoff is at 0.15 Hz, there is no effect of different high-frequency cutoffs on the timing of points or in wave form configuration [33].

8.   How can you tell outward from inward movement when looking at a graphic display of an ACG?

ANS.:   Outward movements are upward movements of a writing arm or oscilloscope beam. Inward movements are shown as downward movements below a baseline.

THE NORMAL APEX CARDIOGRAM

1.   What is the disadvantage of the term *apex cardiogram* (*ACG*)?

ANS.:   a) It usually refers to a method of recording any precordial pulsation and not just to the movement of the "apex" beat. (See p. 125 for other suggested solutions.)

b) The noncardiologist is led at first to believe that an ACG is some sort of an electrocardiogram taken at the site of the LV impulse.

2.   What causes the first outward movement in the normal ACG that begins after the onset of the QRS?

ANS.:   The beginning of LV systolic movement. This is the C point.

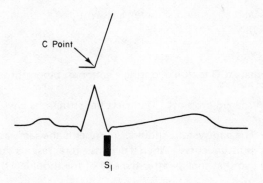

The beginning of contraction of the LV on the ACG is called the C point.

Note: a) The S_1, or first heart sound (due to mitral closure events), occurs about 50 msec (0.05 sec) or less after the onset of the ACG movement. This interval is known as the C—1 interval, i.e., the interval from the onset of LV contraction to the beginning of the S_1. During this time the LV pressure is rising from about 5 mm Hg to overcome left atrial pressure at about 8 mm Hg.

b) The ACG outward movement rises either simultaneously with or slightly before the rise in intraventricular pressure. (In dogs, intramural myocardial tension precedes the intracavitary pressure rise by about 15 msec [9].)

*3.   What is the C—1 interval called by physiologists?

ANS.:   There is no name for it, so we shall have to call it the "preisovolumic contraction period," because as long as LV pressure is not above left atrial pressure, the mitral valve remains open, and blood flows through it into the LV; i.e., the volume is still changing and it is not isovolumic.

Note: The blood flowing from the left atrium across the mitral valve has inertia. By Newton's law of motion, the blood will remain in motion until force is applied to stop it. Therefore, ventricular pressure must exceed atrial pressure for a time before the flow can be brought to rest.

*4.   When in the outward phase of the ACG does the aortic valve open?

ANS.:   Near the peak of the initial outward movement [41]. (If there is an aortic ejection sound, it will occur at this time.)

Note: The period between the closure of the mitral valve and the opening of the aortic valve is called the isovolumic contraction period.

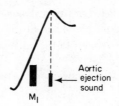

The interval between M₁ and any sound simultaneous with the opening of the aortic valve is isovolumic contraction time.

5.   What does the normal ACG look like during ejection of blood through the aortic valve? Why?

   ANS.:   A sigmoid-shaped drop-off. The heart has struck the chest wall and is now retracting.

   Note: The end-systolic shoulder represents the same as the end-systolic part of the LV pressure curve. When it declines, it represents the beginning of ventricular relaxation, so that shortly after the end of the shoulder, the aortic valve closes.

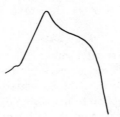

The only reason that this curve does not look like the sustained outward motion of the LV pressure curve is because the kind of transducer used to record it has a shorter time constant (see p. 126) than the ones used to record pressures at cardiac catheterization.

*6.   What marks aortic valve closure and subsequent mitral valve opening on the ACG?

   ANS.:   Either nothing, or a slight notch on the downslope of the sigmoid curve, marks aortic valve closure. Aortic closure marks the beginning of isovolumic relaxation, which ends with opening of the mitral valve. There is a continual drop in downslope from aortic valve closure until the mitral valve opens. The nadir of the ACG isovolumic relaxation phase is called the 0 point. This refers to *opening* of the mitral valve.

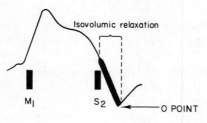

If the mitral valve makes a snapping sound when it opens, as in mitral stenosis, the opening snap will occur near the 0 point of the ACG.

7. What happens to apical movement as the LV rapidly expands while it fills in early diastole?
    ANS.:   As expected, there is an outward movement, which normally is very rapid because
            it represents the phase of early rapid filling of the LV, when about 80% of the total
            diastolic blood volume enters the LV. This early diastolic wave has been called
            the "rapid filling wave." The peak of the rapid filling wave is called the F point.
            (See figure on p. 229.)
8. What ACG movement follows the early filling wave, i.e., during the time of slow filling of
    the "atrioventricle"? What is this movement called?
    ANS.:   A slow rise called the "slow filling wave." (See figure on p. 345.)
9. How does atrial contraction at the end of slow filling in diastole affect the ACG, and what
    is this wave called?
    ANS.:   By suddenly expanding the LV, it produces an outward movement called an A wave
            or an atrial hump. (See figure on p. 115.)

APEX CARDIOGRAM ABNORMALITIES

The following is a list of the ACG abnormalities that can aid in the diagnosis of heart disease.

*Atrial Hump Abnormalities

*1. In LVH or ischemic heart disease, the atrial hump may be
    a) Increased above normal in amplitude. Over 12% or more of the total systolic deflection
       $\left(\dfrac{A}{E \text{ to } O} \text{ or } \dfrac{A}{H} \text{ ratio} \right)$ is abnormal [1]. This abnormal ratio may appear during angina
       or smoking and become normal or disappear altogether with sublingual nitrates.

       Note: The $\dfrac{A}{H}$ ratio may not correlate well with direct left atrial A wave pressures because
       the ACG A wave represents LV volume as well as pressure changes.

          If the $\dfrac{A}{H}$ ratio is over 14%, the atrial hump is almost always palpable if the P–R interval
       is not too short and an apex beat is palpable.
    b) Longer in duration than normal (over 75 msec), probably because atrial contraction is
       prolonged when the atrioventricle loses compliance [4].
       Note: In hypertension, the A wave is more likely to be high than prolonged.
    c) Notched. This has been found in 40% of ACGs taken during early acute myocardial
       infarction [25].
       Note: A short time constant, such as that caused by an air leak, can amplify and peak
       the atrial hump.
*2. Over an aneurysm, the atrial hump is very low [16].
*3. In MS, the atrial hump is usually absent, but if present is very low.
*4. In valvular AS, an $\dfrac{A}{H}$ ratio of over 10% correlates highly with a gradient of 75 mm Hg
     or more.

*Rapid Filling Wave Abnormalities

*1.   In MS, the rapid filling wave is short or absent, so that in early filling, there is often a shallow slope with no distinct change to show the onset of the slow filling phase; i.e., there is usually no distinct F point. When a rapid filling wave is present in significant MS, it is usually very short. The lowest normal duration is probably about 70 msec (see figure on p. 345) [6, 39].

*2.   In severe MR, there is a marked overshoot in the rapid early filling wave. This overshoot may be palpable and is simultaneous with the S_3 (see figure on p. 235).

        With combined MS and MR, a slow early filling wave strongly favors dominant stenosis [2].

        Note: A short time constant of a transducer with an air leak can exaggerate the rapid filling wave. On the other hand, a decrease in venous return, as with a sublingual nitrate, can decrease the amplitude of the rapid filling wave.

*3.   Over a ventricular aneurysm, the rapid filling wave is either absent, very low in amplitude, or shorter in duration than normal. This is probably due to the poor emptying of the sac in systole, with consequent poor filling in diastole.

*Systolic Wave Abnormalities

*Upstroke or C—E Interval Abnormalities

*1.   In left atrial myxomas, large notching may occur on the upstroke [45].

        Note: This same deep notch may occur on the upstroke in patients with MS, probably associated with the sudden deceleration of blood moving into the LV when the ring and pliable valves have reached their upward limit. There is a possibility that a deep notch may mean good mobility of the mitral valves [45].

*2.   In ischemic heart disease, the C—E interval is prolonged. (Top normal is 90 msec.)

        Note: In many reports, this has been called the isometric contraction phase or true isovolumic contraction period. This does not follow the physiologists' definition of isovolumic contraction, which specifies the time between closure of the mitral valve and opening of the aortic valve. Blood is still flowing into the LV between the time it begins to contract (C point) and the closure of the mitral valve (mitral component of the first heart sound, or M_1). The true isovolumic contraction phase would be between the mitral closure sound, M_1, and the E point of the ACG.

        Note: The term *isometric contraction* is wrong because the ventricle changes its dimensions at this time, despite its constant volume. The correct term is *isovolumic*.

*3.   In patients with left bundle branch block and old or recent infarction, the C—E interval corrected for heart rate (by dividing by the square root of the R—R interval) is 0.09 ± 0.03 sec. If no infarction is present by history, ECG, or vectorcardiogram, the corrected C—E interval is 0.14 ± 0.03 sec. Ventricular ejection, as defined by the interval $E—A_2$, corrected for heart rate is longer in those with than in those without infarction (0.284 ± 0.05 sec versus 0.239 ± 0.04 sec) [36].

*4.   If you differentiate the ACG with the use of a differential transducer, the time from the beginning of the QRS to the peak of the first derivative during the preejection phase correlates with an R = 0.81 with the angiographic ejection fraction. The linear equation is:

$$\text{Ejection fraction} = 142 - (0.952 \times R \text{ to peak first derivative}) \text{ [42]}$$

Ejection Slope (E—S_2 Abnormalities)

*1.   In ischemic heart disease

*a) There may be a poor downstroke or no downstroke in systole, but a plateau or even an upward movement known as a late or midsystolic bulge. This is also seen in LVH resulting from any cause.

Note: A steep, long, downward systolic slope can occur if the time constant is too short, as when there is an air leak into the system.

*b) There may be shortening of the early systolic downslope, so that the end-systolic shoulder begins earlier than normal, i.e., before midsystole. If we call the break in systolic slope between the early downslope and the shoulder "B," then the S_1—B is normally longer than B—S_2. If S_1—B is shorter than B—S_2, this is abnormal and may be due to asynergy between normal and abnormal muscle fibers, i.e., the normal muscle shortening at higher velocity completes its contraction phase while the diseased muscle is still contracting [43].

Note: This may occur only during angina, after exercise, or after smoking a cigarette. It can improve or disappear with nitrates or coronary bypass surgery. In some patients with HSS, acute infarction, and the ballooned valve syndrome, the break in slope becomes a midsystolic depression or dip and causes a double systolic impulse.

The late systolic bulge occurs so frequently (in up to 80% of patients with acute myocardial infarction) that one of its causes is thought to be asynergy [25]. Mid- or late systolic bulges are so common when right bundle branch block is combined with anterior divisional block that conduction abnormalities must be considered one of the probable causes of the bulges and perhaps one of the causes of asynergy [5].

*c) Over a ventricular aneurysm there is usually a monophasic wave with a poorly defined B point. It may rise to a peak in late systole.

Note: If you differentiate the ACG, a sharp distinct notch occurs on the downslope that coincides with the aortic valve closure incisura on the carotid pulse. Therefore, the interval from a sharp E point to this notch can be used to measure ejection times [21].

*2.   In constrictive pericarditis, you may see a small outward initial movement to a low E point, followed by a steep descent and wide trough during almost all of systole. A small positive wave follows the trough, to end with a peak just after the S_2 [15].

REFERENCES

1. Benchimol, A., and Dimond, E. G. The apex cardiogram in ischaemic heart disease. *Br. Heart J.* 24:581, 1962.
2. Benchimol, A., Dimond, E. G., Waxman, D., and Shen, Y. Diastolic movements of the precordium in mitral stenosis and regurgitation. *Am. Heart J.* 3:417, 1960.
3. Boicourt, O. W., Nagle, R. E., and Mounsey, J. P. D. The clinical significance of systolic retraction of the apical impulse. *Br. Heart J.* 27:379, 1965.
4. Braunwald, E., and Frahm, C. J. Studies on Starling's law of the heart. *Circulation* 24:633, 1961.
5. Byahatti, V., DePasquale, N. P., and Crampton, R. S. Indirect graphic studies in bilateral bundle branch block. *Chest* 58:223, 1970.
6. Coulshed, N., and Epstein, E. J. The apex cardiogram. *Br. Heart J.* 25:697, 1963.
7. Craige, E., and Schmidt, R. Precordial movements over the right ventricle in normal children. *Circulation* 32:232, 1965.

8. Deliyannis, A. A., Gillam, P. M. S., Mounsey, J. P. D., and Steiner, R. E. The cardiac impulse and the motion of the heart. *Br. Heart J.* 26:396, 1964.

9. Diendone, J. M. Tissue-cavitary difference pressure of dog left ventricle. *Am. J. Physiol.* 213:101, 1967.

10. Dressler, W. *Clinical Aids in Cardiac Diagnosis.* New York: Grune & Stratton, 1970.

11. Dressler, W., Kleinfeld, M., and Ripstein, C. B. Physical sign of tight mitral stenosis. Aid in selection of patients for valvulotomy. *J. A. M. A.* 154:49, 1954.

12. Eddleman, E. E., Jr. Kinetocardiographic changes as a result of mitral commissurotomy. *Am. J. Med.* 25:733, 1958.

13. Eddleman, E. E., Jr., and Langley, J. O. Paradoxical pulsation of the precordium in myocardial infarction and angina pectoris. *Am. Heart J.* 63:579, 1962.

14. Edwards, J. E., Carey, L. S., Neufeld, H. N., and Lester, R. G. *Congenital Heart Disease.* Philadelphia: Saunders, 1965. P. 197.

15. El-Sherif, A., and El-Said, G. Jugular, hepatic, and praecordial pulsations in constrictive pericarditis. *Br. Heart J.* 33:305, 1971.

16. El-Sherif, A., Saad, Y., and El-Said, G. Praecordial tracings of myocardial aneurysms. *Br. Heart J.* 31:357, 1969.

17. El-Sherif, N., and El-Ramly, Z. External left atrial pulse tracings in extreme left atrial dilation. *Am. Heart J.* 84:387, 1972.

18. Epstein, E. J., Coulshed, N., Brown, A. K., and Doukas, N. G. The 'A' wave of the apex cardiogram in aortic valve disease and cardiomyopathy. *Br. Heart J.* 30:591, 1968.

19. Eve, F. C. Measurement of the heart in angular degrees. *Lancet* 1:659, 1941.

20. Feinstein, A. R., Hochstein, E., Luisada, A. A., Perloff, J. K., Rosner, S., Schlant, R. C., Segal, B. L., and Soffer, A. Glossary of cardiologic terms related to physical diagnosis and history. *J. A. M. A.* 209:1693, 1969.

21. Gabor, G., Porubszky, I., and Kalman, P. Determination of systolic time intervals using the apex cardiogram and its first derivative. *Am. J. Cardiol.* 30:217, 1972.

22. Gillam, P. M. S., Deliyannis, A. A., and Mounsey, J. P. D. The left parasternal impulse. *Br. Heart J.* 26:726, 1964.

23. Graham, T. P., Jr., Jarmakani, J. M., and Canent, R. V., Jr. Left heart volume characteristics with a right ventricular volume overload. *Circulation* 45:389, 1972.

24. Holt, J. H., Jr., and Eddleman, E. E., Jr. The precordial movements in adults with pulmonic stenosis. *Circulation* 35:492, 1967.

25. Jain, S. R., and Lindahl, J. Apex cardiogram and systolic time intervals in acute myocardial infarction. *Br. Heart J.* 33:578, 1971.

26. Kastor, J. A., Aronow, S., Nagle, R. E., Garber, T., and Walker, H. Air leaks as a source of distortion in apexcardiography. *Chest* 57:163, 1970.

27. Kjellberg, S. R., Mannheimer, E., Rudhe, U., and Johnsson, B. *Diagnosis of Congenital Heart Disease.* Chicago: Year Book, 1959. P. 411.

28. Mainland, D., and Gordon, E. J. The position of organs determined from thoracic radiographs of young adult males with a study of the cardiac apex beat. *Am. J. Anat.* 68:457, 1941.

29. Manchester, G. H., Block, P., and Corlin, R. Misleading signs in mitral insufficiency. *J. A. M. A.* 191:99, 1965.

30. Mills, R. M., Jr., and Kastor, J. A. Quantitative grading of cardiac palpation. *Arch. Intern. Med.* 132:831, 1973.

31. Morgan, J. R., Rogers, A. K., and Forker, A. D. Congenital absence of the left pericardium. *Ann. Intern. Med.* 74:370, 1971.

32. Nagel, R. E., and Tamara, F. A. Left parasternal impulse in pulmonary stenosis and atrial septal defect. *Br. Heart J.* 29:735, 1967.

33. Pigott, V., and Spodick, D. H. The effects of high frequency filter cut-offs on the apex-cardiogram. *Chest* 59:240, 1971.

34. Rivero-Carvallo, J. M. The left bronchial compression syndrome. *Am. J. Cardiol.* 9:521, 1962.

35. Ronan, J. A., Jr., Steelman, R. B., DeLeon, A. C., Waters, T. J., Perloff, J. K., and Harvey, W. P. The clinical diagnosis of acute severe mitral insufficiency. *Am. J. Cardiol.* 27:284, 1971.

36. Santos, D. E., De La Paz, A., Pietras, R. J., Tobin, J. R., Jr., and Gunnar, R. M. The apex cardiogram in left bundle-branch block. *Br. Heart J.* 31:693, 1969.

37. Shapiro, M. J. Coarctation of the abdominal aorta. *Am. J. Cardiol.* 4:547, 1959.

38. Soloff, L. A., and Zatuchni, J. Cardiac chamber volumes and their significance in rheumatic heart disease with isolated mitral stenosis. *Circulation* 19:269, 1959.

39. Spodick, D. H., and Kumar, S. Rapid filling period of the left ventricle: Measurement by apexcardiography. *Aerosp. Med.* 39:1351, 1968.

40. Stapleton, J. F., and Groves, B. M. Precordial palpation. *Am. Heart J.* 81:409, 1971.

41. Tafur, E., Cohen, L. S., and Levine, H. D. The normal apex cardiogram, its temporal relationship to electrical, acoustic, and mechanical cardiac events. *Circulation* 30:381, 1964.

42. Vetter, W. R., Sullivan, R. W., and Hyatt, K. H. Assessment of quantitative apex cardiography. *Am. J. Cardiol.* 29:667, 1972.

43. Wayne, H. H. *Noninvasive Technics in Cardiology.* Chicago: Year Book, 1973.

44. Wigle, E. D., and Labrosse, C. J. Sudden severe aortic regurgitation. *Circulation* 32:708, 1965.

45. Zitnik, R. S., and Giuliani, E. R. Clinical recognition of atrial myxoma. *Am. Heart J.* 80:689, 1970.

II
Auscultation

6
The Stethoscope

THE BELL CHEST PIECE

1. What is the relation between the tautness (stiffness) of a membrane that collects sound from the chest wall and the ability of the membrane to transmit high or low frequencies?

    ANS.:   The more tautly the collecting membrane is drawn, the higher its natural frequency of oscillation and the more efficient it is at higher frequencies.

2. What is the ideal membrane to apply to a chest wall (if the above statement is true) in order to bring out *low* frequencies?

    ANS.:   As loose and flabby a membrane as possible.

3. How does the use of a bell chest piece fit into these acoustical laws?

    ANS.:   The bell permits one to use the skin as a flabby diaphragm. The skin can only be turned into a sufficiently taut diaphragm if enough pressure is applied to the skin to produce pain.

4. What chest piece diameter picks up the most sound, a very small or a very large one?

    ANS.:   A very large one. The ability of a chest piece to collect sound is proportional to its diameter.

5. What size chest piece diameter picks up low frequencies better, a small or large one?

    ANS.:   A large one.

6. How much pressure should be applied with a bell chest piece?

    ANS.:   Just barely enough to prevent room-noise leak and no more. Any more pressure will tighten the skin and tend to damp out the low frequencies.

7. What is the relation between the internal volume of a stethoscope (air space enclosed by the chest piece and tubing) and the loudness of transmitted sounds?

    ANS.:   Inverse, i.e., the smaller the internal volume, the greater the loudness of the sound.

8. What bell design will give the smallest internal volume and the largest diameter?

    ANS.:   A shallow shell rather than a deep cone.

9. What then is the ideal chest piece for low frequencies?

    ANS.:   A shallow bell with as large a diameter as is consistent with a reasonable seat on the chest wall when only a minimal amount of pressure is applied.

    Note: It is believed by some cardiologists, with no explanation or testing other than their own ears, that a large-diameter corrugated diaphragm applied with light pressure is sometimes best for low frequencies. They still advise having a bell handy, however, both in order to auscultate in small places such as the supraclavicular fossa or between ribs on a bony chest, and because the bell is occasionally superior for certain low frequencies.

---

* indicates material that is for electives or fellows in cardiology, or concerns rare phenomena, of interest primarily to the cardiologist.

10.   What kind of murmurs and sounds are best heard with the bell?
    ANS.:   Murmurs: diastolic murmurs through atrioventricular valves (mitral and tricuspid).
        Sound: the diastolic sounds known as the S_3 and S_4.
            Note: The kettledrum is bell-shaped and is also used to bring out low-frequency,
        booming tones.

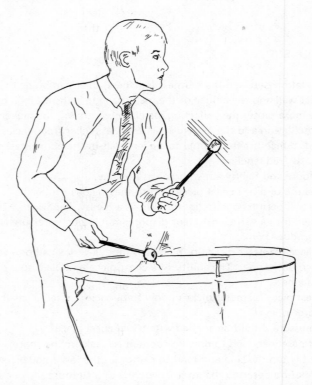

The diastolic rumble and deep, low groan
Needs the bell to magnify it.
For the third heart sound, like the Kettledrum's tone,
There's nothing like a bell, so try it!

    Note: Children can detect frequencies up to 18,000 cycles per second (cps);
    adults, frequencies up to 14,000 cps. However, since cardiac sound does not
    extend much above 1000 cps, loss of ability to hear frequencies over 3000 cps,
    which is the usual type of hearing loss in the older physician, should not interfere
    with hearing any cardiac sounds or murmurs [1, 2].

THE SMOOTH DIAPHRAGM

1.   What is meant by "masking" of sounds?
    ANS.:   The inability to hear a sound well because of interference by another sound occur-
        ring just before it, just after it, or at the same time.

2.   Do low frequencies mask high ones easily?

ANS.:   Yes, unless the lower frequencies are very widely separated from the higher frequencies in pitch or are relatively soft [3, 6].

3.   Do high frequencies mask low ones easily?

ANS.:   No, unless the high frequencies are relatively loud.

4.   What is the purpose of the smooth, stiff diaphragm?

ANS.:   To damp out low frequencies and unmask the high. If the resonance frequency of the diaphragm happens to be the same as that of the murmur, it may actually amplify the murmur.

Note: Amplification of sound may also be due to the summation of reflected or standing waves in tubing. Different tubing lengths therefore can amplify different frequencies [2].

5.   Why not use the bell chest piece as a diaphragm by merely applying pressure, thus eliminating the need for two chest pieces?

ANS.:   The stretched skin is an inefficient diaphragm for filtering out low frequencies. The skin does not become stiff enough to be a good filter. Many bells, however, transmit the high frequencies better than does the diaphragm of the same stethoscope [7]. This is especially true if it is a small-diameter, deep, trumpet-shaped bell [3, 4]. Therefore, if there are not too many low frequencies present to mask the highs, it may be profitable to use the bell to hear high-pitched murmurs.

Note: a) Do not use x-ray film as a substitute for a damaged diaphragm. X-ray film has been shown to be about as good as no diaphragm at all for filtering out low frequencies. It is not stiff enough.

b) A greater degree of pressure variation with the diaphragm has been attained by prestressing a nylon diaphragm by bowing it slightly forward. A small raised area in the center of the diaphragm can further increase the tension by pressure against the skin [8].

c) If the diaphragm is too thick, there is too much loss of amplitude (volume).

6.   Which murmurs and sounds are usually heard well only with the stiff, smooth diaphragm?

ANS.:   Murmurs: the soft aortic and pulmonary diastolic murmur and the soft mitral regurgitation murmur. Sounds: splitting of first or second heart sounds.

Note: The rigid, wooden monaural stethoscope invented by Laennec and still used in some parts of Europe will decrease the loudness of sound in the 60–700 cps range about tenfold. This encompasses the medium- and high-frequency range of cardiac sounds and murmurs.

7.   Why is it very difficult to hear the splitting of heart sounds with a bell?

ANS.:   Because there are so many low frequencies surrounding each component that the ear cannot separate them if the splitting is close. The ear can separate two short, high-frequency sounds placed close to each other more easily than it can separate two prolonged low- or medium-frequency sounds.

*8.   How can a diaphragm help you to localize a murmur?

ANS.:   High-frequency sounds do not spread as widely across the chest wall as do low frequencies. Therefore, the diaphragm may help you to localize sounds to their point of origin [2].

THE TUBING

1.   What frequencies are attenuated (damped) by too long a tubing?

ANS.:   High frequencies. The low frequencies are relatively unaffected by tube length [9].

2.   What is the shortest compromise length that will bring out high frequencies and still not be too short for most people's comfort?

ANS.:   A length of 10 inches.

Note: It has not yet been proved that an additional 3 or 4 inches of length for tall physicians' comfort makes much difference.

*3.   What frequencies are best carried by very narrow or very wide tubing?

ANS.:   Very narrow tubes carry low frequencies best, and high frequencies are best carried by wide tubing.

Note: An internal diameter of 1/8 inch was once recommended as the ideal compromise to carry both low and high frequencies with least loss of each. The average commercial stethoscope has an internal diameter of 3/16 inch, which has been found recently to be even better than 1/8 inch. The Littman, Harvey, Leatham, and the Rappaport and Sprague are 1/8 inch in diameter. The Harvey three-headed stethoscope (one head with a corrugated diaphragm) has a metal headpiece 3/16 inch in diameter.

4.   How can the thickness of tubing affect auscultation?

ANS.:   The thicker the tube, the better is room noise eliminated. A vinyl tube has been found to be better than rubber for this purpose.

5.   Why is dull-surfaced rubber tubing inefficient for stethoscopes?

ANS.:   With this type of tubing, internal frictional resistance is increased.

6.   Which is more efficient, a single tube or a double tube?

ANS.:   The single tube stethoscopes appear at first glance to be more efficient because they eliminate the necessity of binding parallel tubes together in order to prevent collision sounds, and they are more flexible and portable. However, tests have shown that the *double tube is more efficient for high frequencies* because there is less interference from reflected waves [2, 4]. A single tube plus a shallow bell can attenuate the high frequencies by as much as 50 decibels [4]. This is the difference between a shout and a whisper.

AIR LEAKS AND EAR TIPS

1.   How important are air leaks at either the earpieces, changeover valve, or chest piece?

ANS.:   The greatest impairments to the efficiency of stethoscopes are air leaks [5]. Room noise due to air leaks tends to mask high frequencies more than low ones.

2.   How can you test for air leaks at the chest piece or changeover valve?

ANS.:   a) Blow into one tube with the opposite earpiece and tubing occluded. Your fingers will feel the air escaping. Blowing cigarette smoke into the tube will enable you to detect even smaller leaks, but will be very disillusioning because few stethoscopes are built to pass this test.

b) If withdrawing the chest piece quickly from the precordium produces a change in pressure painful to the ear, an air leak, if present, is probably unimportant.

3.   Which kind of earpieces are most likely to cause air leaks, small ones that enter the canal or large ones that merely occlude the external canal?

ANS.:   Small ones are most likely to cause a leak (and so mask high frequencies). Small ones are also the least comfortable.

4.   Why may small ear tips become partially obstructed when being inserted into the ear?

ANS.:   The external auditory meatus points slightly forward, then backward, to make an angle. The usual stethoscope headpieces are designed to point the ear tips slightly anteriorly. If the ear tips are too small, their aperture may impinge partially or completely against the cartilaginous meatus, which points backward [6].

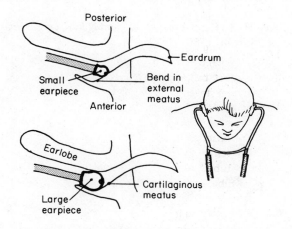

Headpieces are designed to point the ear tips slightly anteriorly. Small ear tips can therefore be partly occluded against the backward-directed meatus.

SUMMARY OF GOOD STETHOSCOPE CHARACTERISTICS

1.   A shallow bell with a large diameter for low frequencies.
2.   A smooth, stiff, thin diaphragm for high frequencies.
3.   A pediatric size bell and diaphragm accessories.
4.   An internally smooth vinyl tubing, not over 10 inches (25 cm) long and 3/16 of an inch in internal diameter.
5.   Double tubing with some method of binding them together.
6.   The largest ear tips possible.
7.   Metal headpieces that can be rotated so that the ear tips can be pointed in the most comfortable direction.

REFERENCES

1. Dawson, J. B. Auscultation and the stethoscope. *Practitioner* 193:315, 1954.
2. Ertel, P. Y., Lawrence, M., Brown, R. K., and Stern, A. M. Stethoscope Acoustics I. The doctor and his stethoscope. *Circulation* 34:889, 1966.

3. Ertel, P. Y., Lawrence, M., Brown, R. K., and Stern, A. M. Stethoscope Acoustics II. Transmission and filtration patterns. *Circulation* 34:899, 1966.
4. Ertel, P. Y., Lawrence, M., and Song, W. How to test stethoscopes. *Med. Res. Eng.* 8:7, 1969.
5. Groom, D. Comparative efficiency of stethoscopes. *Am. Heart J.* 68:220, 1967.
6. Groom, D., and Chapman, W. Anatomic variations of the auditory canal pertaining to the fit of the stethoscope earpieces. *Circulation* 19:606, 1959.
7. Hampton, C. S., and Chaloner, A. Which stethoscope? *Br. Med. J.* 4:388, 1967.
8. Howell, W. L., and Aldridge, C. F. The effect of stethoscope-applied pressure in auscultation. *Circulation* 32:430, 1965.
9. Johnston, F. D., and Kline, E. M. An acoustical study of the stethoscope. *Arch. Intern. Med.* 65:328, 1940.
10. Ongley, P. A., Sprague, H. B., Rappaport, M. D., and Nadas, A. S. *Heart Sounds and Murmurs.* New York: Grune & Stratton, 1960. P. 32.

7

Diagramming and Grading Heart Sounds and Murmurs (The Auscultogram)

A GRAPHIC METHOD for illustrating auscultatory findings is offered here not only as a means of keeping records as conveniently and efficiently as possible but also as an aid to learning auscultation. It has been shown that one such "auscultogram" (see figure) can equal a 629-word description of the auscultatory findings [5]. The graph can tell the story at a glance once the symbols are understood [2].

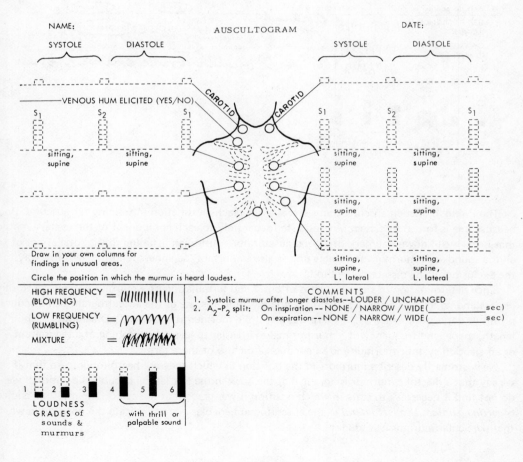

AUSCULTOGRAM

NAME: DATE:

VENOUS HUM ELICITED (YES/NO)

CAROTID   CAROTID

S_1 S_2 S_1 S_1 S_2 S_1

sitting, supine

Draw in your own columns for findings in unusual areas.

Circle the position in which the murmur is heard loudest.

sitting, supine, L. lateral

HIGH FREQUENCY (BLOWING) =

LOW FREQUENCY (RUMBLING) =

MIXTURE =

COMMENTS
1. Systolic murmur after longer diastoles--LOUDER / UNCHANGED
2. A_2-P_2 split: On inspiration -- NONE / NARROW / WIDE (_____ sec)
On expiration -- NONE / NARROW / WIDE (_____ sec)

1   2   3   4   5   6

LOUDNESS GRADES of sounds & murmurs

with thrill or palpable sound

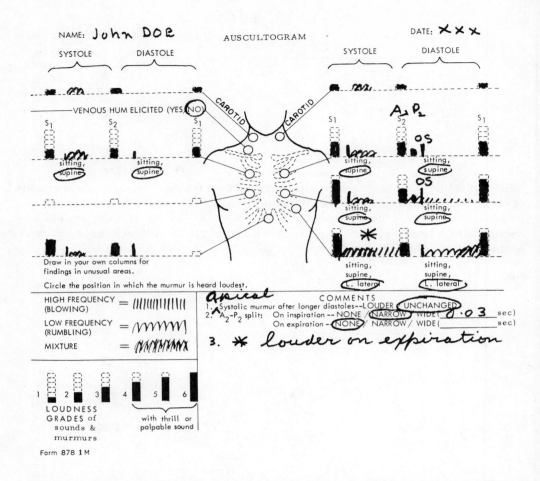

NAME: John DOE   AUSCULTOGRAM   DATE: X X X

The filling in of such auscultograms serves a self-teaching function in training for auscultation because one is forced to dissect out and listen separately to each component of the cycle, a method that is the well-known hallmark of a good auscultator. Although listening to the total effect of all the sounds and murmurs as a single unit is also important, beginners tend to listen this way to the exclusion of the dissection method.

Since determination of the exact sites of onset and termination of a murmur is essential to the understanding of the site of production of the murmur, the use of the auscultogram will discourage primitive descriptions such as: "There was a systolic murmur at the apex." Diagramming the length, shape, and frequency of a murmur makes it easier to learn the meaning of a regurgitant or an ejection systolic murmur and so encourage the use of these terms.

We customarily describe murmurs in the position in which they are heard loudest, so that if we say that a diastolic murmur is "grade 4 at the apex in the left lateral decubitus position," we do not find it necessary to state in which position it was grade 3 at the apex. The multiple choice of *sitting, supine,* and *left lateral* in the auscultogram enables one to indicate the position in which that particular murmur was loudest.

The auscultogram uses widely spaced wavy lines for low frequencies and closely spaced lines for high frequencies, because this is something like the way they look on a phonocardiogram. We believe, therefore, that anyone who sees phonocardiograms will understand these frequency symbols. We add medium, or mixed, frequencies, too, indicated by low-frequency wavy lines with diagonal lines through them. An explanatory example of the frequency symbols is necessary on each auscultogram.

The loudness of sounds and murmurs is indicated by their height relative to a vertical column divided into 6 parts to represent 6 grades of loudness. Drawing sounds and murmurs of different heights is the quickest way of displaying relative as well as absolute differences in loudness. It is analogous to the difference between looking at a complicated column of numbers and looking at a simple bar graph.

Grading amplitude on a scale of 6 is acceptable if we can separate grades 3 and 4. When Freeman and Levine [3], in 1933, introduced the grading of murmurs up to 6, only grades 1, 2, and 6 were described in detail. Grade 6 was a murmur heard with the stethoscope off the chest, and grade 1 could be missed on first applying the stethoscope. Grade 2 was an easily heard, faint murmur. By 1959, Levine [4] had proposed that grade 5 was one that could be heard when the edge of the chest piece (preferably the diaphragm) was applied to the precordium. However, he left the distinction between grades 3 and 4 to be solved by the listener. Although agreement on grades 3 and 4 seems to be impossible because they are both loud murmurs, this problem may be solved by using the thrill as a means of separating them; i.e., if the loud murmur is accompanied by a thrill, it is grade 4 or more. An objection to this system is that since the threshold for appreciation of thrills requires the presence of low frequencies, it appears possible that high-frequency murmurs may be very loud and not become palpable. However, in actual experience, the two typical high-frequency murmurs, those of aortic and mitral regurgitation, have thrills associated with them often enough to convince one that when these murmurs become loud enough, they acquire low frequencies. In 1959, Bruns [1] helped to explain this phenomenon when he showed that according to the vortex theory of the production of murmurs, a high-pitched murmur from a small orifice acquires low frequencies as the orifice enlarges. It may also acquire low frequencies in the direction of flow, i.e., downstream from the source of the murmur.

Note: It is not necessary to add *palpable* to the word *thrill* since all thrills are palpable.

Using palpability to separate grade 3 from grade 4 murmurs has many advantages:

1. It facilitates the teaching of grading out of 6, because grades 3 and 4 are the only stumbling blocks.

2. It teaches the student the relation between a thrill and a murmur, making him realize that a long thrill is never felt in the absence of a murmur. (Widely split components of loud heart sounds and a slight bisferiens pulse may feel like *short* thrills.)

3. It lends itself to the grading of heart sounds.

Despite these advantages, little has been written to support the grading of heart sounds in the same way as one would grade murmurs. Now that we have an easy method of grading, a palpable sound becomes grade 4 or more, and if it is heard with the stethoscope off the chest, it becomes grade 6, the same as for murmurs. A grading chart in one corner teaches the system at a glance, even showing which grades imply palpability.

Note: Thrills and sounds are best perceived with the distal palm. One hand may be more sensitive than the other, so test each hand on a patient with a faint thrill or palpable sound to find your better hand.

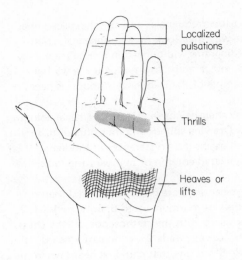

Localized
pulsations

— Thrills

Heaves or
lifts

Although small localized movements are
best perceived by the distal finger pads,
thrills are best felt with the distal palm.

The auscultogram can serve as a means of training the student of cardiology to acquire any
habits of auscultation that a cardiology teaching service desires. For example, by providing a
place on a graph for noting the width and movements of the split with respiration, a constant
reminder is provided. Since we wish to teach our students the value of listening in the neck for
heart sounds and murmurs, we include the neck on our diagram. We also provide a place for
noting the effects of intermittent long diastoles.

The writing and listening should be simultaneous, i.e., with the stethoscope in one hand and a
pen in the other. The auscultogram is for improving the ability to auscultate and to provide an
accurate record; it is not a memory test. It is one of the few times when it is best for a right-
handed physician to carry out his examination from the patient's left side.

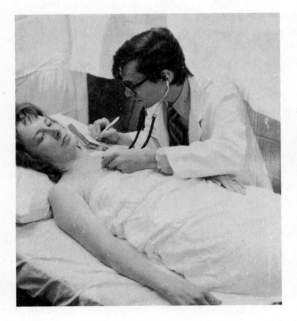

Simultaneous writing and listening is the
key to this method of ear training and
accuracy of recording.

It has been argued that attaching an actual phonocardiogram to the patient's chart is better than a written description of the auscultatory findings. The fallacy of this reasoning is indicated by the following facts:

1. Many soft high-frequency murmurs are difficult to record well on most phonocardiograms.
2. Some patients are too ill to be brought to a phonocardiograph.
3. On the usual phonocardiogram there is no standard grading of amplitude, nor is there any way of showing murmur frequency or quality, site of the microphone, or the position of the patient without using extra symbols. Therefore, writing cannot be eliminated, even on a phonocardiogram.

Thus, it is better to put both a phonocardiogram and an auscultogram on the patient's chart. It is convenient to print auscultogram pads of a size small enough to fit on about half a hospital chart page. A sticky backing makes for easy attachment. The auscultogram illustrated on page 143 is actual size.

REFERENCES

1. Bruns, D. L. A general theory of the causes of murmurs in the cardiovascular system. *Am. J. Med.* 27:360, 1959. Classic article.
2. Constant, J., and Lippschutz, E. J. Diagramming and grading heart sounds and murmurs. *Am. Heart J.* 70:326, 1965.
3. Freeman, A. R., and Levine, S. A. The clinical significance of the systolic murmur. *Ann. Intern. Med.* 6:1371, 1933.
4. Levine, S. A., and Harvey, W. P. *Clinical Auscultation of the Heart.* Philadelphia: Saunders, 1959.
5. Segall, H. N. A simple method for graphic description of cardiac auscultatory signs. *Am. Heart J.* 8:553, 1932–1933.

PHYSIOLOGY OF FIRST SOUND COMPONENTS

1.   Draw a left ventricular (LV) pressure curve.

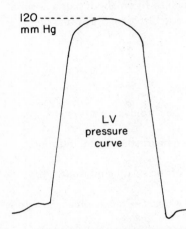

120 - - - - - - - -
mm Hg

LV
pressure
curve

An LV pressure curve begins at a pressure of about 0 mm Hg and rises to the same systolic pressure as in the aorta, i.e., normally about 120 mm Hg.

2.   Draw a left atrial pressure curve on the ventricular curve and show where the mitral valve closes. Why does it close here?

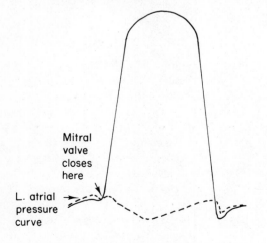

Mitral
valve
closes
here

L. atrial
pressure
curve

The most important component of the S_1, which is the mitral component or M_1, occurs as the result of this valve closure, but the sound should not be thought of as due to the slapping together of leaflets. It is more probably due to sudden cessation of mitral valve flow, setting the entire cardiohemic system into vibration.

---

* indicates material that is for electives or fellows in cardiology, or concerns rare phenomena, of interest primarily to cardiologists.

Boldface type indicates that the term is explained in the Glossary.

ANS.:   The mitral valve closes when LV pressure rises above left atrial pressure which is about 10 mm Hg. If the left atrial pressure at the beginning of ventricular contraction is 10 mm Hg, then as soon as the LV reaches a pressure of slightly over 10 mm Hg, the mitral valve will close.

3.   Draw an aortic pressure curve on the ventricular pressure curve and show where the aortic valve opens.

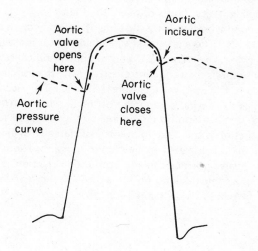

When the LV pressure reaches aortic diastolic pressure (about 80 mm Hg), the aortic valve opens, and an aortic root sound may be produced and become the second component of a split S_1. When aortic recoil power becomes stronger than LV ejection, the aortic valve closes to prevent regurgitation. The S_2 occurs at this time.

4.   When does the aortic valve open if the aortic diastolic pressure is 80 mm Hg?

ANS.:   When the LV pressure exceeds aortic diastolic pressure, i.e., exceeds 80 mm Hg.

   Note: The time between closure of the mitral valve and opening of the aortic valve is the **isovolumic contraction** period.

5.   How do these pressure curves relate to the first heart sound, or S_1?

ANS.:   Events associated with closure of the mitral valve and ejection of blood into the aorta are considered by many cardiologists to be responsible for the two major components of the S_1. Many other cardiologists believe that the second major component of the split S_1 is due to tricuspid valve closure especially if the split is narrow [29].

   Note: The vibration of heart sounds should be attributed to blood flow acceleration or deceleration caused by valve opening or closing [28]. We should not consider the mere slapping together of valve cusps as the cause of the sounds. The first high-frequency component of the S_1 occurs about 20 msec after echocardiographic valve closure and after the crossover of pressure pulses in the LV and atrium [28, 44].

6.   How many components or discrete vibrations can be found in the S_1 of a phonocardiogram?

ANS.:   About four components can be described, depending on the **frequency** response and paper speed of the phonocardiographic equipment used. If low frequencies are being displayed, and the paper speed is such that the heart sound components are spread out, four discrete vibrations can easily be described. If, however, only high frequencies are used, or the paper speed is not very fast, only two or three distinct vibrations will be demonstrated.

7.   Which of the four phonocardiographic distinct vibrations are audible?

ANS.:   The following is a synthesis of many theories:

The second vibration is the first high-frequency component of the S_1 and is always audible. There is general agreement that it is associated with closure of the mitral valve, i.e., it is an M_1. The audibility and cause of the third and fourth distinct vibrations are very controversial. One theory claims that the third vibration is due to tricuspid valve closure, i.e., it is a T_1. According to this theory, the T_1 becomes the second component of the S_1 when narrow splitting is heard and the fourth distinct vibration is audible only when wide splitting is present. The fourth vibration is then due to events associated with ejection into the aortic root and when audible is called an ejection sound, a root sound, or an A_1. An aortic or pulmonary valve opening can also produce an ejection sound that comes even later than the usual fourth vibration. It is often so sharp and short that it is then called an ejection "click." (See figure on p. 157.)

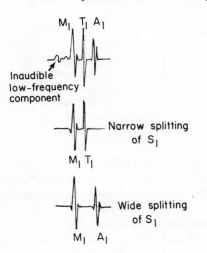

Narrow splitting of S_1 (less than the usual isovolumic contraction time of about 50 msec [0.05 sec]) may be due to M_1, T_1 components. Wide splitting (50 msec or longer) is probably due to the M_1, A_1 components, unless there is a right ventricular volume or pressure overload.

Note: The initial low-amplitude inaudible vibration of S_1 is occasionally due to atrial contraction, but not always, since it sometimes occurs in atrial fibrillation. Nor can it be due to tricuspid valve closure, since it occurs in the presence of prosthetic tricuspid valves. It can become audible in the presence of a mitral prosthetic valve [2]. Therefore, it is probably the result of sudden deceleration of flow across the mitral valve due to ventricular contraction. It is simultaneous with the crossover point between LV and left atrial pressures [27]. The mitral valves probably are in apposition at this point, and when they finally reach their maximum upward movement (about 30 msec later in normal hearts), the M_1 occurs [27].

8. In what percentage of normal subjects is splitting of the S_1 audible?

ANS.:   In about 85%.

*9. What is the latest theory to account for the first important audible component of the split S_1?

ANS.:   The first important component is associated with a change in the rate of pressure rise in the LV, causing a sudden tension of intracardiac structures. This occurs just after the mitral valve closes and does not occur unless the mitral valve closes [35]. Therefore, it may be called "M_1." The M_1 occurs 20—40 msec after the coaptation of the anterior and posterior leaflets as seen on an echocardiogram, or after the cross-over point of left atrial and LV pressure curves [28].

Note: When the mitral valve is removed experimentally, this sound is absent [34]. Thus, we may call this first component M_1, even though it is probably not due to a slapping together of valve leaflets.

*10. What is the latest theory, not yet widely accepted, used to explain the second component of the easily heard, widely split S_1 in subjects with no valvular abnormalities?

ANS.:   The latest theory is that it is caused by a change in the rate of pressure rise in the LV that suddenly tenses aortic root structures just as the aortic valve begins to open [46]. It may therefore be called the "A_1." If it sounds like a click, it has been called a "root click."

Note: The second component of S_1 (seen on phonocardiograms) that is usually too close to the first sound to be audible may well be due to tricuspid valve events. (See figure on p. 154.) Arguments against attributing the usual easily heard second component of a split first sound to tricuspid valve closure are as follows:

a) When the right ventricle (RV) is completely bypassed and destroyed, so that it cannot contract, the two important components of the S_1 are unimpaired.

b) If the LV is completely bypassed and only the RV allowed to beat, there is no S_1.

c) If the heart is explored with a microphone directly on the myocardium, all components of the S_1 become softer over the RV, and there is no amplification of any component of the first heart sound over the RV.

d) In subjects with left bundle branch block (LBBB), the S_1 shows the same degree of splitting and the same number of components despite the marked delay in the onset of S_1 in LBBB [41]. Whenever wide splitting is heard in right bundle branch block (RBBB), the second component can often be shown to be due to an ejection sound [59]. In one series, 40% of patients with RBBB showed no clearly detectable split S_1 (by auscultation), and in another 44%, the usual narrow physiological splitting was observed [54].

e) When a second component of a split S_1 is well separated from the first component, it has often been best recorded within the aorta.

f) In a case of **Ebstein's anomaly** with complete nonfunctioning of the widely regurgitant tricuspid valve, the two components of the S_1 were found to be unimpaired [33].

g) The second major component of the S_1 is simultaneous with the moment of peak acceleration of aortic flow, which is just after opening of the aortic valve.

h) In patients with severe valvular aortic stenosis (AS) with heavy calcification of the valve, there is no split S_1, suggesting that the difficulty in getting blood into the aortic root prevents the second component of S_1 from occurring.

*11.   When is it likely that tricuspid closure *does* contribute to the S_1 in the presence of a normal tricuspid valve?

ANS.:   Whenever the RV has a volume or pressure overload, e.g., in atrial septal defect (ASD) or in pulmonary hypertension. This is supported by the findings that

a) In subjects with an ASD, the second major component of S_1 coincides with the peak of the right atrial C wave.

b) In 75% of children with an ASD, the second component of a split S_1 at the apex is higher than the M_1 [32, 53]. This is an unusual relationship of component loudness in normal children.

c) In one study, among subjects with an ASD, only those with a complete RBBB were found to have a widely split S_1 [30]. (However, whether or not the second component was a pulmonary ejection sound is a moot point.)

Note: a) In at least one report [48], it has even been denied that the second loud component of the split S_1 in ASD is due to T_1, because the investigations, by intracardiac phonocardiography in ASD patients, found that the second component

   1) Was absent in the RV in half the patients tested.

   2) Often occurred after the rise in pulmonary artery pressure.

   3) Showed no constant relationship with the onset of rise in RV pressure.

   4) Showed a constant time relationship with the onset of rise of aortic pressure.

b) In mitral stenosis (MS), a tricuspid component may precede the delayed M_1 [26]. It is easily recorded in MS with pulmonary hypertension because not only is there a high pressure in the RV to make a loud T_1 but the M_1 is delayed in subjects with MS, and so the T_1 is "uncovered." Intracardiac phonocardiography has shown that a right-sided S_1 precedes a left-sided S_1 in about a fourth of patients with MS [11].

c) If the second component of a split S_1 increases on inspiration, you may then be justified in calling it a T_1.

THE M_1 PLUS AORTIC EJECTION SOUND AS A CAUSE OF A SPLIT S_1

1.   How long after the M_1 does the aortic ejection sound (A_1) occur in normal subjects?

ANS.:   The usual A_1 comes at the end of isovolumic contraction, i.e., about 40–60 msec (0.04–0.06 sec) after the M_1 [14]. To help you judge the timing of this normal split of the first sound, note that the 40-msec split takes as long as it does to say "pa-da" as quickly as possible. The 60-msec split can be imitated by saying "pa-ta" as quickly as possible.

Note: Since the normal second component of the S_1 follows the M_1 after an interval that is compatible with the duration of isovolumic contraction, it may be easier to hear a split in S_1 in older subjects because isovolumic contraction times tend to lengthen with age from 30 msec (0.03 sec) in the young to 50 msec (0.05 sec) in the older patients [3].

2.   How can you describe an aortic ejection click, and how does it differ from the usual second component of the split S_1?

ANS.:   The aortic ejection click is an ejection sound that is short and high-pitched, i.e., it sounds like a snap or click. In aortic valvular stenosis it comes later than the usual second component of the split S_1. In the absence of aortic stenosis (AS) it comes at the usual time of the second component of an easily detected split of S_1, i.e., about 50 msec (0.05 sec) from the M_1. (This is imitated by saying "pa-da" as quickly as possible.)

Note: a) The usual split of S_1 can be prolonged if isovolumic contraction is prolonged, secondary to myocardial damage.

b) The differentiation of an M_1 ejection sound interval from an S_4–S_1 is given on page 252, and from a pacemaker click M_1, on page 258.

c) An ejection sound may or may not sound "clicky," even when far from the M_1. Therefore, the terms *ejection sound* and *ejection click* are often used interchangeably, with the understanding that the timing of the sound is more important than its character. If in fact it does happen to sound like a click, there is no reason why it should not be described by that word. On the other hand, it is not logical to call an ejection sound an ejection click if it does not sound like a click.

*3.   What proportion of acute myocardial infarction patients have widely split first sounds in the first three days, i.e., over 60 msec?

ANS.:   About two thirds.

Note: In the uncomplicated acute myocardial infarction, the isovolumic contraction time is not usually prolonged in the first few days because of an excess of catecholamines and sympathetic outflow. However, in the patient with acute infarction who is in failure or who has cardiac damage from a previous infarct, the isovolumic contraction time may well be prolonged and the M_1–A_1 interval widened, even in the first few days.

4.   What are the causes of an aortic ejection sound?

ANS.:   It appears to have two possible causes.

a) It may be a normal phenomenon, due to sudden ejection of blood into the aorta [63]. This "root sound" can become loud and even clicking if the ejection is forceful, as in thyrotoxicosis or aortic regurgitation (AR), or if the ejection is into a stiff system, as in hypertension or **arteriosclerosis**.

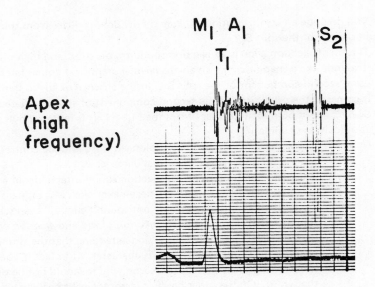

Apex (high frequency)

This phonocardiogram is from a 40-year-old woman with mild hypertension. The third component is probably an aortic ejection sound. This sounded simply like a widely split S_1, probably because the T_1 was too close to the M_1 to be audible.

b) It may be a pathological opening of a stiff aortic valve, as in AS.

5.   What suggests that the aortic ejection click, as in AS, is due to an opening snap of the aortic valve and not merely due to forceful ejection into the aorta?

ANS.:   a) It disappears with severe calcification of the aortic valve, and the louder the sound, the more mobile the valve can be shown to be.

b) It is not a feature of obstruction below the valve (subaortic **hypertrophic subaortic stenosis** [HSS] or discrete subvalvular stenosis), nor is it a feature of supravalvular AS [39].

c) In AS, the rise of pressure in the aorta is too slow to cause a sudden loud vibration unless the AS is mild (see following figure).

d) It occurs later than the normal root ejection sound [63]. Simultaneous intra-arterial micromanometer pressure tracings and phonocardiograms show that the normal ejection sound occurs with the onset of pressure rise in the aorta. The ejection click of AS occurs at the time of the anacrotic notch on the upstroke of the aortic pulse [63]. The ejection click of AS and the anacrotic shoulder have both been shown to be synchronous with the maximum open position of the stiff aortic leaflets.

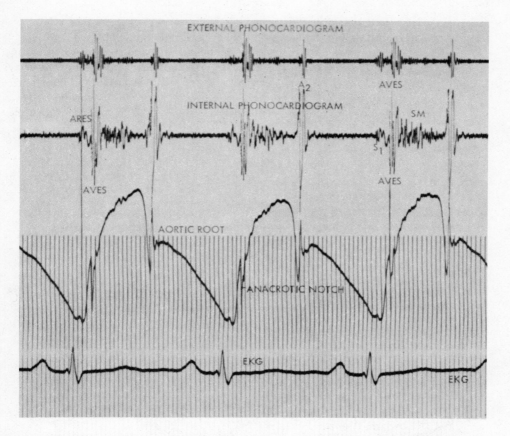

This aortic root tracing from a 16-year-old boy with minimal congenital AS was taken with a catheter tip electromanometer to avoid any delays due to tubing. An aortic root ejection sound (ARES) is present, coincident with the onset of pressure rise in the aortic root. There is no M_1 in this area. An aortic valve ejection sound (AVES) is also present, occurring 40 msec (0.04 sec) later and simultaneously with the anacrotic notch. (From Whittaker, Shaver, Gray, and Leonard [63].)

Note: In AS, the flow, and therefore the murmur, begins after the stiff valve has reached its peak upward doming, which occurs at the time of both the ejection sound and the anacrotic notch. Therefore, the time between the onset of the aortic pressure rise and the anacrotic shoulder represents the time taken to push the valve into its maximum domed position. This time has been found to be about 10 msec shorter with stiff valves than with mobile valves. This explains why anacrotic shoulders are lower in severe AS than in mild AS. The loudness of the ejection click does not correlate with the rate of rise of LV pressure, but does correlate with the distance of excursion of the valve.

It has long been noted that when external carotid tracings are taken simultaneously with phonocardiograms, the normal ejection sound occurs slightly before the upstroke of the carotid, while the later ejection click of AS occurs at the onset of the upward stroke. However, when you take into account the delays in tubing, as well as the distance between the aortic valve and carotid pulse unit, you can appreciate that the normal ejection sound could really come with the onset of carotid pressure rise, while the click of AS really could occur *during* the upstroke of the carotid.

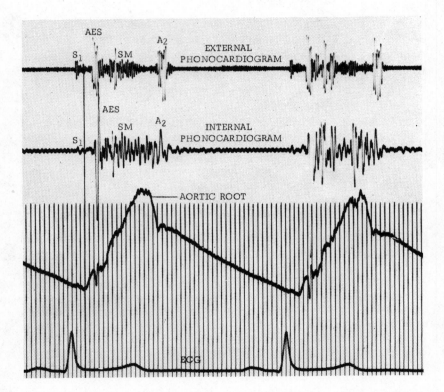

Aortic root tracing from a 23-year-old man with congenital AS taken with a catheter tip electro-manometer (so that there are no tubing delays). The onset of the aortic ejection sound (AES) is coincident with the anacrotic notch, which occurs at the moment of peak doming of the stiff valve, in this case 38 msec from the onset of the aortic pressure rise. (From Whittaker, Shaver, Gray, and Leonard [63].)

6.   Where is the aortic ejection sound best heard?

ANS.:   The normal ejection sound is well heard everywhere on the chest, wherever aortic events are best heard, i.e., anywhere in a straight line or "sash area" from the second right interspace to the apex. (See figure on p. 276.) The ejection click of AS, however, is often best heard at the apex.

7.   Why is the aortic ejection sound of diagnostic help in the presence of AS?
     ANS.:   a) It helps to locate the site of the AS, because only valvular AS characteristically
             has an audible ejection click.
             Note: A small-amplitude phonocardiographic ejection sound may be present
             in any kind of AS and is of no diagnostic help [61]. In some patients with hyper-
             trophic AS, an aortic root sound (as well as a dilated ascending aorta) is occasion-
             ally present [62]. This is not surprising in view of the increased rate of flow into
             the aorta in early systole. This is also the cause of the ejection sounds in AR and
             thyrotoxicosis.
             b) In the presence of known valvular stenosis, the loudness of the sound is propor-
             tional to the mobility of the valve leaflets [19].
             c) The absence of an ejection click in valvular AS implies a calcified aortic valve.
             A calcified valve of that degree is highly correlated with a **gradient** of over
             50 mm Hg [22].
             Note: The absence of an ejection click warns you of two possibilities: either
             there is no valvular stenosis, or there is valvular stenosis with heavy calcification.
             Fluoroscopy can rule out heavy calcification and lead to the conclusion that there
             is no valvular stenosis. Calcification is also likely if the A_2 is poor or absent.

THE PULMONARY EJECTION SOUND

The Ejection Sound in Pulmonary Stenosis

1.   What is responsible for the ejection click in valvular pulmonary stenosis (PS)? Proof?
     ANS.:   The pulmonary valve opening appears responsible for the click, i.e., it is thought
             to be an opening click of the pulmonary valve. The evidence that it is an opening
             snap of the pulmonary valve is as follows:
             a) It is not present in pure infundibular stenosis.
             b) It decreases or disappears with inspiration (even on intracardiac phonocardiog-
             raphy).

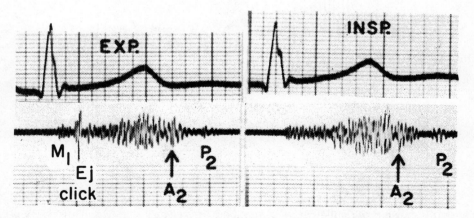

High-frequency tracing from the third left interspace of a patient with PS and a RV pressure of
100 mm Hg. The ejection click that disappears on inspiration shows that the site of obstruction
is at the valve. The A_2–P_2 interval increases slightly from 100–120 msec (0.10–0.12 sec) on
inspiration.

2.   Why does the pulmonary ejection click tend to disappear with inspiration in valvular PS?
ANS.:   The following explanation assumes that the sudden upward movement of a dome-shaped pulmonary valve produces the click. On inspiration, the increased blood drawn into the right atrium causes it to contract more strongly than it does on expiration. The stronger atrial contraction on inspiration at the end of diastole (while the tricuspid valve is still open) raises the pressure in the right ventricle (RV) just before the ventricle contracts. This end-diastolic pressure rise can elevate the RV pressure to a level higher than pulmonary artery pressure. This is easy to understand if you realize that pulmonary artery diastolic pressure in PS may not be much more than 7 mm Hg. Thus, the pulmonary valve will be raised into the domed position at the end of diastole if the end-diastolic pressure in the RV is raised to 8 mm Hg with a strong right atrial contraction.

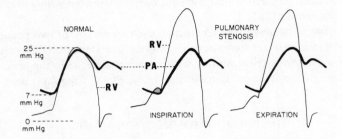

These RV and pulmonary artery pressure tracings show how inspiration can raise the end-diastolic RV pressure above pulmonary artery pressure because of a strong right atrial contraction plus a thick RV.

If the pulmonary valve is already in the domed position at the end of diastole, subsequent RV contraction cannot produce an ejection sound.

On expiration, the end-diastolic pressure in the RV falls, and the pulmonary valve is in the *down* position at the beginning of RV systole. Ventricular contraction can now balloon the pulmonary valve upward to make a click.

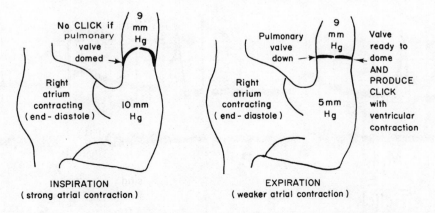

On the left is shown how right atrial concentration is assisted by inspiration in raising RV pressure higher than pulmonary artery pressure. This causes the pulmonary valve to dome up before the RV contracts
On the right is depicted the effect of a reduction in RV diastolic pressure caused by expiration, resulting in a downward position of the pulmonary valve when the RV begins to contract.

Note: Further proof that the pulmonary ejection click in PS is a valvular sound and due to snapping upward of the dome is offered by the following:

a) It can occur before the QRS at the end of diastole if the RV pressure is higher than pulmonary artery pressure due to atrial systole. It can even occur in early diastole at the peak of early rapid ventricular filling, if the RV pressure exceeds pulmonary artery pressure at that time.

b) Echocardiography has correlated the peak opening of the pulmonary valve with the pulmonary ejection click.

c) It occurs simultaneously with the anacrotic notch on the pulmonary artery pressure curve (by intracardiac phonocardiography and simultaneous micro-manometer pressure tracings), at which time the maximum position of pulmonary upward movement occurs, and the ejection murmur begins.

3.   Why does the aortic ejection click not change significantly with respiration?

ANS.:   The end-diastolic pressure in the LV in AS, even when very high (the normal end-diastolic pressure is not much higher than 10 mm Hg), can never exceed the usual diastolic pressure in the aorta (rarely ever lower than 50 mm Hg), and so expiration alone can never place the aortic valve in an upward position at the end of diastole in AS.

*4.   Why may the pulmonary ejection click of PS only show respiratory variation in the sitting position?

ANS.:   If the PS is moderately severe, the pressure in the RV may be high enough at the end of diastole to keep the valve in the domed position even in expiration, and respiration will have no effect on the click. However, in the sitting position, the venous return decreases, which causes a lower RV pressure at the end of diastole and may allow the pulmonary valve to fall to the downward position with expiration.

Note: In very mild PS, there may be a pulmonary ejection click in both inspiration and expiration, with only a little attenuation on inspiration.

5.   Where is the pulmonary ejection click best heard?

ANS.:   Wherever pulmonary sounds and murmurs are best heard, i.e., anywhere along the left sternal border. It may be heard well toward the mid-left thorax if the RV is enlarged.

*6.   What happens to the M_1 to pulmonary ejection click (P_1) interval with respiration, provided the P_1 is still present on inspiration?

ANS.:   The P_1 may be seen to move closer to the M_1 with inspiration as long as the pulmonary valve is moved into even a slightly higher position with inspiration. It may even summate with the M_1 at the apex on inspiration, to make the S_1 louder at this site.

7.   What does the presence of an ejection click tell you about the severity of the PS?

ANS.:   It tends to occur more often in mild to moderate stenosis, i.e., with RV pressures not over 70 mm Hg. Occasionally, however, it can be present with severe enough stenosis to produce a RV systolic pressure of 120 mm Hg [64]. (Normal RV systolic pressure is about 25 mm Hg.)

*8.   Why is there a good correlation between ejection clicks and poststenotic dilatation beyond a valvular stenosis, i.e., dilatation of the pulmonary artery just beyond the valve?

ANS.:   Most patients with ejection clicks have systolic murmurs due to turbulent flow through the stenosed valve. The turbulence causing the murmur can disrupt the elastin structure of the artery just beyond the valve [5, 7]. One theory is based on the principle that turbulent flow increases the forces that tend to drag the lining of a vessel downstream. The distorted endothelial cells then initiate changes in the subjacent layers which can modify the lumen [51].

Low-frequency vibrations, even if inaudible, can cause dilatation of an artery, especially if the artery is young [5].

Note: a) The absence of poststenotic dilatation beyond a purely infundibular PS is unexplained. Perhaps the turbulence that produces the murmur here is dissipated before it can reach the pulmonary artery walls with enough force to destroy the molecular structure.

b) Poststenotic dilatation is so common in the presence of an ejection click that it was originally believed that all ejection clicks were caused by the distention of the dilated segment.

*9.   What is the likely cause of an ejection sound heard in patients with tetralogy of Fallot?

ANS.:   If there is a severe tetralogy (almost pulmonary atresia or pseudotruncus arteriosus), it is an aortic ejection sound due to the dilated and volume-overloaded aorta's receiving an excess of blood. In mild (acyanotic) tetralogy it is probably a pulmonary ejection sound due to pulmonary valve stenosis [36].

Note: a) About half the patients with tetralogy have pure valvular stenosis. The other half have either pure infundibular or mixed infundibular and valvular stenosis. If it is purely valvular and not severe (acyanotic type), not only may there be an ejection sound but also the pulmonary second sound (P_2) may be audible. (The latter is unusual in cyanotic tetralogy.)

b) The rare pulmonary ejection sound with mild tetralogy does not usually decrease with inspiration because the ventricular septal defect (VSD) does not allow the stronger right atrial contraction to increase the RV diastolic pressure, i.e., the right atrium may contract very strongly with inspiration, but its energy is dissipated through the VSD. The click can change with respiration (and even occur in presystole) only if there is resistance to flow from right to left through the VSD due to left ventricular hypertrophy (LVH) from rare concomitant AS.

*10.   Which early clicks are neither aortic nor pulmonary?

ANS.:   a) A persistent truncus arteriosus quadracuspid valve almost always produces an ejection sound, often louder than any of the heart sounds, and is not influenced by respiration [60].

b) The nonejection click of the ballooned valve syndrome (see p. 308) may come so early that it imitates an aortic or pulmonary ejection click. With these early ballooned valve clicks, however, a systolic regurgitant murmur can nearly always be elicited [23].

c) Ventricular septal defects often close spontaneously by being covered over by a pouch or small septal aneurysm. This aneurysm can produce an early systolic click [47].

Note: These clicks are loudest on expiration, usually localized to the left lower sternal border, and are not loud. They are usually present with the pansystolic murmur of the pinhole VSD. These Q to click intervals are in the range of 100—130 msec, much the same as that of pulmonary or aortic ejection clicks.

Ejection Sounds in Pulmonary Hypertension

1.   Why is an ejection sound heard in pulmonary hypertension?
     ANS.:   Two theories are as follows:
         a) It may be a pulmonary valve click if the pulmonary valves are made stiff by
            their rings stretching, i.e., the high pressure in the pulmonary artery may cause
            a dilated pulmonary artery root, which stretches the valve ring. The taut valves,
            opening at a very rapid rate, may produce the click.
         b) The click is produced by sudden tension of the relatively inelastic annulus of
            the pulmonary artery. This theory has been given support by these findings:
            1) An ejection click can be produced by tying a ring loosely around the pul-
               monary artery and suddenly expanding the artery [20].
            2) Palpation of the pulmonary artery during surgery on a patient with pulmo-
               nary hypertension may reveal a sudden checking of the fibrous annulus
               during systole.
         Note: The pulmonary ejection click noted in bilateral pulmonary artery
         stenosis may have a similar etiology to that heard in pulmonary hypertension [8].
2.   How does a pulmonary hypertension ejection sound differ from a PS ejection sound?
     ANS.:   In pulmonary hypertension the ejection sound is
         a) Often heard better lower down on the chest.
         b) Rarely changed by respiration.
         *c) Simultaneous with the upstroke of a pulmonary artery pressure tracing.
         *d) Usually later than 60 msec after the M_1 (Q—P_1 over 140 msec).

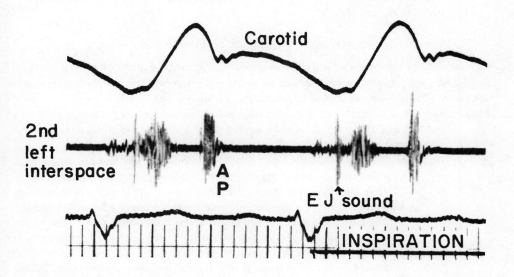

This high-frequency phonocardiogram and simultaneous carotid tracing is from a patient with
severe pulmonary hypertension secondary to a VSD (**Eisenmenger syndrome**). Note that the
pulmonary ejection sound does not diminish with inspiration.

The Q to Ejection Click Interval

*1.   What happens to isovolumic contraction time with increasing PS? Why?

ANS.:   It becomes shorter, because as the PS becomes more and more severe,

a) The rate of RV pressure rise becomes faster and faster [21].

b) The pulmonary diastolic pressure becomes lower and lower.

Note: a) The $Q-P_1$ (Q to ejection click) interval in mild PS, i.e., with RV not over 60 mm Hg, is about 110 msec or more. The Q—P in severe PS, i.e., RV pressure 120 mm Hg or more, is about 60 to 100 msec.

This refers to the rate-corrected $Q-P_1$; i.e., the interval must be corrected to a heart rate of 60 by dividing by the square root of the cycle length, or R—R interval [15].

b) If the stenosis is severe, the ejection sound may merge with the M_1. Then its presence can only be detected by its respiratory variation in loudness [21].

c) The earliness of the aortic ejection click does not correlate with the degree of AS.

*2.   What happens to the $Q-P_1$ interval or the M_1-P_1 interval with pulmonary hypertension?

ANS.:   It becomes longer, because isovolumic contraction is prolonged as the RV takes longer to reach the high pulmonary diastolic pressure.

Note: In patients with ASD, there is a good correlation between the $Q-P_1$ or $M-P_1$ interval and the degree of pulmonary hypertension. If the $Q-P_1$ is over 140 msec, or the M_1-P_1 over 60 msec, the pulmonary artery pressure is probably over 80 mm Hg.

Ejection Sounds in Idiopathic Dilatation of the Pulmonary Artery

1.   How can you explain the ejection click in idiopathic dilatation of the pulmonary artery if there is no high pressure in the artery to tense the valve ring, and the pulmonary valve is not stenosed and therefore unable to produce an opening snap?

ANS.:   Idiopathic dilatation of the pulmonary artery implies a damaged artery with marked loss of elasticity. A jerky expansion of this damaged and lax pulmonary artery may cause a click.

Note: a) A sudden expansion of a dilated pulmonary artery was the only reasonable explanation for the click in a patient with an absent pulmonary valve and dilated pulmonary artery in whom intracardiac phonocardiograms showed the ejection murmur preceding the click by 50 msec [1].

b) The clicks of idiopathic dilatation of the pulmonary artery tend to be far from the M_1, also suggesting a distal event, such as dilatation of a lax pulmonary artery, as a cause of the click.

c) Simultaneous pulse tracings and intracardiac phonocardiograms show that the ejection click in idiopathic dilatations occur slightly later than the onset of rise of pulmonary artery pressure.

2.   What lesion produces a rapid ejection into a dilated pulmonary artery without an ejection click?

ANS.:   An **atrial septal defect** (ASD) produces a rapid flow through the pulmonary artery, but there is often no audible ejection click unless pulmonary hypertension is present or the pulmonary artery is markedly dilated. If the dilatation is due only to an extra volume, without destruction of the pulmonary artery tissue to reduce its elasticity, there is no mechanism to produce the ejection click.

Note: With most ASDs, a sound is recorded on the phonocardiogram at the time of an ejection sound. It is louder than the first component of the split S_1 at the apex in patients with ASDs so often that it has been proposed as a helpful diagnostic clue to the presence of an ASD [32]. This second component of the split is generally considered to be a tricuspid component (T_1). Although it has been timed on echocardiograms with closure of the tricuspid valve, there is still no proof that it may not sometimes be a pulmonary ejection sound (P_1). The T_1/M_1 loudness ratio has not correlated well with either the degree of pulmonary hypertension or the pulmonary systemic flow ratio.

THE LOUDNESS OF THE M_1

1.   What factors besides the chest-wall shape or thickness control the loudness of M_1?

ANS.:   a) The rate of rise of ventricular pressure. The faster the rise, the louder the M_1 [17]

b) The timing of mitral valve closure in relation to onset of ventricular contraction. The longer the LV must contract before it can close the mitral valve, the louder the M_1 [55].

c) The position of the mitral valve at the time of the beginning of ventricular contraction. If the mitral valve is closed or almost closed, the M_1 will be soft.

d) The stiffness of the AV valve. A slightly stiff valve produces a loud M_1, but as the valve becomes too stiff to move much, the M_1 is diminished.

Ventricular Pressure Rise and M_1 Loudness

1.   What is the physiologist's way of expressing the rate of rise of pressure?

ANS.:   Delta P/delta t = change of pressure/change of time. This is usually shortened to dP/dt.

2.   What is the relationship between dP/dt of the LV and the M_1 loudness?

ANS.:   The greater the dP/dt (i.e., the faster the rate of the LV pressure rise), the louder the M_1.

Note: The loudness of the S_1 correlates well with the closing velocity of the mitral leaflets on the echocardiogram.

3.   What can cause an increased dP/dt of the LV and therefore make the M_1 louder?

ANS.:   a) Increased contractility due to positive inotropic agents (catecholamines, sympathetic stimulation, digitalis, or thyroxine). Sympathetic stimulation is probably the cause of the loud M_1 in sinus tachycardia.

b) Increase in diastolic volume or pressure (**Starling effect**).

4. What can decrease the dP/dt of the LV and therefore make the M_1 softer?

ANS.: Any myocardial damage such as that due to myocardial infarction or chronic cardiomyopathy.

Note: These soft first sounds are often described as muffled, because they have lost much of their high frequencies. For some unknown reason, the M_1 is more likely to be softer in posterior than in anterior myocardial infarction [49]. The M_1 is said to be soft in acute myocardial infarction also because the acutely infarcted area tends to balloon outward paradoxically with systole, so that part of the energy developed by the LV is absorbed by the elastic distention of the infarcted area. This latter argument is weakened by the finding that in most patients with **aneurysms** the S_1 is not softer than in those patients with a previous infarction and no aneurysm [37]. Also in some patients with anteroseptal aneurysms the M_1 may actually be loud. This has been explained by the fact that a sudden tensing of the tissue of a ventricular aneurysm (suspended between two rubber stoppers in a tank of water) can produce as loud a sound as tensing of mitral valve leaflets, especially in the low-frequency range [12].

Timing of Mitral Valve Closure and M_1 Loudness

1. How does the timing of the mitral valve closure at the beginning of systole affect M_1 loudness?

ANS.: The greater the delay in closure of the mitral valve relative to the onset of ventricular contraction, the louder the M_1. This is because *the LV accelerates as it contracts.* This means that the longer the ventricle contracts before it closes the mitral valve, the more time there is for acceleration and the higher will be the dP/dt at which the valves will close.

2. What produces a delay in timing of mitral closure relative to onset of ventricular contraction?

ANS.: The gradient or pressure difference across the valves at the moment that ventricular contraction begins as when there is a short P–R interval or when there is MS. The higher the pressure in the left atrium, the longer the ventricle has to contract before it can close the mitral valve.

3. Why does a short P–R interval cause a loud M_1?

ANS.: The P represents atrial contraction, which raises left atrial pressure as it flings the mitral valves open. The R represents ventricular contraction. The short P–R interval allows ventricular contraction to occur so quickly after the atrium has contracted that left atrium has not had time to relax, and atrial pressure is still at a high level when the pressure in the LV exceeds it, to close the mitral valve [55]. This means that the ventricle has had a chance to accelerate to a rapid dP/dt part of its pressure curve by the time it closes the mitral valve. See the following figure for Q 4.

4. Why does a long P–R interval cause a soft M_1?

ANS.: The delayed LV contraction allows the left atrial pressure a chance to drop to low levels by the time the LV begins to contract. Thus, LV pressure will exceed left atrial pressure at the very early slow part of its acceleration curve [55].

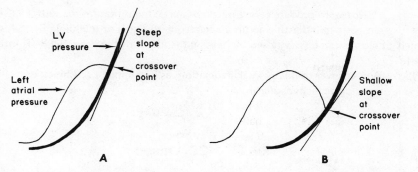

(A) If the P—R interval is short, the LV contracts before the left atrium has had a chance to relax and drop its pressure. Therefore, the LV pressure will not exceed left atrial pressure until it has contracted for a long enough time to accelerate to a stage of rapid pressure rise by the time the mitral leaflets are closed. This produces an abrupt deceleration of forward flow and a loud sound.

   (B) If the P—R interval is long, the LV contracts later than at A, so that the left atrium has had time to drop to a low pressure when the LV pressure exceeds it. The pressure crossover point is on the slow part of the LV acceleration curve, and the valves are closed at a relatively slow rate, producing a soft sound.

> *Note:* a) The paradox of a short P—R interval and a normal or soft M_1 is seen in the Wolff-Parkinson-White (W-P-W) syndrome, type B, where the pre-excitation activates the RV first, thus causing the LV to contract later, as if there were a long P—R interval.
>
> b) The paradox of a long P—R interval and a loud S_1 is seen in MS and in Ebstein's anomaly. In the latter, the M_1 may actually be very soft, but the second component of the S_1 may be loud, short, and clicking because it is due to closure of a large deformed tricuspid septal valve leaflet. Since the septal leaflet has been likened to a large sail flapping in the breeze, this loud T_1 has been called the "sail sound" [13]. It may come either soon after the M_1 or so late that it occurs in midsystole. It is presumably late because of the very slow initial rise in RV pressure. The sail sound has been shown to occur at the transition between the slow and rapid rise of RV pressure. It often increases with inspiration and will usually be associated with a very late tricuspid opening snap.

*5.   How does the position of the mitral valves at the time that LV pressure exceeds left atrial pressure control the loudness of the M_1?

   ANS.:   If the valves are open anywhere from fully to even a third of their full opening capacity, then, all else being equal, the position of the valves should not have much effect on the loudness of M_1. S_1 loudness does not correlate well with the degree to which the valve is open when the LV begins to contract [55]. This is because the time for a valve to move from fully open to closed is so rapid that there is not enough time for a significant LV acceleration to occur. If, however, the mitral valves are closed or very nearly closed at the time the LV exceeds left atrial pressure, then no matter what the LV dP/dt is at the time, the M_1 sound will be soft or absent. In other words, the relative position of the mitral valves at the time LV pressure exceeds left atrial pressure controls loudness of the M_1 in an "all-or-none" fashion; i.e., if they are more than slightly open, it matters little how much more open they are. If they are nearly closed or closed, the M_1 will be soft or absent.

Note: In sudden, severe mitral or aortic regurgitation the mitral valve may be closed in mid-diastole and is associated with a soft or inaudible S_1 [38, 40].

6.   Which situations can be diagnosed by hearing the effect of the changing P—R interval on the M_1?

ANS.:   Any **atrioventricular (AV) dissociation**, as in complete **AV block** or as in some ventricular tachycardias.

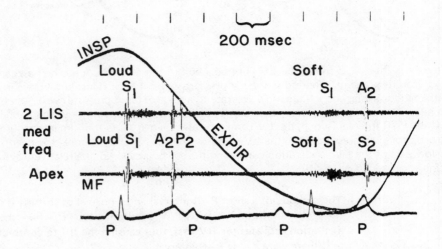

This medium-frequency (MF) phonocardiogram is from a patient with complete AV block, i.e., the P waves and QRS complexes are independent, thus causing the P—R intervals to vary. Note the loud S_1 after the short P—R (first one) and the soft one after the long P—R both at the apex and second left interspace (2 LIS).

Note: a) Wenckeback periods also have gradually longer P—R intervals until complete AV block occurs, and a beat is dropped. The gradually longer P—R interval has been said to cause a softer and softer first sound until a pause occurs. This is not likely to be a constant finding, because if the longest P—R is very long, e.g., about 360 msec, the valves may reopen due to continued pulmonary venous return, and so produce a loud first sound. If, also, the changes are small, such as from 120—140 msec, no perceptible M_1 changes may occur.

b) The first heart sound will not change despite complete AV block if
  1) There are no P waves; e.g., if the atria are fibrillating or fluttering.
  2) There is a poor effect of atrial contraction, as in very severe heart failure [55].

c) There is no correlation between ejection fraction and M_1 loudness in AV dissociation. The maximum ejection fraction occurs at a P—R interval of 180—200 msec. As the P—R becomes either longer or shorter than this range, the ejection fraction decreases [4].

*7.   In atrial fibrillation, how will the different lengths of diastole and absence of atrial con-
      traction control the loudness of the M_1 if the valves are normal?

    ANS.:   Since there is nothing to place the mitral valves into a closed position before
      ventricular contraction, only changes in LV contractility can affect the loudness
      of the M_1. A series of short cycles can cause an increase in contractility (treppe
      effect) and will produce a loud M_1. A short diastole, on the other hand, will
      modify the loudness by causing a decrease in LV stretch and a decrease in the
      Starling effect. A series of short diastoles followed by a long one should there-
      fore produce a loud M_1 (treppe plus Starling effect [16]).

        Note: The loudest M_1 in atrial fibrillation occurs when it coincides in timing
      with the occurrence of an S_3 [52]. Why this occurs is uncertain.

8.   Why does the M_1 in severe AS tend to be soft?

    ANS.:   a) Atrial contraction not only reopens the mitral valve at the end of diastole, but
      also always causes an immediate partial closure movement, probably due to a
      Bernoulli effect or eddy-current effect. The backward flipping motion is
      easily seen on an echocardiogram. The strong atrial contraction caused by loss
      of compliance of the LV may so enhance the atriogenic mitral valve closure
      effect, that the valves may be in a nearly closed position by the time the ven-
      tricular pressure reaches left atrial pressure.

        b) The high end-diastolic pressure generated in the LV by the powerful atrial con-
      traction may push the mitral valves upward into the nearly closed position
      while the atria are relaxing.

        c) When the systolic gradient exceeds 50 mm Hg, LV contractility has been shown
      to decrease, especially in patients over age 40 [56].

        Note: In hypertensive persons with a strong enough left atrial contraction to
      produce a sound (S_4) as it forces blood into the LV and makes the latter expand,
      decreasing venous return with leg tourniquets can make the S_4 migrate toward
      the M_1. As it does so, the M_1 becomes louder. This is difficult to understand.
      One possibility is that as the atrial pressure is lowered, it contracts in a more
      peristaltic fashion, so that it causes a progressively later rise in peak left atrial
      pressure [6]. Thus, when the LV contracts (from a progressively lower end-
      diastolic pressure), it has to contract for a longer time to reach a higher left atrial
      pressure.

*9.   Why does LBBB affect the loudness of the M_1?

    ANS.:   It causes a decrease in the loudness because

        a) The dP/dt of early contraction is often decreased in LBBB [10]. This is proba-
      bly because initial conduction is entirely septal and suggests that the main LV
      mass may not participate in preisovolumic contraction, i.e., in pre-M_1 contrac-
      tion.

        b) The onset of left ventricular contraction may be delayed so that the effect is
      the same as that of a long P—R interval.

*10. How does thyrotoxicosis affect the M_1 loudness?

    ANS.:   It makes it louder.

        Note: Even when the heart rate is slowed by reserpine, the M_1 is still loud.

*11. How can S_1 loudness during normal heart rates suggest the cause of paroxysmal tachy-cardias?

ANS.: If the S_1 is very loud, it suggests a short P—R, normal QRS type of preexcitation and therefore a Lown-Ganong-Levine syndrome with episodes of atrial tachycardia.

THE M_1 IN MITRAL STENOSIS

1. What can cause a forward gradient (see p. 262) across a mitral valve?

ANS.: Torrential flow across the mitral valve, as in mitral regurgitation (MR), may cause a gradient in early and mid-diastole, while a stenotic valve, even with less-than-normal flow, can cause a gradient across the mitral valve throughout all of diastole. (See p. 343 for illustration of mitral valve gradient.)

2. How does a forward gradient across the mitral valve at the end of diastole affect the M_1? Why?

ANS.: It makes the M_1 loud, because the gradient at the end of diastole requires the ventricle to reach a higher pressure before it can close the valve. This gives the LV more time to accelerate.

3. What does a stiff mitral valve, as in mitral stenosis (MS), do to the quality of the M_1? Why?

ANS.: It makes the M_1 short and snapping. The resistance of the fibrotic and tethered edges to movement may cause the still flexible body or belly of the valves to billow upward with a sudden motion, like that of a snapping sail.

4. What is the short, snapping M_1, secondary to MS, often called?

ANS.: The closing snap of MS.

Note: The apical impulse in MS has often been characterized as "tapping." Since this really implies a palpable first sound, it should not be used to describe a movement or impulse.

5. When will a stiff mitral valve produce no unusually loud, snapping M_1?

ANS.: When the whole structure is very stiff and immobile due either to calcium or fibrosis.

Note: If, under these circumstances, the M_1 is loud, it will not be short or snapping, because the loudness will not then be due to the usual mechanism of the loud M_1 in MS.

*6. How does the M_1 loudness vary in MS if atrial fibrillation is present?

ANS.: At least three types are seen:

Type 1: If the MS is mild, and the large anterior or septal leaflet is mobile (a good opening snap is heard), the variation is the same as with the normal valve, except that there is less tendency for the M_1 to become louder with long diastoles. The frequent absence of increasing loudness after long diastoles may be due to the equalization of atrial and ventricular pressures at the end of long diastoles.

Type 2: If the valves are heavily calcified or fibrotic (no opening snap is present), the M_1 is dependent entirely on end-diastolic volume and preceding R—R intervals. Thus, the S_1 becomes louder proportionately to the length of the previous diastole and inversely to the length of the R—R preceding the previous diastole.

Type 3: If the valves are moderately stenosed, the S_1 loudness varies inversely with the duration of the previous diastole; i.e., the shorter the previous R—R interval, the louder the M_1 [50].

7.   How can the site of the loudest M_1 tell you if a "closing snap" is present?

   ANS.:   Unlike the opening snap, the M_1 of MS is almost always loudest at the apex. If an M_1 is loudest at the left lower sternal border, it is unlikely to be due to MS.

*8.   How does the apex cardiogram suggest that the M_1 of MS has a different mechanism than the normal M_1?

   ANS.:   The normal M_1 is simultaneous with a notch on the upstroke of the apex cardiogram. In MS, the major loud, snapping sound occurs later than the notch, which is deeper than normal and simultaneous with a soft component of S_1 [45]. This suggests that the major loud component of the M_1 in MS is indeed a "closing snap" and not the usual M_1.

   Note: A left atrial myxoma may also have a deeper notch than normal on the upstroke of the apex cardiogram coincident with the M_1, and this lesion often mimics MS by auscultation.

*THE M_1 IN MITRAL REGURGITATION

*1.   When can mitral regurgitation (MR) entirely eliminate the flow across the mitral valve during the last part of diastole?

   ANS.:   In sudden, severe MR, the LV in diastole cannot dilate rapidly enough in response to the sudden increase in volume load to maintain normal diastolic pressures [38]. The LV diastolic pressure may rise rapidly enough to equal or even momentarily exceed the left atrial pressure in the presence of severe MR such as that due to ruptured chordae. Therefore, the pressure in this relatively nonelastic, overloaded LV will rise so high by mid- or late diastole as to close the mitral valves in mid- or late diastole. This will make the M_1 soft or inaudible.

   Note: It is theoretically improbable that a measurable reversed gradient could occur across the mitral valve in diastole for more than a moment if the ventricular pressure rise is due entirely to flow from the left atrium, for as soon as the pressure rises high enough in the LV to close the mitral valve, forward flow and LV pressure rise cease. A slight momentary reversed gradient probably must occur, however, in order to close the mitral valve.

   Sudden, severe AR, however, such as when a sinus of Valsalva ruptures, can easily cause a reversed gradient between LV and left atrium and so eliminate the M_1.

*2.   What happens to the rate of rise of ventricular pressure in the preisovolumic contraction period (before the mitral valve closes) if a ventricular leak such as a VSD or MR is present?

   ANS.:   The rate of pressure rise and, therefore the loudness of the M_1, should be decreased [57]. In actual fact, however, only about half the patients with MR have a soft M_1 because

   a) The extra diastolic stretch of the volume overload compensates for the leak and allows a rate of rise of pressure even faster than normal [18]. Therefore, if the LV is not damaged, the M_1 may even be loud.

   b) Many patients with dominant MR have MS and an opening snap, and in these patients, a closing snap may make the M_1 loud.

*THE Q—1 INTERVAL

*1.   What is meant by the Q-1 interval?

ANS.:   The time from the onset of the QRS complex to the M_1, i.e., the $Q—M_1$ interval. (The upper limit of normal is 70 msec.)

*2.   What important factors prolong the Q—1 interval?

ANS.:   Left bundle branch block, hypertension, a poorly functioning myocardium, a high atrial pressure (as in MS and MR), or a shunt flow through a VSD or a patent ductus arteriosus [24].

   Note: a) There is a close correlation between the prolongation of the Q—1 interval and the size of the left-to-right shunt through a VSD [24].

   b) There is a poor correlation between the Q—1 interval and the severity of MS, although almost all subjects with significant MS have a Q—1 beyond the upper limit of normal, and successful mitral surgery will shorten the Q—1 interval [25, 31].

*3.   How does the Q—1 vary with various diastolic lengths in atrial fibrillation in (a) MS and (b) normal subjects?

ANS.:   a) In MS, the shorter the previous diastole, the higher the left atrial pressure and the longer the Q—1.

   b) In normal subjects, the Q—1 intervals change very little with varying diastoles.

*4.   In atrial fibrillation, how long does it take for the left atrium to empty enough to drop its pressure low enough to equal LV pressure with (a) no MS, (b) mild MS, and (c) severe MS?

ANS.:   a) With even the shortest diastoles, the pressures will equalize.

   b) In about 700 msec, the pressures will equalize.

   c) In about 1 sec, the pressures will equalize.

   Note: a) This provides a method of judging the severity of the MS. If the Q—1 never becomes longer after 700-msec cycles, it is mild. If the Q—1 requires at least 1-sec cycles to stabilize, it is probably severe [58].

   b) How the Q—1 is used together with the opening snap to judge the severity of the MS is discussed on p. 220 [57].

   c) The C—1 interval probably correlates better than the Q—1 with the severity of the MS. (See the following section.)

*THE C—M_1 (C—1) INTERVAL

*1.   What is meant by the C—1 interval?

ANS.:   It is the interval between the onset of ventricular contraction on the apex cardiogram and the mitral closure sound. This is the preisovolumic contraction period.

   Note: a) Some factors that control the C—1 interval are:

   1) The ability of the LV to contract rapidly and strongly (ventricular contractility or inotropism).

   2) The heart rate. The faster the rate, the shorter the C—1.

   3) The stiffness or resistance of the mitral valve.

   4) The height of the left atrial pressure.

b) You can use the C—1 interval in helping to diagnose the presence or absence of MS, because if the C—1 interval is less than 30 msec, MS is very unlikely. If, on the other hand, the C—1 interval is over 50 msec, MS is very likely [42].

*2.   How can the C—1 interval be used to estimate the mean left atrial pressure?

ANS.:   The greater the MS, the longer the LV must contract before it can close the mitral valve. Isovolumic contraction time, i.e., the time between the M_1 and the opening of the aortic valve (roughly the E point on the apex cardiogram), is unchanged by MS. The ratio of $\dfrac{C-1}{C-E}$ correlates with the degree of MS with an r of approximately 0.85 [9]. The C—E interval is unchanged by the presence of MR as long as MS is predominant [43].

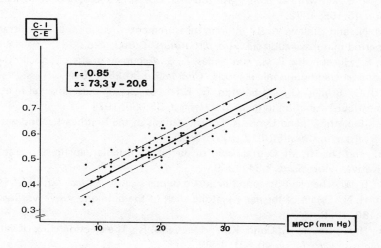

The longer the C—1 is relative to the C—E, the higher the mean pulmonary capillary pressure (MPCP) and the more severe the mitral stenosis. (From Comhaire and Uyttenhove [9].)

REFERENCES

1. Ahuja, S. P., and Coles, J. C. Further observations on the genesis of early systolic clicks. *Am. J. Cardiol.* 17:291, 1966.

2. Armstrong, T. G., and Gotsman, M. S. Initial low frequency vibrations of the first heart sound. *Br. Heart J.* 35:691, 1973.

3. Aronow, W. S. Isovolumic contraction and left ventricular ejection times. *Am. J. Cardiol.* 26:238, 1970.

4. Bashour, T. T., Naughton, J. P., and Cheng, T. O. Systolic time intervals in patients with artificial pacemakers. *Am. J. Cardiol.* 32:287, 1973.

5. Boughner, D. R., and Roach, M. R. Effect of low frequency vibration on the arterial wall. *Circ. Res.* 29:136, 1971.

6. Brockman, S. K. Dynamic function of atrial contraction in regulation of cardiac performance. *Am. J. Physiol.* 204:597, 1963.

7. Bruns, D. L., Connolly, J. E., Holman, E., and Stofer, R. C. Experimental observations on post-stenotic dilatation. *J. Thorac. Cardiovasc. Surg.* 38:662, 1959.

8. Cheng, T. O. Early systolic ejection click associated with supravalvular pulmonary stenosis. *Am. J. Cardiol.* 18:2, 1966.

9. Comhaire, F., and Uyttenhove, P. Evaluation of mitral stenosis. *Am. Heart J.* 81:443, 1971.

10. D'Cunha, G. F., Friedberg, H. D., and Jaume, F. The first heart sound in intermittent left bundle branch block. *Am. J. Cardiol.* 27:447, 1971.

11. Di Bartolo, G., Nunez-Dey, D., and Bendezu-Prieto, J. Left heart studies in mitral stenosis with special reference to intracardiac phonocardiography. *Am. J. Cardiol.* 10:93, 1962.

12. Dock, W. The genesis of diastolic heart sounds. *Am. J. Med.* 50:178, 1971.

13. Fontana, M. E., and Wooley, C. F. Sail sound in Ebstein's anomaly of the tricuspid valve. *Circulation* 46:155, 1972.

14. Frank, M. N., and Kinlaw, W. B. Indirect measurement of isovolumetric contraction time and tension period in normal subjects. *Am. J. Cardiol.* 10:800, 1962.

15. Gamboa, R., Hugenholtz, P. G., and Nadas, A. S. Accuracy of the phonocardiogram in assessing severity of aortic and pulmonic stenosis. *Circulation* 30:35, 1964.

16. Gibson, D. G., Broder, G., and Sowton, E. Effect of varying pulse interval in atrial fibrillation on left ventricular function in man. *Br. Heart J.* 33:388, 1971.

17. Gould, L., Belletti, D., and Lyon, A. F. The genesis of the first heart sound with varying P–R intervals. *Dis. Chest* 52:817, 1967.

18. Gould, L., and Shariff, M. Comparisons of the left ventricular, aortic, and brachial arterial first derivative. *Vasc. Surg.* 3:34, 1969.

19. Hancock, E. W. The ejection sound in aortic stenosis. *Am. J. Med.* 40:569, 1966.

20. Hultgren, H. N. Origin of the early systolic click of the pulmonary artery. *Stanford Med. Bull.* 14:183, 1956.

21. Hultgren, H. N., Reeve, R., Cohn, K., and McLeod, R. The ejection click of valvular pulmonic stenosis. *Circulation* 40:631, 1969.

22. Hunt, D., Baxley, W. A., Kennedy, J. W., Judge, T. P., Williams, J. E., and Dodge, H. T. Quantitative evaluation of cineaortography in the assessment of aortic regurgitation. *Am. J. Cardiol.* 31:696, 1973.

23. Hutter, A. M., Jr., Dinsmore, R. E., Willerson, J. T., and DeSanctis, R. W. Early systolic clicks due to mitral valve prolapse. *Circulation* 44:516, 1971.

24. Karnegis, J. N., and Wang, Y. The Q–1 interval of the phonocardiogram. *Am. J. Cardiol.* 11:452, 1963.

25. Kelly, J. J., Jr. Diagnostic value of phonocardiography in mitral stenosis: Mode of production of first heart sound. *Am. J. Med.* 19:862, 1955.

26. Lakier, J. B., Bloom, K. R., Pocock, W. A., and Barlow, J. B. Tricuspid component of first heart sound. *Br. Heart J.* 35:1275, 1973.

27. Lakier, J. B., Fritz, V. U., Pocock, W. A., and Barlow, J. B. Mitral components of the first heart sound. *Br. Heart J.* 34:160, 1972.

28. Laniado, S., Yellin, E. L., Miller, H., and Frater, R. W. M. Temporal relation of the first heart sound to closure of the mitral valve. *Circulation* 47:1006, 1973.

29. Leatham, A. Heart murmurs, mechanism, intensity, and pitch. *Lancet* 2:757, 1958. Classic article.

30. Leatham, A., and Gray, I. Auscultatory and phonocardiographic signs of atrial septal defect. *Br. Heart J.* 18:193, 1956.

31. Lee, Y., Scherlis, L., and Singleton, R. T. Mitral stenosis, hemodynamic, electrocardiographic and vectorcardiographic studies. *Am. Heart J.* 69:559, 1965.

32. Lopez, J. F., Linn, H., and Shaffer, A. B. The apical first heart sound as an aid in the diagnosis of atrial septal defect. *Circulation* 26:1296, 1962.

33. Luisada, A. A., Kurz, H., Slodki, S. J., MacCanon, D. M., and Krol, B. Normal first heart sounds with nonfunctional tricuspid valve of right ventricle. *Circulation* 35:119, 1967.

34. Luisada, A. A., and MacCanon, D. M. Functional basis of heart sounds. *Am. J. Cardiol.* 16:631, 1965.

35. Luisada, A. A., and MacCanon, D. M. The physiologic basis of the heart sounds. *Dis. Chest* 49:258, 1966.

36. Martin, C. E., Reddy, P. S., Leon, D. F., and Shaver, J. A. Genesis, frequency, and diagnostic significance of ejection sound in adults with tetralogy of Fallot. *Br. Heart J.* 35:402, 1973.

37. McGinn, F. X., Gould, L., and Lyon, A. F. The phonocardiogram and apexcardiogram in patients with ventricular aneurysm. *Am. J. Cardiol.* 21:467, 1968.

38. Meadows, W. R., VanPraagh, S., Indreika, M., and Sharp, J. T. Premature mitral valve closure. *Circulation* 28:251, 1963.

39. Oakley, C. M., and Hallidie-Smith, K. A. Assessment of site and severity in congenital aortic stenosis. *Br. Heart J.* 29:367, 1967.

40. Oliver, G. C., Jr., Gazetopoulos, N., and Deuchar, D. C. Reversed mitral diastolic gradient in aortic incompetence. *Br. Heart J.* 29:239, 1967.

41. Oravetz, J., Wissner, S., Argano, B., and Luisada, A. A. Dynamic analysis of heart sounds in right and left bundle branch blocks. *Circulation* 36:275, 1967.

42. Oreshkov, V. I. Q—1 or C—1 interval in the diagnosis of mitral stenosis. *Br. Heart J.* 29:778, 1967.

43. Oreshkov, V. I. Isovolumic contraction time and isovolumic contraction time index in mitral stenosis. *Br. Heart J.* 34:553, 1972.

44. Parisi, A. F., and Milton, B. G. Relation of mitral valve closure to the first heart sound in man. *Am. J. Cardiol.* 32:779, 1973.

45. Perosio, A. M. A., Silva, M. A. C., and Ricci, G. J. The first heart sound: Its relation with the apex cardiogram. *Am. J. Cardiol.* 32:283, 1973.

46. Piemme, T. E., Barnett, G. O., and Dexter, L. Relationship of heart sounds to acceleration of blood flow. *Circ. Res.* 18:303, 1966.

47. Pieroni, D. R., Bell, B. B., Krovetz, L. J., Varghese, P. J., and Rowe, R. D. Auscultatory recognition of aneurysm of the membranous ventricular septum associated with small ventricular septal defect. *Circulation* 44:733, 1971.

48. Plass, R., Schmidt, K. H., and Guenther, K. H. Intracardiac sounds and murmurs in atrial septal defect. *Am. J. Cardiol.* 28:173, 1971.

49. Price, W. H., and Brown, A. E. Alterations in intensity of heart sounds after myocardial infarction. *Br. Heart J.* 30:835, 1968.

50. Ravin, A., and Bershoff, E. The intensity of the first heart sound in auricular fibrillation with mitral stenosis. *Am. Heart J.* 41:539, 1951.

51. Rodbard, S., Ikeda, K., and Montes, M. An analysis of mechanisms of post stenotic dilatation. *Angiology* 18:349, 1967.

52. Rytand, D. A. The variable loudness of the first heart sound in auricular fibrillation. *Am. Heart J.* 37:187, 1949.

53. Sanchez, J., Rodriguez-Torres, R., Lin, J. S., Goldstein, S., and Kavety, V. Diagnostic value of the first heart sound in children with atrial septal defect. *Am. Heart J.* 78:467, 1969.

54. Segall, H. N., and Sharp, A. Heart sounds in bundle branch block. *Jap. Heart J.* 8:468, 1967.

55. Shah, P. M., Kramer, D. H., and Gramiak, R. Influence of the timing of atrial systole on mitral valve closure and on the first heart sound in man. *Am. J. Cardiol.* 26:231, 1970.

56. Simon, H., Krayenbuehl, H. P., Rutishauser, W., and Preter, B. O. The contractile state of the hypertrophied left ventricular myocardium in aortic stenosis. *Am. Heart J.* 79:587, 1970.

57. Surawicz, B., Mercer, C., Chlebus, H., Reeves, J. T., and Spencer, F. C. Role of the phonocardiogram in evaluation of the severity of mitral stenosis and detection of associated valvular lesions. *Circulation* 34:759, 1966.

58. Tavel, M. E., Feigenbaum, H., and Campbell, R. W. A study of the Q-1 interval in atrial fibrillation with and without mitral stenosis. *Circulation* 31:429, 1965.

59. Van Bogaert, A. A new concept on the mechanism of the first heart sound. *Am. J. Cardiol.* 18:253, 1966.

60. Victorica, B. E., Krovetz, L. J., Elliott, L. P., VanMierop, L. H. S., Bartley, T. D., Gessner, I. H., and Schiebler, G. L. Persistent truncus arteriosus in infancy. *Am. Heart J.* 77:13, 1969.

61. Vogel, J. H. K., and Blount, S. G. Clinical evaluation in localizing level of obstruction to outflow from left ventricle. *Am. J. Cardiol.* 15:782, 1965.

62. Weintraub, A. M., Perloff, J. K., Conrad, P. W., and Hufnagel, C. A. Poststenotic dilatation of the aorta with muscular subaortic stenosis. *Am. Heart J.* 68:741, 1964.

63. Whittaker, A. V., Shaver, J. A., Gray, S., III, and Leonard, J. J. Sound-pressure correlates of the aortic ejection sound. *Circulation* 39:475, 1969.

64. Yahini, J. H., Dulfano, M. J., and Toor, M. Pulmonic stenosis. *Am. J. Cardiol.* 5:744, 1960.

9

The Second Heart Sound

1. What produces the normal second heart sound (S$_2$)?

    ANS.: Events associated with closure of the aortic and pulmonary valves.

    Note: The exact cause of the sound is unknown. Valve closure itself probably produces no noise. It is thought that closure of the aortic and pulmonary valves causes a deceleration of forward flow, and that this sudden deceleration somehow causes the sound [60]. The aortic component of the second sound, for example, has been shown in dogs to occur simultaneously both with the peak deceleration of forward flow in the aorta and with the aortic incisura.

2. Which valve normally closes first, the aortic or pulmonary?

    ANS.: The aortic valve. (It is crucial to commit this to memory.) The sequence is A, P, i.e., aortic and pulmonary, as in Atlantic & Pacific. The A comes first, as in the alphabet. We shall call the aortic component of the second sound A$_2$ and the pulmonary component, P$_2$.

3. What is the old meaning of A$_2$ and P$_2$ (to which we shall *not* refer in this book)?

    ANS.: A$_2$ used to mean the total S$_2$ in the "aortic area" (second right interspace). P$_2$ used to mean the total S$_2$ in the "pulmonary area" (second left interspace). We now use A$_2$ to mean only the *aortic component* of the S$_2$, and P$_2$ to mean the *pulmonary component* of the S$_2$.

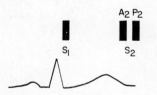

A$_2$ is the aortic valve closure component of the S$_2$. P$_2$ is the pulmonary valve closure component of the S$_2$. Note that the S$_2$ occurs near the end of the T wave of the ECG; i.e., the T wave is a systolic event.

---

* indicates material that is for electives or fellows in cardiology, or concerns rare phenomena, of interest primarily to cardiologists.

Boldface type indicates that the term is explained in the Glossary.

EXPLANATION OF NORMAL SPLITTING SEQUENCE OF S$_2$

1.   Draw a separate ventricular pressure curve and aortic pressure curve.

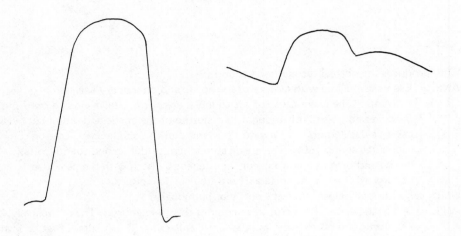

2.   Superimpose the aortic pressure curve on the ventricular pressure curve.

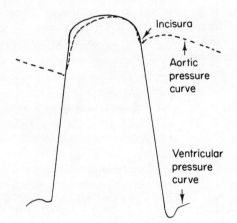

Note that when the LV pressure rise exceeds aortic pressure, the aortic valve will open and produce a single chamber effect or an "aortoventricle." The point at which ejection is finished and the aortic and LV pressure curves separate is called the incisura and is simultaneous with the aortic second sound, or A$_2$.

3. At what pressure in the left ventricle (LV) would you expect the aortic valve to open, assuming a normal blood pressure of 120/80 mm Hg?

    ANS.:   When pressure in the LV rises to just above aortic diastolic pressure, i.e., at about 80 mm Hg the aortic valve will open.

4. After the aortic valve opens, what is the difference in pressure between the LV and the aorta?

    ANS.:   Almost none. The LV and aorta are in reality almost a single pressure chamber as soon as the aortic valve opens. (It may be called an "aortoventricle" at this time.) Only in the presence of aortic stenosis (AS) is there a significant pressure difference (**gradient**) between the aorta and the ventricle.

    Note: In actual fact, there is a slight positive gradient between the LV and aorta during the first two-thirds to three-quarters of systole. This can only be accurately measured by special electromanometer type of catheters. It has been called an impulse gradient.

5. What do we call the notch on the aortic pressure tracing that occurs roughly at time of aortic valve closure? How does it relate to the heart sounds?

    ANS.:   In the external carotid tracing taken by putting a pressure-sensitive pickup on the neck, it is called the *dicrotic notch*. In aortic pressure tracings, it is called the *incisura*. The incisura is simultaneous with the A_2 if aortic root pressure tracings are used for timing. (See figure on p. 155.)

6. At what pressure does the A_2 occur, i.e., does it occur at aortic systolic, diastolic, or some intermediate pressure?

    ANS.:   The aortic valve closes when the force of ventricular ejection decreases, and the peripheral resistance plus the elastic recoil of the expanded aorta overcomes the decreasing pressure in the LV. This occurs at just below aortic systolic pressure, or about a fourth of the way down between aortic systolic and diastolic pressure; e.g., if the systolic pressure in the aorta is 120 mm Hg, the A_2 probably occurs at a pressure of about 110 mm Hg. (See figure on p. 149.)

    Note: The pulmonary artery pressure tracing also has a dicrotic notch or incisura where the P_2 occurs. The normal pulmonary artery pressure is about 25/10 mm Hg.

*7. How does actual aortic valve closure relate in time to the incisura and the A_2?

    ANS.:   The actual closure of the aortic and pulmonary valves has been shown to occur slightly before their respective incisuras and sounds. This is because forward flow (due to inertia of the ejected blood) is still continuing even after LV pressure has dropped below aortic pressure and the valve has closed. In one study, forward flow even continued for a short time after the onset of the sound [43].

    Note: The duration of forward flow after aortic pressure exceeds LV pressure is controlled by the impedance of the system of blood flow and the vessels into which flow is occurring. That is, it comprises the forces that tend to resist forward flow, namely, the size of the vascular bed (capacitance), resistance of the vascular bed, the compliance or distensibility of the vascular bed into which the blood is ejected, and the inertia of the mass of blood flowing into the vascular bed. Thus, if impedance is low, forward flow will continue for a long time after the pressure crossover point, and the A_2 or P_2 will occur very late [53].

8.   If the aortic valve closes at a pressure of about 100 mm Hg, and the pulmonary valve closes at about 20 mm Hg, why should the aortic closure occur first?

ANS.:   There are several possible explanations.

a) The conduction system of the heart feeds the LV before the right ventricle (RV). Therefore, contraction begins slightly earlier in the LV than in the RV.

b) The sounds are simultaneous in time with the incisura of the pulmonary artery and aorta. The timing of the incisura in turn has been shown to be related to the impedance to flow; e.g., the less the arteriolar resistance and elastic recoil and the greater the capacity of the pulmonary arteries, the longer will forward flow occur, and the later the incisura will occur on the pressure curve of the pulmonary artery or aorta [55]. The pulmonary vascular resistance is a tenth that of the systemic resistance. The elastic recoil of the normal pulmonary artery is probably less than that of the aorta, and capacitance of the pulmonary vascular bed is greater than that of the aorta. Therefore, the forward flow continues longer in the pulmonary circuit than in the aortic circuit after their respective pressure crossovers and valve closures have occurred. This would cause the pulmonary pressure and closure sound (P_2) to occur later than the aortic incisura and A_2 [54].

Note: In truncus arteriosus, the single valve should theoretically be incapable of causing a split S_2. However, when the cusps are abnormal, or exceed three in number, the S_2 is likely to be split and may even increase in width on inspiration. The cause of this split is unknown. It seems to be the "true reduplicated second sound" that all split sounds were called before they were recognized as coming from aortic and pulmonary valves separately. It may be double movement of the valves due to a different impedance of the pulmonary and aortic circuit. Split P_2s have been recorded in some normal subjects; the cause of this is also unknown.

PHYSIOLOGY OF THE NORMALLY MOVING SPLIT

1.   Does the normal split of S_2 widen on inspiration or expiration?

ANS.:   It widens on inspiration, so that the A_2P_2 becomes A_2—P_2.

2.   Does the split movement of the S_2 occur due to the movement of the A_2 or to movement of the P_2?

ANS.:   Both. The P_2 moves out, away from the A_2, and the A_2 moves inward, away from the P_2.

3.   Which component moves more, the A_2 or the P_2?

ANS.:   The P_2. In all age groups, but especially over age 40, there are normal subjects in whom the A_2 does not move at all [25]. When it does move, it can contribute up to 30% of the total movement [25].

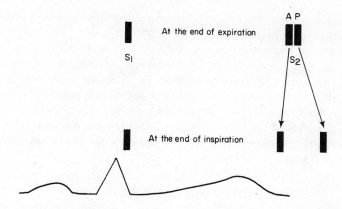

The P_2 outward movement contributes more to the inspiratory widening of the S_2 than does the inward movement of the A_2.

4.   Why does the P_2 come later with inspiration?

ANS.:   There are at least two explanations:

a) The RV becomes larger with inspiration [54]. This is because inspiration lowers intrathoracic pressure, i.e., makes it more negative, and this acts to draw more blood from the superior and inferior vena cava into the right side of the heart. The lungs act like a bellows; i.e., when they expand, they act like a suction apparatus, which sucks blood in from the inferior and superior vena cava into the right atrium and ventricle. This increased RV volume on inspiration delays pulmonary closure because when a ventricle increases its volume and has only one outlet for systole, it takes longer to eject that extra volume.

b) On inspiration, the pulmonary impedance falls [54]. (See p. 177 for explanation.) This causes a delay in pulmonary valve closure.

5.   Why does the A_2 come earlier with inspiration?

ANS.:   Because the LV becomes smaller with inspiration [53]. This is because inspiration, by enlarging the chest volume, also enlarges the volume capacity of the lungs so much that they cannot draw as much blood from the RV as they could contain. In other words, the lungs do not fill from the RV in proportion to their increase in blood space potential during inspiration. This excessive increase in lung capacity withholds some blood from the LV.

Note: There is another explanation given to account for the A_2 movement with respiration. The increased blood that comes into the RV on inspiration crosses over to the LV by the time expiration occurs. This enlarges the LV and delays the A_2 on expiration. By the time the next inspiration occurs, this extra blood has been ejected, and now only a small amount of blood reaches the LV, and the A_2 moves away from the P_2. That this is not the only reason for the movement of A_2 is shown by the fact that even after apnea, inspiration results in a decreased LV stroke volume [46].

*6.   At exactly what point of inspiration or expiration does the maximum widening and narrowing of the split A_2–P_2 occur?

ANS.:   a) Maximum widening occurs at the peak of inspiration.

b) Maximum narrowing occurs almost equally between mid- and end-expiration [39].

7.   Does the normally moving split phenomenon, i.e., widening on inspiration and narrowing on expiration, refer to held expiration and inspiration, or to moving respiration?

ANS.:   It refers to moving and quiet respiration.

Note: Held expiration results in a steady state in which the split remains fixed somewhere between the width on inspiration and expiration, with the A_2 coming first, as usual.

LOUDNESS OF COMPONENTS OF S_2

The Psychology and Physics of Loudness

1.   What is the difference between intensity, loudness, and amplitude of a sound or murmur?

ANS.:   Intensity refers to the energy of the sound, whereas loudness refers to the subjective sensation produced by that energy on the ear. Amplitude refers to the size of the waves or movement produced by the sound energy. On a phonocardiogram, amplitude refers to the height of the sound or murmur.

2.   Is the greatest amplitude or loudness of the components of S_2 in the low-, medium-, or high-**frequency** range?

ANS.:   In the low- and medium-frequency range.

3.   Since the bell is best for bringing out low and medium frequencies, why is it usually better to listen to the splitting of S_2 with the diaphragm?

ANS.:   The diaphragm separates the two components of the split better. Soft, high-frequency components are masked by louder and longer low and medium frequencies unless they are markedly separated in pitch or in width. Since the diaphragm damps out the louder low and medium frequencies, one sacrifices volume for clarity. Therefore, if one of the components of S_2 is very soft, the bell may actually bring it out better.

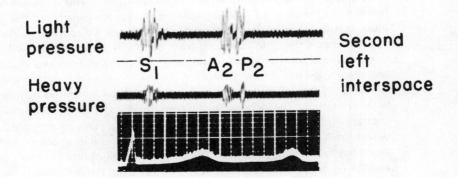

Light pressure

Heavy pressure

S_1 A_2 P_2

Second left interspace

With light pressure, the low- and medium-frequencies dominate and cause the split sounds (about 50 msec [0.05 sec] apart) to run together. Heavy pressure, by turning the skin into a diaphragm, attenuates the reverberations of the low and medium frequencies and helps to separate the components of the split.

Sites of A_2 and P_2 Loudness

1. What was originally meant by the expression "A_2 is louder than P_2?"
    ANS.:   The A referred to the "aortic area" (second right interspace), and the P meant "pulmonary area" (second left interspace). It meant that the entire S_2 in the second right interspace is louder than the entire S_2 in the second left interspace.
2. What is wrong with using the expression "A_2 is louder than P_2," or vice versa?
    ANS.:   Now that the A_2 and P_2 mean the aortic and pulmonary components of the S_2, an altogether different meaning would be implied. These expressions are now used only by physicians who are not in the habit of differentiating the components of the S_2.

    If you consider the S_2 as a single entity (whether split or not), it may normally be louder, in both children and adults, in *either* the second left or right interspace [64]. This means that the expression "A_2 is louder than P_2" (meaning the total S_2 in the second right versus the second left interspace) can have no clinical significance.
3. Which *component* of the S_2 is best heard in normal subjects at the second left interspace (formerly called the "pulmonary area")? What is the clinical significance of this?
    ANS.:   Not only is the A_2 louder than the P_2 in the second left interspace in 70% of normal subjects in all age groups but also, in subjects over age 20, *the A_2 is always normally louder than the P_2 in the second left interspace* [47]. Even with severe pulmonary hypertension, as in **Eisenmenger reactions**, the A_2 is often louder than the P_2 in the second left interspace. This, and the fact that the P_2 is often best heard in the third or fourth left interspace, rules out the second left interspace as truly a "pulmonary area." Since this term is misleading, we encourage the use of *second left interspace* instead.

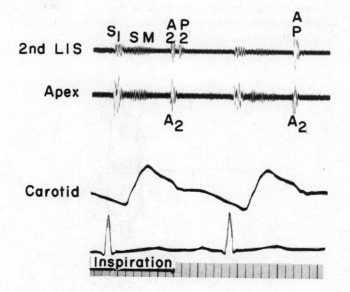

This simultaneous carotid pulse tracing and phonocardiogram is from a normal 16-year-old with a normal split of S_2 on inspiration. Note that (1) only the A_2 would be audible at the apex, and (2) the A_2 has a greater amplitude than the P_2 at the second left interspace (2nd LIS).

4.   Where is the A_2 normally heard on the chest wall?

ANS.:   Anywhere that one would normally listen to heart sounds.

5.   Where is the P_2 normally heard on the chest wall?

ANS.:   In adults, the P_2 is normally heard only a few centimeters to the left of the sternum, as well as over the sternum. In infants and young children, or in the young adult with a thin chest wall and a narrow anteroposterior chest diameter, it may also be heard at the apex.

Note: This implies that if the P_2 is also heard to the right of the sternum or at the apex in a thick-chested adult, the P_2 is probably louder than normal. When the P_2 is louder than the A_2 in the second left interspace, it is almost always also heard at the apex. When the P_2 is unexpectedly heard at the apex, you will usually find that the RV is enlarged, and the apex beat is not due to the LV but entirely to the RV. Thus, in **atrial septal defects** (ASDs) it is expected that the large RV would make the P_2 audible at the apex, even though there may be no pulmonary hypertension.

6.   Where is the S_2 splitting most often appreciated on the chest wall?

ANS.:   At the second or third left interspaces parasternally.

Note: a) In the obese patient, the split S_2 is often best appreciated at the *first* left interspace [40].

*b) The split second sound may be best heard to the right of the sternum in dextroversion, dextrocardia, congenitally corrected transposition of the great vessels (or uncorrected transposition), and in persistent truncus arteriosus [61].

7.   Where is the aortic component of S_2 usually best heard in normal subjects of all ages?

ANS.:   At the second and third left interspaces. This is probably because the aortic valve is situated behind the sternum, close to this area. This further denies that the second right interspace is truly an "aortic area," as it is usually called in most of the auscultation literature.

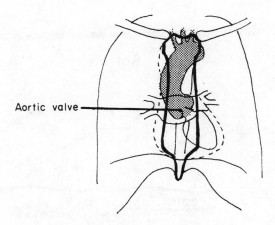

Aortic valve ———

The root of the aorta with its aortic valve is behind the middle of the sternum.

Causes of a Loud A_2 or P_2

1. What tends to make the aortic component louder than normal?

    ANS.:   a) Conditions that raise aortic systolic pressure, e.g., systemic hypertension and **coarctation** of the aorta. These conditions often produce a drumlike quality, or "tambour" S_2.

    b) Conditions that produce a hyperkinetic systemic circulation, e.g., youth, thyrotoxicosis, and aortic regurgitation.

    c) Conditions that place the aorta close to the anterior chest wall, e.g., a thin chest, **transposition of the great vessels** (uncorrected or congenitally corrected), and **tetralogy of Fallot**.

    Note: In tetralogy of Fallot, the S_2 is single and consists entirely of the A_2 because the P_2 is attenuated by

    1) A deformed pulmonary valve when there is valvular stenosis.

    2) The anterior placement of the aorta relative to a posteriorly placed pulmonary artery.

    3) The low pulmonary artery pressure resulting from the diversion of RV blood through the high subaortic **ventricular septal defect** (VSD) directly into the aorta.

2. Besides a thin chest wall, what tends to make the P_2 louder than normal?

    ANS.:   a) Conditions that cause pulmonary hypertension even if the pulmonary flow is normal or low, as in **primary pulmonary hypertension**; or in the pulmonary hypertension secondary to mitral stenosis (MS), pulmonary emboli, or shunts with **Eisenmenger** reactions.

    b) Conditions that produce hyperkinetic pulmonary hypertension, as in ASD or VSD. (See p. 198 for explanation of hyperkinetic pulmonary hypertension.) In VSD with normal or slightly elevated pulmonary artery pressures, the P_2 may be accentuated slightly but it is difficult to detect this because it may still be softer than the A_2 in the second left interspace; and even if it is louder, it is not heard at the apex. This is because the volume overload on the left heart accentuates the A_2 and also enlarges the LV, so that pulmonary events cannot be transmitted well to the apex.

    Note: The increased pulmonary flow due to an ASD does not necessarily make the P_2 louder than the A_2 in the absence of a pulmonary artery pressure of at least 50 mm Hg [36]. If pulmonary stenosis (PS) is present with the ASD, the P_2 will probably be less than 50% of the A_2 on expiration and will usually split to 60 msec or more [35].

*3. Is the absolute loudness of the S_2 a good sign of pulmonary hypertension in MS patients?

    ANS.:   Only if it is loud. A soft S_2 is often present despite severe pulmonary hypertension. A P_2 louder than the A_2 in the second left interspace is also a good sign of pulmonary hypertension, but does not tell you the degree of pulmonary hypertension present.

4.   Why does the A_2 tend to be loud in hyperkinetic states such as thyrotoxicosis or aortic regurgitation (AR)?

ANS.:   The intensity of the A_2 is increased if the aortic valve closes when the aorta is energetically recoiling from the violent stretch due to the increased volume flung into it during systole. This is because the loudness of the A_2 is proportional to the energy involved when the closure of the aortic valves decelerates the forward flow through the valve.

Note: With severe AR the A_2 may be soft, presumably because of the absence of adequate valve substance to cause a sudden deceleration of forward flow.

5.   How does inspiration affect the loudness of each component of the S_2?

ANS.:   The P_2 commonly becomes louder, because extra blood in the pulmonary artery on inspiration raises its pressure slightly. The A_2, on the other hand, becomes softer, because inspiration decreases aortic pressure and also puts the aorta farther from the stethoscope.

Note: All sounds become softer on inspiration if you listen over the upper chest, where excess lung space is interposed between stethoscope and heart on inspiration.

6.   Why does aortic pressure decrease on inspiration?

ANS.:   a) Intrathoracic pressure drops on inspiration, i.e., it becomes more negative. Since the aorta is an intrathoracic organ for much of its course, its pressure will also drop.

b) On inspiration, the lungs withhold some blood from the left ventricle.

Causes of a Softer A_2 or P_2

1.   What can make either the A_2 or the P_2 softer than normal, besides the effect of respiration and abnormal chest shapes and thickness?

ANS.:   a) Conditions that lower systolic pressure, e.g.,
        1) Systemic hypotension will soften the A_2.
        2) Pulmonary stenosis, with its low pulmonary artery pressure, especially if there is a right-to-left shunt through an ASD or VSD, will soften the P_2.
    Note: In tricuspid atresia the P_2 is soft or absent, presumably because the pulmonary circuit is not receiving sufficient volume.

b) Conditions that distort the **semilunar valves**, e.g., calcification or sclerosis or fusion of the cusps, as in AS or PS.

Note: a) In PS, the pulmonary valve is thick and leathery. It is often adherent at its base to the surrounding pulmonary artery. This not only makes the P_2 soft, but also adds to its lateness, because the RV pressure must drop considerably below pulmonary artery pressure before it can move the relatively immobile valve.

*b) A massive pulmonary embolus that touches the pulmonary valve will make the P_2 soft even in the presence of pulmonary hypertension.

*c) Conditions that place the pulmonary artery farther from the stethoscope, e.g., transposition of the great vessels, congenitally corrected or not, will soften the P_2 even in the presence of pulmonary hypertension.

*d) Supravalvular AS can soften the A_2. The reason here is unknown, but fibrous attachments to the aortic valves may partly account for it. In supravalvular PS, the P_2 is either normal or increased in loudness [42].

*2.   If increased pulmonary flow produces a loud P_2, and valvular PS produces a soft P_2, what happens to the P_2 intensity in a patient with both a VSD and PS?

ANS.:   The PS dominates, and the P_2 is usually soft [19].

Note: If only a single S_2 is heard following the murmur of PS, you can tell that a P_2 is actually present without the help of a phonocardiogram by using exercise, leg-raising, or squatting to return more blood to the pulmonary artery, so that its pressure is slightly raised.

*3.   How does an easily heard P_2 in *mild* tetralogy help you to predict the site of the PS?

ANS.:   An easily heard P_2 strongly suggests valvular PS.

Note: If a P_2 is heard in tetralogy, any ejection click present is probably pulmonary and not aortic. A P_2 is only likely to be heard in tetralogy that is mild, i.e., acyanotic.

Relative Loudness, Pitch, and Duration of S_1 and S_2

1.   When is it difficult to distinguish an S_1 from an S_2 by stethoscope alone?

ANS.:   When systole equals diastole in duration. This is called "ticktack" rhythm (like the ticking of a clock) or embryocardia (like the fetal heart sounds in a pregnant woman).

2.   What causes ticktack rhythm?

ANS.:   Anything that prolongs systole relative to diastole, as in severe AR or anything that shortens diastole more than it does systole as in tachycardias. As the heart rate increases, both systole and diastole shorten but diastole is shortened relatively more than systole.

3.   How may the relative loudness of the S_1 and S_2 help to distinguish one from the other?

ANS.:   The S_2 is normally louder than the S_1 at the second right or left interspace, i.e., at the **base of the heart**, possibly because here is where the aortic and pulmonary valve structures are closest to the chest wall. At the apex, the S_1 is usually louder than the S_2.

Note: The apex area is not as reliable as the base for distinguishing an S_1 from an S_2 by loudness, because with a long P–R interval or with myocardial damage, the S_1 may be very soft.

4.   If the S_1 is louder than the S_2 at the bases, what does this suggest?

ANS.:   It suggests that there is an extra-loud S_1 present, as in MS, or that there is an extra-soft S_2, as in AS with a calcified aortic valve.

5.   How can you tell at the bedside which heart sound is the S_2 when relative loudness is of no help?

ANS.:   a) The S_2 is higher pitched and shorter than the S_1. The S_1 is relatively muffled. This is implied in the "lub-dup" often used to mimic the sound of the S_1–S_2.

b) Palpate the carotid while listening with the stethoscope. The S_1 will come just before the carotid impulse. Imagine the carotid as having the same relationship to the S_1 as an early systolic murmur would have; i.e., if we use the letter C to represent the carotid impulse, then the rhythm goes "1-C-2, 1-C-2." This is due to the slight delay between ventricular contraction and the carotid impulse's reaching the neck.

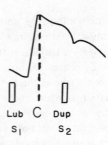

Lub C Dup
S_1 S_2

The tap of the carotid pulse on your fingers is felt *after* and *not with* the first heart sound.

c) Place the stethoscope or finger over the apex beat, and note the outward impulse that occurs during systole. It should bulge outward with or just after the S_1. The stethoscope itself can be seen to rise during systole and will tell you which is the S_1. The S_1 will appear to "produce" the rise in apical impulse.

d) If you can hear inspiratory splitting of one sound at the left sternal border and therefore know which is the S_2 there, then inch toward the apex, keeping the rhythm intact by moving the stethoscope exactly in time with the heart sounds.

NARROW AND WIDE SPLITTING DEFINED

*1.   What do physiologists often call heart sounds in contradistinction to heart murmurs?
        ANS.:   Transients.

*2.   What is the smallest time interval between transients that the ear is capable of distinguishing as two separate sounds?
        ANS.:   20 msec. This narrow interval can only be distinguished as separate sounds if they are very short and high in frequency, as, for example, the sound of a camera shutter or a snare drum. For practical purposes, a split of 20 msec merely sounds like an impure or dirty sound rather than a sharp and clean one. This means that the narrowest split of heart sounds that the ear can clearly separate is about 30 msec.

3.   What is meant by a wide split of S_2?
        ANS.:   There are three ways of defining a wide split.
        a) One that splits widely on inspiration, i.e., to at least 60 msec (0.06 sec), even if it is single on expiration.
        b) A persistent split of S_2 on expiration that widens still more on inspiration.
        c) A split that is slightly wide on held expiration, i.e., at least 40 msec (0.04 sec).
        Note: The concept of wide and narrow splitting is best understood if you practice the vocal imitation of splitting widths as follows: a normal narrow split on inspiration is 30—40 msec (0.03—0.04 sec). Imitate this by rolling the tongue as in a French *dr* or *tr*. A slightly wide split is 50—60 msec (0.05—0.06 sec). Say "pa-da" quickly. A wide split is 70—80 msec (0.07—0.08 sec). Say "pa-ta" quickly. Articulate both the p and the t sharply. A very wide split is 90—100 msec (0.09—0.10 sec). Say "pa-pa" as quickly as possible.

THE WIDELY SPLIT S$_2$

1. What conditions can cause wide splitting of S$_2$ as a result of delay in pulmonary valve closure?

    ANS.:   Delays of P$_2$ are caused by:

    a) Conditions that cause electrical delay of activation of the right ventricle, e.g., right bundle branch block (RBBB).

    b) Conditions that cause an increased volume in the RV in comparison with the LV, e.g., at least a moderately sized ASD or moderate amount of pulmonary regurgitation (PR), either congenital or as a result of pulmonary valve surgery.
    Note: For some unknown reason the S$_2$ in even severe congenital PR may occasionally be narrowly split.

    c) Conditions that cause outflow tract obstruction to the RV, e.g., valvular or infundibular PS.

    d) Conditions that cause either acute dilatation of the RV in response to a sudden rise in pulmonary artery pressure, as in massive pulmonary embolism, or chronic dilatation, such as that occurring in the late stages of chronic pulmonary embolism or primary pulmonary hypertension [14].

    e) Conditions that decrease the elastic recoil and increase the capacitance of the pulmonary artery, e.g., idiopathic dilatation of the pulmonary artery [44, 50].
    Note: The reason for the lack of wide splitting in some patients with idiopathic dilatation of the pulmonary artery is unknown, but may be due to relatively less loss of elastic tissue. The exceptionally broad P$_2$ in some patients with idiopathic dilatation is also unexplained.

    f) Conditions that cause RV failure and so prolong **isovolumic contraction** of the RV, as in severe primary pulmonary hypertension.

    *g) Bilateral pulmonary artery branch stenosis [16, 27].

*2. What has been shown to cause the delay of P$_2$ in patients with ASD or VSD?

    ANS.:   The Q–P$_2$ interval is lengthened because

    a) There is a delay in the onset of RV contraction. The interval from Q to the onset of RV contraction (electromechanical interval) in VSDs may be prolonged by as much as 60 msec above the normal of 40–60 msec. This has not been confirmed in ASDs.
    Note: The electromechanical interval is prolonged with increasing age and is relatively independent of heart rate. It is almost not measurable under age 1 year and is less than 5 msec by age 4. It reaches about 30 msec by age 14.

    b) The preejection period in ASDs is prolonged [63].

    c) The ejection period of the RV is prolonged; i.e., the time during which the pulmonary valve is opened is prolonged [63]. This means that the impedance of the pulmonary circuit is probably decreased. (See p. 198 for explanation of impedance.)

Note: a) In uncomplicated ASDs, the interval from Q to the end of total ventricular systole (to the bottom of the ventricular pressure curves) is the same in both ventricles [33]. However, the Q to the pulmonary incisura is longer than the Q to the aortic incisura, and the P_2 is as far from the A_2 as their respective incisuras. Therefore, in ASDs, the P_2 comes late because the incisura comes late. The cause of the late incisura is thought to be low impedance of the pulmonary vascular bed. The dilatation of the main pulmonary artery (increased capacitance) and the lower pulmonary resistance generally found in patients with ASDs both decrease impedance. Also the high velocity of flow into the pulmonary artery is more difficult to halt. In over 75% of postoperative ASD patients, the wide splitting of the S_2 persists. This suggests that the theory implicating a dilated pulmonary artery in causing delay of the incisura might be correct, since the pulmonary artery remains dilated after corrective surgery.

  b) If a VSD shunts into the right atrium, the S_2 split is often not wide. The reason is unknown.

  c) There is no significant relationship between the width of the split in ASD patients and the size of the shunt [11].

3. Will a RBBB pattern, i.e., an S in lead I, and an R' in V1, with *no prolongation* of the QRS, cause a wide split of S_2?

  ANS.: No. There must be terminal delay or slowing of conduction, as in incomplete or complete RBBB, in order to produce a widely split S_2.

4. When can a wide split occur due to early closure of A_2?

  ANS.: a) In **tamponade** the early occurrence of A_2 is due to a markedly disproportionate decrease in the size of the LV in comparison with the RV on inspiration [23]. (The $Q-P_2$ does not change with inspiration in tamponade. The $Q-A_2$, on the other hand, shortens, due to a marked decrease in LV volume.)

  *b) In the presence of a left atrial tumor, usually a myxoma, due to underfilling of the LV [30].

  *c) In severe mitral regurgitation (MR). There is evidence that LV events may start earlier than usual in moderately severe to severe MR, i.e., the interval from Q to the onset of LV contraction is shortened [9]. This shifts all left ventricular events "to the left." Mild MR does not cause a widely split S_2.

  Note: a) It has been assumed in the past that the widely split S_2 in severe MR is due to an early A_2 secondary to shortening of the ejection time because of the presence of two outlets for systole. This is unreasonable because

    1) There may be two outlets, but there is also more volume to be ejected.

    2) The S_2 is not widely split in mild to moderate MR.

    3) Left ventricular ejection times are normal in MR unless the output is decreased at rest.

  b) It is important to know that MR can produce a widely split S_2 because

    1) A wide split not only tells you that the MR is at least moderately severe but also tells you that you must not assume that a widely split S_2 with MR is due to an A_2—opening snap. (How to tell the difference between an A_2-P_2 and an A_2—opening snap is discussed on pp. 215–218.)

    2) The rare silent MR may only be suspected by hearing an unexplained widely split S_2.

5. In tamponade, why does the LV decrease in size so markedly in comparison with the RV during inspiration?

ANS.:   The increase in RV volume during inspiration stretches the entire pericardium. This also restricts the expansion of the left atrium, so that it cannot stretch with the blood it receives from the pulmonary veins. During inspiration, the left atrial pressure may actually be higher than the pulmonary venous pressure, and blood may flow backward into the pulmonary veins, so that less blood than normal reaches the LV. This results in a wide split on inspiration.

Note: a) The extra-wide split during inspiration is manifested only for a few beats during the beginning of inspiration [5].

*b) You can prove by phonocardiogram that the RV cannot accommodate the extra volume brought to it by inspiration, as in constrictive pericarditis, by measuring the distance from S_1 to P_2 in both inspiration and expiration. If it is not longer on inspiration, the RV has not been able to accommodate the extra volume.

*6. What is the *widest* normal split in (a) held expiration and (b) the expiratory phase of normal respiration?

ANS.:   a) On held expiration, the widest normal split is about 40 msec. Roll the tongue as in the French *tr* to imitate this.

b) Normal expiration may end with a split that is 40-msec wide, but this is very rare, especially in a normal subject over age 20.

Note: At all ages, from 1 to 80, normal expiration produces a single S_2 in over 85% of subjects. Over age 50, the S_2 closes in expiration in 95% of normal subjects in the recumbent position [2]. The greatest difference in the split of the S_2 between inspiration and expiration in normal subjects on quiet respiration is about 50 msec. In some normal children, exceptionally wide splitting is found (80 msec on inspiration). The reason is unknown [18].

*7. What should happen to the width of the split of S_2 when both ventricles are volume-overloaded by a rupture of a sinus of Valsalva into the right atrium or RV?

ANS.:   This produces a volume overload of both ventricles and a volume overload to both ventricles widens the split S_2, no matter what the cause.

THE A_2–P_2 IN PULMONARY STENOSIS

1. Why will a stenotic RV outflow tract or valve cause a delay of RV emptying?

ANS.:   a) In PS, RV pressure is much higher than pulmonary artery pressure. Thus, it takes an extra-long time for the RV pressure to drop down to the closing pressure of the pulmonary artery valve. (See figure on p. 263.)

b) The outflow tract may undergo secondary hypertrophy and contract late, producing a kind of "wringing-out" action that prolongs total ventricular systole; i.e., the inflow tract or main body of the RV contracts first and is followed by contraction of the **infundibulum**, or RV outflow tract. The greater the infundibular stenosis, the greater the delay between inflow and outflow tract contraction.

*2. Is there less delay in RV emptying in valvular or supravalvular PS?

ANS.: In supravalvular PS, there is usually less delay, because there is a high pressure between the valve and the supravalvular obstruction. In supravalvular PS or in unilateral pulmonary artery stenosis, the A_2-P_2 split is usually normal or narrow [16, 42].

Note: In bilateral pulmonary artery branch stenosis the split S_2 is wide [14]. This has been attributed to the very low incisura found in these patients. The very low incisura is unexplained.

*3. Does the PS seen in severe tetralogy of Fallot produce a wide split of S_2?

ANS.: The majority of cardiologists who have recorded the split have found a markedly delayed P_2 (80–120 msec from the A_2). In actual practice, the P_2 is rarely audible in severe tetralogy of Fallot. Intracardiac phonocardiography with the microphone in the pulmonary artery, however, has shown the delayed P_2 [19]. Also, after shunt operations that increase pulmonary flow, it has been seen to be very delayed.

Note: About a third of cyanotic adults with tetralogy have an audible P_2. The reason is unknown [26].

*4. What kind of sounds can obscure the awareness of a widely split S_2, as in PS?

ANS.: A long systolic murmur that continues into or through the A_2 along the left sternal border. This occurs with the murmur of VSD or with severe PS.

Note: You can easily tell if the murmur is obscuring an A_2 by

a) Exploring the split S_2 away from the maximal murmur area.

b) By comparing simultaneous phonocardiograms at the apex, where the aortic component will be seen (because it is far from where the murmur is maximum in VSD and PS), and at the left sternal border, where only the P_2 may be seen.

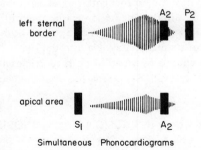

Simultaneous Phonocardiograms

At the apex, the easily recorded A_2 may be heard despite the murmur, which is much softer in that area.

5. How can the A_2-P_2 interval tell you the probable RV pressure in PS?

ANS.: In general, the more severe the obstruction and the higher the RV pressure, the longer the A_2-P_2 interval.

Note: Thus, for RV pressures of less than 80 mm Hg, the A_2-P_2 intervals have been found to vary among different subjects from 55–95 msec. For RV pressures from 80–120 mm Hg, the A_2-P_2 range was found to be 50–125 msec. For RV pressures over 120 mm Hg, the range was 85–175 msec [22].

Correcting for the R—R interval might narrow the ranges slightly, because there is some tendency for A_2—P_2 intervals to be narrower with faster heart rates; i.e., asynchrony in the normal heart is reduced with less blood in the heart, as with sitting or standing, or in atrial fibrillation after shorter R—R intervals. If you do not have a calculator or a slide rule to give you the square roots for correction, you can use the following rough method of calculating the right ventricular pressure:

If the A_2—P_2 interval is 40 msec or less, the RV pressure ranges from normal to about 45 mm Hg. If the A_2—P_2 is 50 msec, the RV pressure has a wide range of from normal to about 55 mm Hg. If the A_2—P_2 is 60 msec, the right ventricular pressure is no longer likely to be normal, but ranges from about 45 mm Hg to about 80 mm Hg. If the A_2—P_2 is 80 msec, the range of RV pressure is from 60 to about 120 mm Hg. If the A_2—P_2 is 100 msec, the range is from 70 to 160 mm Hg.

*6.   What is meant by the contractile type of infundibular obstruction? How does this affect the A_2—P_2 interval?

ANS.:   If the infundibulum is hypertrophied (usually secondary to valvular PS), contraction of the infundibulum may occur later than that of the body of the RV. This prolongs contraction of the total RV. Thus, it takes longer for RV pressure to drop below pulmonary artery pressure, delaying closure of the pulmonary valve.

The A_2—P_2 interval in the contractile form of infundibular obstruction is always 100 ± 2 msec on expiration, whether the stenosis is mild or severe. Therefore, a wide A_2—P_2 interval could be present in a contractile form of infundibular stenosis with only a moderate gradient.

*7.   When is the wide split of S_2 in PS relatively fixed?

ANS.:   a) With mild PS and marked dilatation of the pulmonary artery [55].

b) With severe PS and marked right ventricular hypertrophy (RVH) [55].

THE FIXED SPLIT OF S_2

1.   What is meant by a fixed or relatively fixed split of S_2?

ANS.:   If it changes less than 20 msec (0.02 sec) with respiration, it is called a fixed or relatively fixed split.

2.   What can cause a fixed or relatively fixed split of S_2?

ANS.:   a) Heart failure, because

1) It does not permit much of a change in the volume of the ventricles with respiration because breathing with congested lungs is shallow.

2) It prevents the ventricles from responding to changes of volume and pressure [41]. The heart in failure is relatively insensitive to changes in filling pressure; e.g., a rise in LV end-diastolic pressure of a few millimeters of mercury in the normal ventricle can almost double cardiac output. In the failing ventricle, the output rises only slightly or not at all.

b) ASDs.

c) VSDs. In uncomplicated moderate to large VSDs, inspiration can probably elevate RV pressure and so decrease the shunt from left to right and not allow the LV to become smaller on inspiration [7]. An obviously moving split on the phonocardiogram of a patient with a VSD usually implies a small shunt (less than 2:1 pulmonary/systemic flow ratios) and a pulmonary artery systolic pressure of less than 50 mm Hg [28].

d) Pulmonary stenosis in some patients.

*e) Pulmonary embolism. In massive pulmonary embolism or with the late sequelae of chronic pulmonary embolism, when the pulmonary artery pressure is at least two-thirds of systemic pressure [15].

f) Idiopathic dilatation of the pulmonary artery. In 6 of 8 patients with idiopathic dilatation of the pulmonary artery in one series, the split was relatively fixed [29].

Note: A relatively fixed split is a variation of normal children and young men, especially in the supine position [37]. The reason is unknown. If the split is fixed with the patient supine, it will not be fixed in the sitting position, and vice versa [37].

3. Does complete RBBB produce a fixed split?
   ANS.:   No [51].

The Fixed Split of S_2 in ASD

1. Why is the S_2 splitting in ASD relatively fixed?
   ANS.:   In ASD the LV does not become smaller on inspiration and may even become larger. This is because on inspiration caval blood is drawn into the right atrium, where pressure then rises. The left-to-right shunt through the ASD is therefore decreased by the increased pressure in the right atrium. This nonshunted left atrial blood passes instead through the mitral valve into the LV and thus tends to keep LV volume constant during inspiration [6].

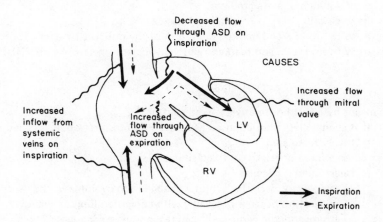

The increased inflow into the right atrium on inspiration (vertical solid arrows) causes a decreased flow through the ASD and thus increased flow through the mitral valve.

Note: a) If the left-to-right shunt is *markedly* decreased on inspiration due to a poorly compliant RV, the LV volume may even *increase* with the large inflow of blood from the left atrium during inspiration.

*b) There is physiological proof that the shunt from the left to right atrium in ASD is decreased by inspiration. Oxygen saturation in the pulmonary artery has been shown to be less during inspiration in subjects with ASD [4]. It has been found that a 50% decrease in left-to-right shunt can occur with inspiration.

*2.   Does the P_2 move normally with respiration in the presence of an ASD?

ANS.:   On quiet respiration, it moves less than normally or not at all. The $Q-P_2$ interval moves less than 20 msec in ASDs on quiet inspiration [4]. (In normal subjects the $Q-P_2$ will almost always be lengthened by at least 20 msec and in most cases, by about 40 msec.) With deep inspiration, however, the P_2 in ASDs can move almost normally, as shown by the following evidence that deep inspiration can increase the flow into the RV:

a) A tricuspid diastolic flow murmur due to torrential flow through the valve is often heard only on deep inspiration.

b) The P_2 may become louder on deep inspiration both on external and intracardiac phonocardiograms [20].

*3.   How does the A_2 move in ASDs?

ANS.:   Either not at all or slightly toward the P_2 on inspiration.

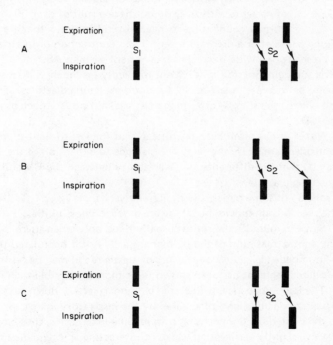

If, as in A, the A_2 moves forward on inspiration exactly the same amount as the P_2, the split will be absolutely fixed on respiration. This is uncommon. Usually, even when the A_2 moves forward with inspiration, it does not move as much as does the P_2 as in B and C.

*4.   When can the split of the S_2 in ASDs be narrow rather than wide?

ANS.:   a) In some subjects with an ASD, the split S_2 may be narrow for unknown reasons. It is unrelated to the size of the shunt. It should be noted, however, that a narrow split on inspiration that remains split on expiration, especially in the sitting position, is an excellent sign of a relatively fixed split, because if a split is narrow on inspiration, it should *close* on expiration. A narrow split that is not fixed should close in the sitting position.

b) Tachycardias will also narrow the splitting in ASDs and make it especially indicative of fixed splitting if you note that the split remains open on expiration in the sitting position [11].

Note: a) The faster heart rates in children may be the reason why A_2–P_2 intervals tend to be narrower in younger subjects. In infants with ASDs and congestive failure, however, wide splitting is the rule [11].

b) It is not surprising that in ASD patients, even a narrow split of S_2 remains open in the sitting position, since it has been shown that in uncomplicated left-to-right ASD shunts, the shunt flow increases in the upright position [10].

c) In ASD patients, there is often more variation of the split S_2 with respiration in the sitting than in the supine position, and the longer the subject sits, the more variation there may be.

d) Even though ASDs are noted for causing wide splitting of S_2, the majority of patients with ASD do not have a split of over 60 msec [19]; some normal young subjects have inspiratory splits that are wider than this.

*5.   How can a long pause after a premature ventricular contraction or in atrial fibrillation suggest the presence of a wide fixed split in a patient with an ASD?

ANS.:   After a long pause, the split widens markedly (as much as 40 msec). This may be due to an increase in left-to-right shunt during long diastoles. The normal heart also widens the split S_2 after long diastoles, but not so much as in the presence of an ASD.

Note: It has often been postulated that the left-to-right shunt in diastole is controlled largely by the relative resistance to expansion of the RV and LV. It may be that the difference in distensibility between the RV and LV is exaggerated by a long diastole.

*6.   Why is the split S_2 of some patients with PS relatively fixed?

ANS.:   The reason is unknown, but there are at least 3 possibilities:

a) Since in mild PS, the split is usually fixed only when there is marked poststenotic dilatation of the pulmonary artery, it is postulated that the decrease in impedance caused by the loss of elastic recoil may be responsible. The dilated segment has been shown to be more distensible than normal [44]. The low impedance of the large pulmonary artery during expiration may be paradoxically slightly increased by the inspiratory increase of ejection into the dilated portion, causing it to recoil a little faster, thus closing the pulmonary valve slightly earlier than usual, counteracting any tendency to a later P_2 on inspiration.

b) The markedly hypertrophied RV often has much fibrosis and may not be able to respond as well as a more normal RV to the increased volume brought to it by inspiration.

c) Shortening of RV isovolumic contraction time as a result of the more powerful right atrial contraction that occurs during inspiration may also contribute to the poor movement of P_2.

Note: If an ASD is diagnosed, suspect a combination of an ASD and PS when the split on expiration is 60 msec or more, and the P_2/A_2 loudness ratio is less than one-half at the left sternal border in a high-frequency phonocardiogram.

DIFFERENTIAL DIAGNOSIS OF THE WIDE FIXED SPLIT

1. What may mimic a wide fixed split of S_2?
   ANS.: a) A paradoxical split in complete left bundle branch block (LBBB), especially with some heart failure. (The paradoxical split is explained on p. 200.)
   b) The A_2 followed by an opening snap. (The six ways of distinguishing an A_2–P_2 from an A_2–opening snap are detailed on pp. 215–218.)
   c) A very wide split in which normal movements of the A_2–P_2 are difficult to perceive by auscultation. It is much easier to perceive movement of two sounds when they are close together than when they are very far apart. The answer to this dilemma is to make the two sounds approach one another by bringing less blood back to the heart, as with sitting or standing.

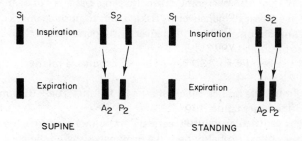

It would be difficult to perceive movement of the split in the supine position shown in the S_2 on the left, and you might call it a relatively fixed split until the patient sits or stands up.

2. Why does the split S_2 in the normal subject tend to narrow on sitting or standing?
   ANS.: This is because when both ventricles receive less blood (due to pooling in the abdomen and the legs) the RV responds by ejecting its blood relatively faster than does the LV [38].

3. How can sitting a patient up help to distinguish the supine expiratory splitting of S_2 in a normal young patient from the relatively fixed split of a patient with an ASD?
   ANS.: The normal patient will usually have increased respiratory variation on sitting, and the split will close on expiration [2, 12, 37]. The sitting ASD patient will maintain the split on expiration, even though respiratory variation may increase in this position also.
   *Note: To complicate matters, however, about 15% of normal children do not have more respiratory variation in the sitting than the supine position. They may have splits that appear to be fixed in the sitting but not in the supine position [12].

*4. What happens to the splitting of S_2 after a Valsalva maneuver during the period immediately following and then a few seconds following release? How can you use this maneuver to detect the presence of an ASD?
   ANS.: Immediately on release, the split widens by over 20 msec [4]. This is because the Valsalva maneuver dams up venous blood behind the RV, causing a high venous pressure. On release of this blood, the RV has extra filling for a few beats, in contrast to the LV, which actually contains less blood for a few beats because the lungs had been partially emptied.

A few seconds after the release of the Valsalva, the split S_2 becomes very narrow or single. This is due to the dammed-up blood now reaching the LV after a few beats, by which time the RV is receiving only a normal amount of blood. This puts a comparatively greater volume into the LV than into the RV for a few beats, thus narrowing the split.

In ASDs, however, the atria act almost as a single chamber, so that any rise in right atrial pressure is reflected also in a rise in left atrial pressure. Thus, on release of the Valsalva, any increased venous blood that rushes into the RV will also cause more blood to enter the LV, and there will be only slight immediate widening (not over 20 msec) and no delayed narrowing of the S_2 [4].

After surgery on an ASD, the wide relatively fixed split may persist for at least a year. The post-Valsalva effect will, however, indicate the true situation [62].

Note: You can overcome difficulties in a patient's understanding of how to perform a Valsalva maneuver by asking him to push against your hand pressed against his abdomen. He will inadvertently perform a Valsalva maneuver in the process of doing this [24].

5.   What abnormalities besides an ASD can not only produce a relatively fixed split of S_2 but also a *wide* split?

ANS.:   a) Right bundle branch block plus heart failure. The RBBB makes the split wide, and the heart failure fixes it.

b) **Right ventricular failure** secondary to pulmonary hypertension. The wideness of the split is probably due to a prolonged isovolumic contraction time in the failing RV.

*c) Some moderately large VSDs. The widening here is partly due to a delayed P_2 [7].

*d) Partial anomalous pulmonary venous drainage into the right atrium.

Note: Although this anomaly can cause all the same physical, ECG, and x-ray signs as an ASD, the effect of respiration on the split of S_2 can often enable you to distinguish the two lesions. If the splitting is normal, the differentiation is easy [21]. Some subjects with partial anomalous pulmonary venous drainage, however, have relatively fixed splits due to a prolongation of P_2 on *expiration*. A phonocardiogram showing a prolongation of the $Q–P_2$ interval on expiration can help the differentiation. This should be done during a prolonged expiration, to allow maximum filling of the right atrium via the anomalous pathway [31].

*6.   How can you distinguish the wide, fixed split and loud P_2 of right ventricular failure from that of ASD with pulmonary hypertension?

ANS.:   a) Exercise will widen the split still further only in RV failure, because it delays the P_2. This is probably because the rise in pulmonary artery pressure with exercise will increase the isovolumic contraction time of the failing RV and leave the isovolumic contraction of the normal LV relatively unchanged or even shorter.

b) Phonocardiograms at rest can show that in RV failure, inspiration causes the $Q–P_2$ either to remain the same or to be prolonged, without any change in the $Q–A_2$. In ASDs, a deep inspiration will cause not only the $Q–P_2$ to be prolonged but also the $Q–A_2$. A phonocardiogram showing a split S_2 with prolongation of the $Q–A_2$ on inspiration is diagnostic of an ASD even when there is severe pulmonary hypertension, as in an Eisenmenger reaction.

THE NARROWLY SPLIT S$_2$

1. List the causes of a narrowly split S$_2$.
   ANS.:   a) Conditions that increase the volume of the LV, but without an extra outlet
      (a VSD or MR is an extra outlet), i.e., **patent ductus arteriosus** (PDA) and AR.
   b) Conditions that cause electrical delay of LV conduction: LBBB and some
      types of **Wolff-Parkinson-White** (W-P-W) **preexcitation** that imitate LBBB by
      causing premature depolarization of the RV.
   c) Conditions that selectively prolong isovolumic contraction time of the LV,
      such as coronary disease.
   d) The aging process. As a person grows older, the isovolumic contraction time
      of the LV becomes slightly longer [56]. There is also some suggestion that the
      P$_2$ comes slightly earlier; i.e., the Q–P$_2$ interval shortens [52].
   e) Conditions that increase impedance of the pulmonary vasculature, i.e., pulmo-
      nary hypertension. (In late stages the split widens probably due to RV failure.)
   *f) Shortening of RV systole due to underfilling of the RV secondary to a right
      atrial tumor, usually an **atrial myxoma** [30].
   g) Conditions that cause a significant gradient across the outflow of the LV (i.e.,
      AS), so that there is a delay in LV pressure's dropping below aortic pressure.
   Note: *a) The delay in A$_2$ in AS is not due to prolonged LV contraction. From
      the Q wave to the end of LV systole, i.e., from the Q to the beginning
      of the fall in LV pressure (end of LV systole) on a LV pressure curve,
      is *shorter* than from Q to the end of RV systole in all degrees of AS [32].
   b) A gradient of about 70 is considered by most centers to require surgery
      if any of the AS symptoms triad, namely, dyspnea, angina, or syncope,
      are present to a significant degree. If there is heart failure or myocardial
      damage, a gradient of 50 is generally considered significant enough to
      require surgery.
   *c) Marked poststenotic dilatation may further delay A$_2$ by decreasing the
      impedance beyond the valve [44].

2. Why do patients with an uncomplicated **PDA** have an increased LV volume load without a
   similar increase in RV volume load?
   ANS.:   See glossary description of PDA.

*3. Why is the split S$_2$ often narrow and occasionally even reversed in systemic hypertension?
   ANS.:   a) Myocardial damage superimposed on systemic hypertension can lengthen the
      Q–A$_2$, probably by selectively prolonging LV isovolumic contraction time.
   b) Hypertension can prolong the Q–A$_2$ more than the Q–P$_2$, probably by selec-
      tively delaying the *onset* of LV contraction (electromechanical interval).
      Hypertension may also slightly prolong ejection time.
   c) Many hypertensive persons are in the older age groups. In these groups, aging
      not only further prolongs LV ejection time, thus delaying the A$_2$, but also
      causes a shortening of the Q–P$_2$ interval, thus bringing the P$_2$ earlier. The A$_2$
      in the elderly often does not move at all.

4. In about what percentage of normal subjects is S$_2$ single on quiet inspiration (a) under age
   50 and (b) over age 50?
   ANS.:   S$_2$ is single
   a) In about 30% of subjects under age 50.
   b) In about 60% of subjects over age 50 [2].

5.   What causes a split second sound to appear to be single on auscultation besides being too narrow, i.e., less than 30 msec (0.03 sec)?

ANS.:   a) Too deep an inspiration may interpose too much lung between the stethoscope and heart, causing one of the S_2 components (usually the P_2) to disappear.

b) The first component of the split may be so loud that it masks a soft component following it. This is known as *forward masking*.

*c) If a split with a soft P_2 is followed by a loud, high-pitched opening snap, the P_2 may not be heard. This is known as *backward masking*.

6.   How can you tell that an S_2 is split on inspiration even if you do not hear two distinct components?

ANS.:   If the S_2 is clean and sharp on expiration and becomes impure or wide and rough on inspiration, then it probably has opened up slightly on inspiration (to about 20 msec [0.02 sec]).

7.   What cardiac abnormalities cause only the A_2 component of a wide split to be heard?

ANS.:   Severe PS with decreased pulmonary arterial flow may cause the late P_2 to be inaudible. Decreased pulmonary arterial flow with PS not only occurs when heart failure is present but also when there is a right-to-left shunt. When an ASD is present (trilogy of Fallot) or a VSD is present (tetralogy of Fallot), severe PS plus the right-to-left shunt bypassing the lungs will cause the P_2 to become inaudible.

8.   What kinds of respiration will obscure awareness of whether the split moves?

ANS.:   a) Too deep an inspiration will interpose too much lung between the stethoscope and the heart, making one or both S_2 components disappear.

b) Too shallow an inspiration may not open the S_2 at all.

c) Rapid respiration will not allow time for the hemodynamic changes to occur that produce splitting on inspiration and narrowing on expiration.

9.   How can you control the respiration of a patient so that there are enough cardiac cycles on inspiration and expiration to distinguish normal from abnormal splitting?

ANS.:   Ask the patient to follow your arm, raising it for inspiration and lowering it for expiration; i.e., you may "conduct" his respiration so that there are at least two or three cycles during each phase of respiration. Be certain that the patient does not breathe too deeply, or he will make too much chest noise or even close his glottis at the end of inspiration, producing either a Valsalva or a **Müller maneuver**.

Note: Using your arms to direct breathing allows you to close your eyes while listening and also allows you to demonstrate the phases of respiration to large groups when group listening is taking place through multiple stethophones or loudspeakers.

THE S_2 SPLIT IN PULMONARY HYPERTENSION

1.   What are the three general types of pulmonary hypertension?

ANS.:   a) Hyperkinetic, i.e., due to excess volume flow, as in large left-to-right shunts. The pulmonary arterioles can dilate to accommodate up to three times normal cardiac output before the pulmonary artery pressure must rise.

b) Vasoactive, i.e., due to pulmonary arteriolar constriction, as in response either to hypoxia or to a high left atrial pressure as in patients with MS.

c) Obstructive, i.e., due to fixed lumen obliteration, as in pulmonary emboli, or narrowing, as in medial hypertrophy in some ASDs, PDAs, or VSDs with bidirectional shunting (Eisenmenger reaction). Fixed lumen obliteration also occurs with endocardial and medial hypertrophy in primary pulmonary hypertension.

2. In which of the preceding causes of pulmonary hypertension do you expect (a) normal or narrow splitting, i.e., opening from 20—60 msec (0.02—0.06 sec) on inspiration and closing on expiration, (b) wide splitting, or (c) no splitting?

ANS.: a) Normal or narrow splitting is expected in some subjects in the early stages of primary pulmonary hypertension and with the pulmonary hypertension of most subjects with PDA or MS [58]. The increased impedance due to the high resistance and tense pulmonary artery should cause an early P_2, so that the S_2 should be single. However, the dilated pulmonary artery, so often found in patients with pulmonary hypertension, decreases the impedance to pulmonary flow and may be the cause of the separation to normal degrees on inspiration.

*Note: The level of pulmonary hypertension does not correlate with the width of the splitting in MS (ranges from 20—60 msec) or in MR (ranges from 40—70 msec) [58].

b) Wide splitting is expected in ASDs, in massive pulmonary embolism and in some patients with severe primary pulmonary hypertension with prolonged RV isovolumic contraction time.

c) No splitting is expected in VSDs with an Eisenmenger reaction, but in VSDs with hyperkinetic pulmonary hypertension, the S_2 may be either single or split normally [58].

*Note: Although a single S_2 in VSDs does not tell you whether or not the pulmonary hypertension is too fixed to be operable, the split S_2 usually implies that an operation is feasible.

3. How much obstruction is necessary before an acute pulmonary embolism can produce wide, relatively fixed splitting of S_2?

ANS.: Almost the entire pulmonary tree on both sides must be obstructed. If, however, there is already pulmonary hypertension from previous disease, a further embolus to one branch may cause wide, fixed splitting.

*Note: a) Moderate exercise can bring out the wide splitting in borderline cases and exaggerate it still more in advanced obstruction. In severe obstruction, the split may be almost 80 msec. Since it is relatively fixed, it may be mistaken for an opening snap but standing the patient up or applying venous tourniquets to the legs will narrow the split S_2 and widen an S_2-opening snap interval.

b) This wide split often narrows with lysis of the embolus over three to six days.

c) The cause of the wide split in acute pulmonary embolism is due to a shortened $Q—A_2$ and a normal $Q—P_2$. The early A_2 is probably due to shortening of LV systole, partly by catecholamines and partly by a reduced LV stroke volume. A prolonged isovolumic contraction time of the RV due to the sudden pulmonary hypertension may keep the $Q—P_2$ normal.

4.   What is an ASD, VSD, or PDA with bidirectional shunting called?

     ANS.:   An Eisenmenger situation, syndrome, or reaction. The pulmonary hypertension may be so severe that only right-to-left shunting occurs.

           Note: When a VSD is the cause of the pulmonary hypertension, it is often called an Eisenmenger *complex,* because this is the original lesion described by Eisenmenger in 1897.

5.   How does the S_2 of a VSD with an Eisenmenger reaction differ from the wide S_2 split of the usual VSD?

     ANS.:   The S_2 becomes single on both phases of respiration [58]. This is so because only a large VSD could produce an Eisenmenger reaction, and such a large communication between ventricles tends to make them function as a single chamber.

           Note: Unless the right ventricle hypertrophies to meet a high pulmonary artery pressure, the two ventricles do not act as a single chamber. Therefore, the rare single ventricle with only hyperkinetic pulmonary hypertension may have an appreciably split S_2.

6.   How does the S_2 differ among the three different levels of Eisenmenger syndromes, i.e., VSD, ASD, or PDA?

     ANS.:   In VSDs, the S_2 is single; in ASDs, it is split and fixed (often widely split); in PDAs, it is normally or narrowly split and when split, it moves normally [58].

           Note: a) Early in the course of development of an ASD Eisenmenger reaction, the high resistance beyond the pulmonary valve may narrow the split S_2. As the RV begins to fail, its isovolumic contraction time prolongs and the split becomes wide again.

           b) The A_2/P_2 ratio can be used to suggest the presence of hyperkinetic pulmonary hypertension in a subject with a VSD. In a VSD with normal pulmonary artery pressure, the A_2 at the second left interspace is generally louder than the P_2 that follows it. Therefore, if the P_2 is louder (more easily seen on a phonocardiogram), pulmonary hypertension is probably present.

THE REVERSED OR PARADOXICALLY SPLIT S_2

Physiology and Etiologies

1.   What is meant by a reversed or paradoxical split of S_2?

     ANS.:   A split in which the order of components is P_2A_2 instead of the normal A_2P_2.

2.   Can too early a P_2 cause a reversed split?

     ANS.:   A reversed split caused by such a phenomenon must be very rare (see p. 205). A reversed split is nearly always caused by a delayed A_2.

3.   What can delay A_2 enough to cause paradoxical splitting?

     ANS.:   a) Conduction defects that delay depolarization of the left ventricle, such as complete LBBB and some types of Wolff-Parkinson-White preexcitation that imitate LBBB [45, 66].

           Note: The type of W-P-W preexcitation that acts like LBBB is the one in which the initial conduction (delta wave) passes to the RV muscle first. This is known as type B, because the QRS points posteriorly.

b) A marked systolic gradient across the aortic valve, causing a delay in the fall of LV to below aortic pressure, as in severe AS. (See p. 263.)

Note: Poststenotic dilatation can contribute to the delay in A_2 perhaps by producing a loss of elastic recoil, as well as by increasing the capacitance of the aorta.

*c) Marked volume loads on the LV, e.g., severe AR or a large PDA.

*d) Acute ventricular dysfunction, as in acute myocardial infarction, acute myocarditis, or during angina pectoris.

*e) Hypertension, plus myocardial damage.

*f) Severe chronic ischemic heart disease.

4.   What causes the widest reversed split?

ANS.:   Complete LBBB, i.e., with a QRS of 120 msec (0.12 sec) or longer. This is also the commonest cause of a reversed split and the only one that will be easily recognized by the noncardiologist.

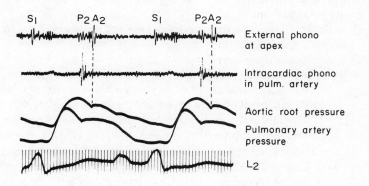

These simultaneous intra-arterial and phonocardiogram tracings are from a 59-year-old man in heart failure due to an idiopathic cardiomyopathy. Because of LBBB, the incisura of the pulmonary artery and its simultaneous P_2 comes before the aortic incisura and its simultaneous A_2. (His pulmonary artery systolic pressure was 35 mm Hg; his LV pressure, 120 mm Hg; and his cardiac index, 2.4.) These are catheter-tip electromanometer tracings, so that there are no tubing delays.

*5.   What produces the delayed A_2 in LBBB, prolongation of isovolumic contraction, a short ejection phase, or a delay in onset of ventricular contraction?

ANS.:   Isovolumic contraction is usually prolonged. This has been shown in subjects with intermittent LBBB [8, 48]. Prolongation of the electromechanical interval, i.e., Q to onset of ventricular contraction (Q–C), is prolonged in some but not in others. When the main left bundle is cut in dogs, the Q–C is always prolonged [65].

Note: In transposition of the great vessels, the RV is the systemic ventricle. Therefore, a RBBB acts the same as a LBBB without a transposition and can cause a reversed split [67].

6. What is the significance of a reversed split in congenital or rheumatic AS?

ANS.: In either type of AS it implies that the gradient is at least 60 mm Hg or more. This is more reliable in congenital than in rheumatic stenosis, because in the latter, myocardial damage may add extra delays to the A_2 by delaying the onset of the aortic valve opening, i.e., the isovolumic contraction time may be prolonged.

Note: In hypertrophic subaortic stenosis (HSS) there may be day-to-day variation in S_2 splitting, so that splitting could change from normal to single to reversed.

The highest incidence of audible reversed splits apparently occurs in severe HSS, probably because there is no calcification of the valve to make the A_2 disappear [59].

*7. When do reversed splits occur in patients with ischemic heart disease in the absence of LBBB?

ANS.: It is rare to observe reversed splitting in chronic coronary disease [13]. It does, however, occur

a) During acute angina or after exercise in the presence of significant coronary obstruction [17].

b) During the first three days of acute myocardial infarctions in about 15% of patients [57].

c) In patients over 70 with coronary disease and usually with enough heart damage to produce an S_3 [3].

d) If such patients are hypertensive.

Note: a) Reversed splits occur in hypertensive patients only if they have myocardial damage as well. Proof of this is that the reversed split can appear with the development of early failure and disappear after digitalis is given [1].

b) The split reversal is so narrow in coronary disease problems that often a phonocardiogram has to be used to detect it. One may hear a pure S_2 on inspiration and an impure sound on expiration as the only sign of reversal. The delay of A_2 in patients with coronary disease is usually due to a prolonged preejection period, i.e., there is a delay in the onset of opening of the aortic valve.

8. What is the significance of expiratory splitting of S_2?

ANS.: It means either

a) A wide split.

b) A narrow or wide fixed split.

c) A paradoxical split.

Note: Since only 5% of normal subjects over age 50 have expiratory splitting of S_2, when found in this age group, it is probably abnormal. In the young, a wide split may be normal.

9. What can be confused with paradoxical splitting of S_2?

ANS.: a) The S_2—opening snap. (This is discussed in detail on p. 216.)

*b) A widely split A_2–P_2 in atrial fibrillation. After short diastoles, there is narrow splitting. Inspiration, by its vagolytic effect on the A–V node, may cause a faster rate. Therefore, the split may narrow on inspiration because of the shorter R—R intervals. The widening on expiration and narrowing on inspiration will act like a reversed split [34].

Eliciting and Recognition of Reversed Splits

1.   What should make you suspect paradoxical or reversed splitting?

ANS.:   A split that widens on expiration and narrows on inspiration implies that the P_2 comes first.

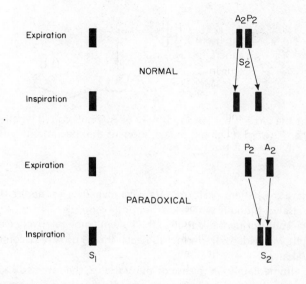

If the split narrows on inspiration, the P_2 must come first, and the split S_2 is reversed.

2.   How can you confirm by stethoscope alone that a wide split actually is reversed so that the A_2 is last, even when the respiratory movements are so erratic that respiratory widening cannot be recognized?

ANS.:   a) At the apex, the A_2 is either the only sound heard — or the louder component of the S_2 if both are heard there. Therefore, you should gradually move your stethoscope from the left sternal border toward the apex as you listen to the split second sound. The component of the split, which either disappears at the apex or becomes softer at the apex, will be the P_2. If it is the second component that does this, then you know that it was A_2–P_2, and the wide split is probably due to something like a RBBB. If, on the other hand, you hear the first component becoming softer or disappearing relative to the second component, then the order was P_2–A_2, and you are probably eliciting LBBB.

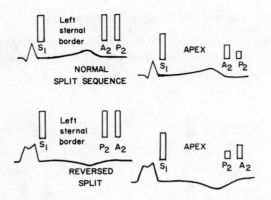

If the split is fixed at the left sternal border, it may be difficult to tell whether it has a normal or paradoxical sequence. Toward the apex, the component that becomes relatively softer must be the P_2.

b) Have the patient perform a Valsalva maneuver for about 10 sec. During a Valsalva, blood is withheld from both ventricles. Thus, if you can still hear the split during the Valsalva, the P_2 will come relatively early, and the reversed split will widen. In normal subjects, the S_2 usually becomes narrow during the Valsalva.

Immediately on release of the Valsalva, the reversed split S_2 narrows, because more blood comes back to the right side, and the P_2 comes closer to the A_2. In normal subjects, the sudden return of blood into the RV causes an immediate widening of the S_2 split.

A few beats after the release of the Valsalva, the reversed split widens again markedly. In normal subjects, on the contrary, the split narrows as the excess pulmonary blood reaches the LV after traversing the lungs.

*3. How can you confirm by phonocardiogram alone that a reversed split is present?

ANS.: Simultaneous phonocardiograms at the second left interspace and apex will show the louder component, or even the only component, of S_2 at the apex to be simultaneous with the second component at the sternal border.

Note: You can confirm by a simultaneous phonocardiogram and pulse tracing that the split is reversed by timing the split with the carotid tracing. We know that the aortic component of S_2 is almost simultaneous with the dicrotic notch (except for a slight delay in the carotid tracing). Therefore, any component coming before the aortic component is likely to be a P_2.

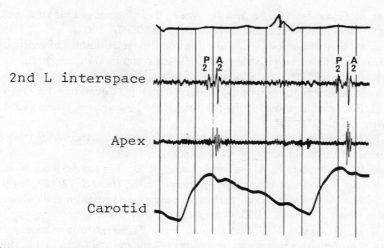

2nd L interspace

Apex

Carotid

Note that (1) the two components of S_2 come before the carotid dicrotic notch, and (2) the second component of the S_2 is coincident with the only sound at the apex, which is always the A_2.

*4.   What is meant by nonparadoxical reversed splitting?

ANS.:   The order is P_2A_2, but it splits more widely on inspiration than on expiration. It can occur in the presence of LBBB in a patient with a cardiomyopathy or acute myocardial infarction. It is apparently due to an excessively early P_2 on inspiration. It can only be diagnosed by simultaneous phonocardiograms or pulse tracings, but can be suspected if a patient with a known LBBB has an apparently normal movement with a widely split S_2 [49].

REFERENCES

1. Abbott, J. A., and Whipple, G. H. Paradoxic splitting of the second heart sound in systemic hypertension. *Dis. Chest* 46:304, 1964.

2. Adolph, R. J., and Fowler, N. O. The second heart sound: A screening test for heart disease. *Mod. Concepts Cardiovasc. Dis.* 39:91, 1970.

3. Agnew, T., Bucher, H., McDonald, L., and Seymour, J. Delayed closure of the aortic valve in ischaemic heart disease. *Br. Heart J.* 29:775, 1967.

4. Aygen, M. M., and Braunwald, E. The splitting of the second heart sound in normal subjects and in patients with congenital heart disease. *Circulation* 25:328, 1962.

5. Beck, W., Schrire, V., and Vogelpoel, L. Splitting of the second heart sound in constrictive pericarditis with observations on the mechanism of pulsus paradoxus. *Am. Heart J.* 64:765, 1962.

6. Berry, W. B., and Austen, W. G. Respiratory variations in the magnitude of the left to right shunt in experimental interatrial communications. *Am. J. Cardiol.* 14:201, 1964.

7. Blazek, W. V., and Bliss, H. A. The second heart sound in uncomplicated ventricular septal defect. *Med. Clin. North Am.* 50:111, 1966.

8. Bourassa, M. G., Boiteau, G. M., and Allenstein, B. J. Hemodynamic studies during inter-mittent left bundle branch block. *Am. J. Cardiol.* 10:792, 1962.

9. Bourassa, M. G., and Campeau, L. Duration and time relationships of ventricular ejection in valvular lesions. Montreal Heart Institute. Personal communication, 1969.

10. Bruce, R. A., and John, G. G. Effects of upright posture and exercise on pulmonary hemo-dynamics in patients with central cardiovascular shunts. *Circulation* 16:776, 1957.

11. Castle, R. F. Variables affecting the splitting of the second heart sound in atrial septal defect. *Am. Heart J.* 73:468, 1967.

12. Castle, R. F., Hedden, C. A., and Davis, N. P., II. Variables affecting splitting of the second heart sound in normal children. *Pediatrics* 43:183, 1969.

13. Caulfield, W. H., Jr., Smith, R. H., and Franklin, R. B. The second heart sound in coronary artery disease. A phonocardiographic assessment. *Am. Heart J.* 77:187, 1969.

14. Cobbs, B. W., Jr. The second heart sound in pulmonary embolism and pulmonary hyperten-sion. *Am. Heart J.* 71:843, 1966.

15. Cobbs, B. W., Jr., Logue, R. B., and Dorney, E. R. Fixed splitting of the second heart sound. A useful sign of massive pulmonary embolism. *Circulation* 36(Suppl.):11, 1967.

16. D'Cruz, I. A., Augustsson, M. H., Bicoff, J. P., Weinberg, M., Jr., and Arcilla, R. A. Stenotic lesions of the pulmonary arteries. *Am. J. Cardiol.* 13:441, 1964.

17. Dickerson, R. B., and Nelson, W. P. Paradoxical splitting of the second heart sound. *Am. Heart J.* 67:410, 1964.

18. Ehlers, K. H., Engle, M. A., Farnsworth, P. B., and Levin, A. R. Wide splitting of the second heart sound without demonstrable heart disease. *Am. J. Cardiol.* 23:690, 1969.

19. Feruglio, G. A., and Gunton, R. W. Intracardiac phonocardiography in ventricular septal defect. *Circulation* 21:49, 1960.

20. Feruglio, G. A., and Sreenivasan, A. Intracardiac phonocardiogram in thirty cases of atrial septal defect. *Circulation* 22:1087, 1959.

21. Frye, R. L., Marshall, H. W., Kincaid, O. W., and Burchell, H. B. Anomalous pulmonary venous drainage of the right lung into the inferior vena cava. *Br. Heart J.* 24:696, 1962.

22. Gamboa, R., Hugenholtz, P. G., and Nadas, A. S. Accuracy of the phonocardiogram in assess-ing severity of aortic and pulmonic stenosis. *Circulation* 30:35, 1964.

23. Golinko, R. J., Kaplan, N., and Rudolph, A. M. The mechanism of pulsus paradoxus during acute pericardial tamponade. *J. Clin. Invest.* 42:249, 1963.

24. Hamby, R. I., Meron, J. M., and Roberts, G. S. Valsalva maneuver made easy. *Am. Heart J.* 82:838, 1971.

25. Harris, A., and Sutton, G. Second heart sound in normal subjects. *Br. Heart J.* 30:739, 1968.

26. Higgins, C. B., and Mulder, D. G. Tetralogy of Fallot in the adult. *Am. J. Cardiol.* 29:837, 1972.

27. Honey, M. Delayed closure of the pulmonary valve. *Lancet* 5:318, 1966.

28. Kardalinos, A. The second heart sound. *Am. Heart J.* 64:610, 1962.

29. Karnegis, J. N., and Wang, Y. The phonocardiogram in idiopathic dilatation of the pulmonary artery. *Am. J. Cardiol.* 14:75, 1964.

30. Kaufmann, G., Rutishauser, W., and Hegglin, R. Heart sounds in atrial tumors. *Am. J. Cardiol.* 8:350, 1961.

31. Kraus, Y., Yahini, J. H., Shem-Tov, A., and Neufeld, H. N. Splitting of the Second Heart Sound in Partial Anomalous Pulmonary Venous Connection with Intact Interatrial Septum. In *Proceedings of Fourth Asian-Pacific Congress of Cardiologists.* New York: Academic, 1969. P. 147.

32. Kumar, S., and Luisada, A. A. Mechanism of changes in the second heart sound in aortic stenosis. *Am. J. Cardiol.* 28:162, 1971.

33. Kumar, S., and Luisada, A. A. Second heart sound in atrial septal defect. *Am. J. Cardiol.* 28:168, 1971.

34. Leachman, R. D., Talat, A., and Cokkinos, V. P. Narrowed splitting of the second heart sound on inspiration in patients with giant left atrium. *Chest* 60:151, 1971.

35. Leatham, A., and Gray, I. Auscultatory and phonocardiographic signs of atrial septal defect. *Br. Heart J.* 18:193, 1956.

36. Macieira-Coelho, E., and Guimaraes, C. Phonocardiography in atrial septal defects of the ostium secundum type. *Cardiologia* 44:78, 1964.

37. MacKenzie, J. C., Rosenberg, M. E., Kroll, G., and Brandfonbrener, M. Postural variation in second sound splitting. *Chest* 63:56, 1973.

38. Moss, W. G., and Johnson, V. Differential effects of stretch upon the stroke volumes of the right and left ventricles. *Am. J. Physiol.* 139:52, 1943.

39. Nandi, P. S., Pigott, V. M., and Spodick, D. H. Sequential cardiac responses during the respiratory cycle: Patterns of change in systolic intervals. *Chest* 63:380, 1973.

40. Nelson, W. P., and North, R. L. Splitting of the second heart sound in adults forty years and older. *Am. J. Med. Sci.* 56:805, 1967.

41. Perloff, J. K., and Harvey, W. P. Mechanisms of fixed splitting of the second heart sound. *Circulation* 18:998, 1958.

42. Perloff, J. K., and Lebauer, E. J. Auscultatory and phonocardiographic manifestations of isolated stenosis of the pulmonary artery and its branches. *Br. Heart J.* 31:314, 1969.

43. Piemme, T. E., Barnett, O., and Dexter, L. Relationship of heart sounds to acceleration of blood flow. *Circ. Res.* 18:303, 1966.

44. Roach, M. R. Changes in arterial distensibility as a cause of poststenotic dilatation. *Am. J. Cardiol.* 12:802, 1963.

45. Rodriguez-Torres, R., Yao, A. C., and Lynfield, J. Significance of split heart sounds in children with Wolff-Parkinson-White syndrome. *Bull. N.Y. Acad. Med.* 44:511, 1968.

46. Ruskin, J., Bache, R. J., Rembert, J. C., and Greenfield, J. C., Jr. Pressure-flow studies in man: Effect of respiration on left ventricular stroke volume. *Circulation* 48:79, 1973.

47. Sainani, G. S., and Luisada, A. A. "Mapping" the precordium. *Am. J. Cardiol.* 19:788, 1967.

48. Sakamoto, T., Uozumi, Z., Kawai, N., Yamada, T., Inoue, K., Horikoh, U., and Ueda, H. QRS dependence of the split interval of the second heart sound in complete right and left bundle branch block. *Jap. Heart J.* 8:459, 1967.

49. Sakamoto, T., Yamada, T., Uozumi, Z., Kawai, N., Inoue, K., and Ueda, H. Methoxamine induced "non-paradoxical" reversed splitting. *Jap. Heart J.* 8:642, 1967.

50. Schrire, V., and Vogelpoel, L. The role of the dilated pulmonary artery in abnormal splitting of the second heart sound. *Am. Heart J.* 63:501, 1962.

51. Shafter, H. A. Splitting of the second heart sound. *Am. J. Cardiol.* 6:1013, 1960.

52. Shah, P. M., and Slodki, S. J. The Q-II interval. *Circulation* 29:551, 1964.

53. Shaver, J. A., Nadolny, R. A., O'Toole, J. D., Thompson, M. E., Reddy, P. S., Leon, D. F., and Curtiss, E. I. Sound pressure correlates of the second heart sound. *Circulation* 49:316, 1974.

54. Shuler, R. H., Ensor, C., Gunning, R. E., Moss, W. G., and Johnson, V. The differential effects of respiration on the left and right ventricles. *Am. J. Physiol.* 137:620, 1942.

55. Singh, S. P. Unusual splitting of the second heart sound in pulmonary stenosis. *Am. J. Cardiol.* 25:28, 1970.

56. Slodki, S. J., Hussain, A. T., and Luisada, A. A. The Q-II interval. III. A study of the second heart sound in old age. *J. Am. Geriatr. Soc.* 17:673, 1969.

57. Stock, E. Auscultation and phonocardiography in acute myocardial infarction. *Med. J. Aust.* 1:1060, 1966.

58. Sutton, G., Harris, A., and Leatham, A. Second heart sound in pulmonary hypertension. *Br. Heart J.* 30:743, 1968.

59. Tavel, M. E. Clinical phonocardiography. *J. A. M. A.* 203:123, 1968.

60. VanBogaert, A. Role of the valves in the genesis of normal heart sounds. *Cardiologia* 52:330, 1968.

61. Victorica, B. E., Gessner, I. H., and Schiebler, G. L. Phonocardiographic findings in persistent truncus arteriosus. *Br. Heart J.* 30:812, 1968.

62. Wang, Y. Wide fixed splitting of the second heart sound and right ventricular diastolic over-load. *Circulation* 36(Suppl.):11, 1967.

63. Weinstein, P. B., Leighton, R. F., Goodwin, S. G., and Wooley, C. F. Mechanism for splitting of the second heart sound in atrial septal defect. *Circulation* 36(Suppl.):11, 1967.

64. Weisse, A. B., Schwartz, M. L., Heinz, A., Cyrsky, F. T., and Webb, N. C. Intensity of the normal second heart sound components in their traditional auscultatory areas. *Am. J. Med.* 43:171, 1967.

65. Wennemark, J. R., Blake, D. F., and Keydie, P. Cardiodynamic effects of experimental bundle branch block in the dog. *Circ. Res.* 10:280, 1962.

66. Zuberbuhler, J. R., and Bauersfeld, S. R. Paradoxical splitting of the second heart sound in the Wolff-Parkinson-White syndrome. *Am. Heart J.* 70:595, 1965.

67. Zuberbuhler, J. R., Bauersfeld, S. R., and Pontius, R. G. Paradoxic splitting of the second sound with transposition of the great vessels. *Am. Heart J.* 74:816, 1967.

MECHANISM AND TIMING

1. Draw a simultaneous normal LV and left atrial pressure curve. At what point on the curve does the mitral valve open?

   ANS.: The mitral valve opens when left ventricular (LV) pressure drops below left atrial pressure. The normal peak left atrial pressure is about 10 mm Hg. Therefore, when LV pressure drops to about 9 mm Hg, the mitral valve should open.

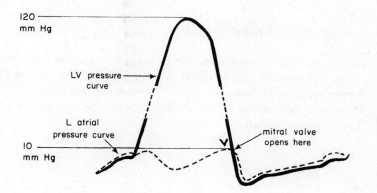

Note that the left atrial V wave rise is abruptly interrupted by LV pressure's falling below left atrial pressure and opening the mitral valve.

2. Draw a LV, left atrial, and simultaneous aortic pressure curve. What left-sided event produces a sound just before the mitral valve opens?

   ANS.: Closure of the aortic valve produces the A_2 about 100 msec (0.10 sec) before the mitral valve opens. This 100 msec interval takes about as long as it takes to say "pa-pa" as quickly as possible.

---

* indicates material that is for electives or fellows in cardiology, or concerns rare phenomena, of interest primarily to cardiologists.

Boldface type indicates that the term is explained in the Glossary.

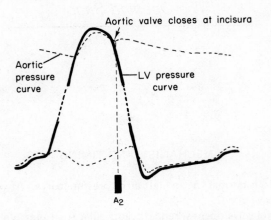

The A_2 is simultaneous with the aortic valve incisura and occurs shortly before the LV pressure drops below left atrial pressure, to open the mitral valve. The interval between the aortic valve closure (A_2) and the opening of the mitral valve is the isovolumic relaxation time.

3.   Is mitral valve opening ever heard normally?
    ANS.:   No.
4.   What is usually necessary before the opening of the mitral valve becomes audible?
    ANS.:   At least some mitral stenosis (MS), with stiffening of the edges of the valve or
        commissures by fibrosis or calcium. The valve may act like a sail that billows
        downward into a dome and ends with a snap only when its edges are held stiffly
        by fibrosis or calcium.

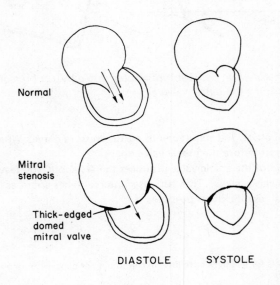

This concept of the cause of the opening snap is one in which the belly of the stenotic mitral valve (mostly the anterior leaflet) bulges downward with a jerk to produce a clicking or snapping sound as it opens. Therefore, it also must close with a snap as it domes upward.

Note: a) Torrential flow through the mitral valve can on rare occasions produce an opening snap (OS) in the absence of MS. It has been recorded on rare occasions in ventricular septal defects (VSDs), patent ductus arteriosus, tricuspid atresia, thyrotoxicosis, after a Blalock-Taussig operation for tetralogy and in mitral regurgitation due to the ballooned valve syndrome [9, 11]. It has even been recorded in some presumably normal children with innocent ejection murmurs.

b) In congenital MS in infants, there is rarely an OS because congenitally abnormal leaflets are usually not pliable.

5. Why is the audible opening of the mitral valve called an opening snap (OS)?

ANS.: Because most of the time it is a short, high-frequency (see **frequency**), crisp click or snap.

6. Which leaflet is responsible for the OS?

ANS.: The anterior leaflet must be the one to have mobility in order to produce an OS, because it is three times broader than the posterior leaflet, so that even though MS tends to convert the two semi-independent leaflets into a continuous funnel-like sleeve, the belly of the anterior leaflet contributes most to the sounds.

Note: An OS can occur with dominant mitral regurgitation (MR) as long as the regurgitation is due to a thickened, rolled, immobile posterior (mural) leaflet and as long as the anterior (septal) leaflet still has a mobile belly [12].

7. What do we call the interval between the closing of the aortic valve and the opening of the mitral valves?

ANS.: The isovolumic relaxation period.

Note: Formerly, this was known as the isometric relaxation period because there was thought to be only a change of tension or pressure without a change of dimension. In actual fact, the dimensions of the ventricle do change, in that some parts are expanding while others are contracting. Therefore, it is not isometric, although the volume does remain the same, i.e., it is isovolumic.

8. What do cardiologists call the interval between the aortic closure sound and the OS sound?

ANS.: The A_2—OS interval, or, simply, the 2—OS interval.

Note: When there is a tricuspid OS, one must necessarily say the "P_2 to the tricuspid OS interval." When no specific mention of which side of the heart is made, the 2—OS interval refers to the A_2 to mitral OS interval, since a tricuspid OS is relatively rare.

RELATION BETWEEN THE 2—OS AND SEVERITY OF MITRAL STENOSIS

1. What controls the duration of isovolumic relaxation, or the 2—OS interval?

ANS.: a) The pressure in the left atrium at the time the mitral valve opens.

b) The heart rate. The more rapid the heart rate, the shorter the 2—OS interval, because isovolumic relaxation is faster under the influence of the same sympathetic tone or catecholamines that cause the faster rate.

c) The stiffness of the mitral valve (due mostly to calcium) [15].

d) The rate and strength of relaxation of the myocardium, i.e., the state of myocardial function or inotropic state (contractility) of the myocardium.

e) The pressure at which the aortic valve closes (near systolic pressure).

2.   What is the relationship between the degree of MS and the height of the V wave in the left atrium?

ANS.:   The greater the stenosis, the greater the obstruction to flow and thus the slower and more incomplete will be the emptying of the left atrium. Therefore, the greater the MS, the higher the V wave.

Note: This will only be clear if you recall that the V wave is built up during ventricular systole when the mitral valve is closed. If the V wave begins to build up from a high pressure, that wave will rise even higher. If the left atrium did not empty well in diastole due to MS, the V wave will start to build up from an already high pressure.

3.   Does a high left atrial pressure make the 2—OS interval shorter or longer? Why?

ANS.:   Shorter, because the LV pressure does not have to fall so far to open the mitral valve.

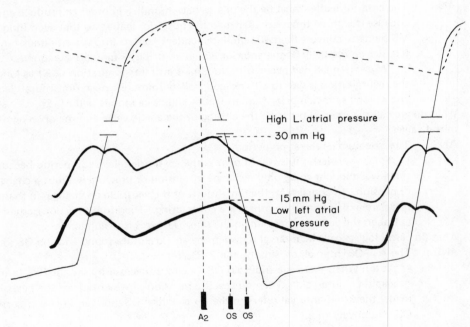

Note that the distance between the A₂ and the OS is shorter with the higher left atrial pressure.

Note: Other causes of a high V wave, such as MR, do not necessarily cause an early OS, probably because the OS in MS occurs not at the peak but on the downstroke of the V wave, and if MR is also present, the OS may occur far down on the downstroke of the V wave [17]. Even though the descent of the mitral cusps begins at the crossover of LV and left atrial pressures, the descent of the mitral valves may take another 25—70 msec to reach its maximum excursion. The OS occurs at the moment of maximum excursion of the mitral valve. It is probably this valvular descent before the OS that expands the left atrial capacity and allows the beginning of the Y descent to occur before the OS.

4.   Will a very stiff mitral valve make an earlier or later OS, i.e., will the 2—OS interval be shortened or lengthened? Why?

ANS.:   Lengthened, because the stiffer the valve, the lower the LV pressure will have to fall below atrial pressure before it can "suck" the valve open [15]. Stiffness here refers not to the degree of stenosis but to the degree of *mobility* of the bellies of the valves. Stenosis refers to the size of the opening, which is controlled by the degree of fusion of the edges.

5.   Besides a stiff mitral valve, list the causes of a late OS aside from a mild degree of MS.

ANS.:   a) Bradycardia. This prolongs isovolumic relaxation time.

b) Poor myocardial function due to either damage or aging due to prolongation of isovolumic relaxation time. (Isovolumic relaxation time increases strikingly with age [8].)

c) Aortic regurgitation (AR). This may be due to the aortic regurgitant jet's striking the underbelly of the anterior mitral leaflet and holding it up excessively long as it tries to move down to reach its maximum open position. (AR may even eliminate an OS.)

d) A low left atrial pressure due to a large left atrium and severe failure with low flow.

e) High aortic pressure. If the aortic valve closes at a high pressure, the LV pressure has to drop further before it can drop below left atrial pressure to open the mitral valve.

Note: At an aortic pressure above 130 mm Hg, the 2—OS interval will be unreliable in telling the degree of MS [2]. (Remember that the aortic valve closes at near aortic systolic pressure.)

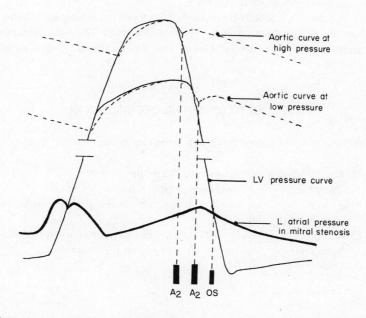

Aortic curve at high pressure

Aortic curve at low pressure

LV pressure curve

L atrial pressure in mitral stenosis

A₂   A₂ OS

Note that the higher the aortic pressure, the longer the A₂—OS interval.

6.   Which is more reliable in predicting the degree of MS, a narrow or a wide 2—OS? Why?

   ANS.:   A narrow 2—OS is more reliable. This is because there is not much besides a tight MS or a tachycardia that can narrow a 2—OS interval, but there are at least five causes besides mild MS for a wide 2—OS.

   Note: a) Unequivocally tight MS is suggested by a resting 2—OS of 50 msec or less [21].

   The lowest normal isovolumic relaxation time (measured from the aortic incisura to the LV—left atrial pressure curve crossover) is 55 msec [1]. Since the mitral OS is later than the crossover of pressure by about 40 msec, the shortest 2—OS interval with almost normal left atrial pressures would be about 95 msec.

   b) A supine leg-raising postexercise 2—OS of 80 msec or more suggests mild MS (mean left atrial pressure not over 12 mm Hg). If the 2—OS after exercise is 50 msec or less, the stenosis is severe (mean left atrial pressure of at least 25 mm Hg) [7].

7.   Will a long diastole of atrial fibrillation produce a long or short 2—OS? Why?

   ANS.:   A long 2—OS. More diastolic time to empty the left atrium allows its pressure to drop. The next systole will begin and end with a lower left atrial pressure, thus making a long 2—OS.

8.   Without a phonocardiograph, how can you tell a late from an early OS?

   ANS.:   a) If you say "pa-pa" as quickly as possible, you will be separating the sounds by about 100 msec (0.10 sec) or more. This is a late OS distance from the second heart sound.

   b) If you say "pa-da" as quickly as possible, you ought to be able to separate the sounds by about 50—70 msec (0.05—0.07 sec). This is a narrow 2—OS and suggests moderate to tight MS.

   Note: You should time yourself on a phonocardiogram. Some physicians say "pa-pa" so slowly that the syllables are really 120 msec apart, which is the distance of an S_2 to an S_3. (See p. 186 for imitations of intervals between 30 and 100 msec.)

THE LOUDNESS OF THE OPENING SNAP

1.   Besides an obese or emphysematous chest, what can cause a soft or absent OS despite significant MS?

   ANS.:   a) Too calcified a mitral valve for the bellies to move.

   Note: Fibrosis alone is rarely responsible for a soft OS.

   b) An extremely low flow, due either to myocardial failure or to the exceptional severity of the stenosis.

   c) A large right ventricle (RV) (usually due to pulmonary hypertension or tricuspid regurgitation), pushing the LV away from the chest wall.

   d) Moderate to severe AR.

2. Why will severe pulmonary hypertension in a patient with MS produce a soft OS aside from the buffering effect of a large RV?

    ANS.:   Because there are then two causes for a low flow: the obstruction at the mitral valve and obstruction at the pulmonary arterioles.

    Note: A reduced flow occurs with pulmonary hypertension, probably because an elevation of RV pressure may not completely compensate for the high resistance produced by pulmonary arteriolar constriction.

3. What proofs are there that very low flow can prevent the appearance of an OS?

    ANS.:   Digitalis has been known to bring out an OS that was previously absent. Standing can cause a soft OS to disappear. Raising the legs can cause an OS to become louder.

4. Does mitral commissurotomy eliminate the OS?

    ANS.:   Probably in not more than half the cases.

5. Why may AR prevent or soften an OS?

    ANS.:   Perhaps because the regurgitant stream strikes the underbelly of the anterior leaflet of the mitral valve and holds it up enough to prevent a rapid opening movement. Therefore, AR could theoretically make the OS both late and soft.

    Note: When a patient with AR sits up, you may hear a soft OS for the first time. This is probably because the decreased venous return of the sitting position reduces the amount of AR, and the mitral valve can open with a jerk.

HOW TO TELL AN A_2–P_2 FROM A 2–OS

1. Where on the chest wall is the OS best heard?

    ANS.:   Between the apex and the left sternal border. This is not too surprising when one considers that the anterior leaflet of the mitral valve, which creates most of the sound, makes its motion in a line that points almost directly at the left sternal border.

    Peculiarly, it can often be heard at the second right interspace, even if it is only moderately loud at the left lower sternal border.

    Note: Like all sounds and murmurs, when the OS is loud, it can be heard anywhere on the chest wall. It may even be up to grade 6 in loudness.

2. Is the range of the 2–OS interval different from that of the A_2–P_2 interval?

    ANS.:   No. They may both be from 30–100 msec (0.03–0.10 sec).

3. How does the quality, frequency, or duration of an OS differ from that of a P_2?

    ANS.:   They do not differ. They may both be short, with many high frequencies. Occasionally, the OS may have mostly low frequencies, especially if the valve is heavily calcified or fibrosed.

4. Which is likely to be best heard at the left lower sternal border, the P_2 or the OS?

    ANS.:   Either one.

5. When may a P_2 be well heard at the apex?

    ANS.:   a) In thin-chested young people.

    b) If the RV is so large that it usurps the site of the usual apex beat.

    c) If it is louder than normal.

6. Is a P_2 ever louder at the apex than at the left sternal border?

    ANS.:   No.

7.   When is an OS louder at the apex than at the left sternal border?
     ANS.:   As a rule only when the LV is dilated, or if a rib has been removed in previous
             heart surgery. This places the stethoscope almost directly on the heart at the
             apex.
                 *COROLLARY 1: If the second component of a split S$_2$ is louder at the apex
                 than elsewhere, it is probably an OS.*

8.   How does the effect of respiration affect the loudness of the P$_2$ and of the OS?
     ANS.:   Inspiration makes the P$_2$ louder (more blood is drawn into the right side of the
             heart with inspiration) and makes the OS softer (blood is withheld from the left
             atrium on inspiration, so that less blood flows through the mitral valve).
                 Note: Since all sounds will tend to become softer on inspiration high on the
                 chest the P$_2$ can only be expected to become louder on inspiration at the left
                 lower sternal border.

9.   How does the effect of lung expansion between stethoscope and heart add or subtract from
     the effect of inspiration on the OS?
     ANS.:   It adds to it; i.e., it exaggerates the inspiratory decrease in the loudness of the OS.

10. When will an A$_2$ be confused with an OS?
     ANS.:   If there is a reversed or paradoxical split due to left bundle branch block (LBBB),
             so that the A$_2$ follows the P$_2$. This is because in LBBB, the reversed split may be
             wide and
             a) Both an A$_2$ and an OS become louder on expiration.
             b) Not only does a reversed split widen on expiration, but a 2—OS interval also
                appears to widen on expiration.
                 Note: Only the paradoxical split found in LBBB is widely split enough to be
                 confused with a 2—OS.

11. What makes the 2—OS interval appear to widen on expiration?
     ANS.:   It actually does not widen on expiration, i.e., it is an illusion. The slight move-
             ment of the pulmonary component on expiration is toward the aortic component
             and therefore away from the OS. This gives the illusion of a wide splitting of the
             2—OS interval.

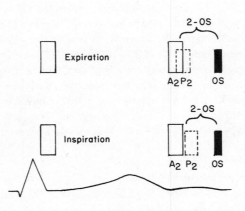

Note that respiration will give the impression of a reversed split, because the P$_2$ moves away from
the OS on expiration and toward the OS on inspiration.

Note: a) A sinus arrhythmia may contribute to widening of the 2—OS on expiration by slowing the heart rate on expiration.

b) Even though the left atrial pressure rises on expiration and should make the 2—OS shorter, the aortic pressure also rises on expiration and so keeps the 2—OS about the same.

COROLLARY 2: A widely split S_2 on inspiration that tends to become wider on expiration is an OS in the absence of a complete LBBB.

COROLLARY 3: If the second component of an S_2 becomes louder on expiration at the left lower sternal border in the absence of a LBBB, it is probably a mitral OS.

12. Can an A_2, P_2, and OS ever be heard as three distinct sounds in one place?

ANS.: Yes, a triple S_2 can often be heard along the left sternal border in MS. This can be recognized by listening for a snare-drum effect or a "trill" with the second sound. This snare-drum triple S_2 is most likely to be heard during inspiration, when the P_2 pulls away from the A_2. But occasionally the OS is so soft that it can only be heard on expiration, and if the split second sound A_2—P_2 happens to remain split on expiration, you will only hear the snare-drum or trill effect on expiration.

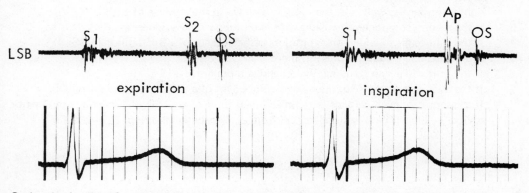

On inspiration, the S_2 split opened up into its A_2 and P_2 components. Together with the OS, a triple second sound is heard that produces a snare-drum effect.

Note: A loud OS can make it difficult to appreciate S_2 splitting unless the split is wide. This is known as backward masking [3].

COROLLARY 4: A triple second sound, with the three sounds close enough together to sound like a snare drum, implies the presence of an OS.

13. What effect does standing have on the 2—OS interval? Why?

ANS.: It widens it. The pooling of blood in the legs decreases venous return to the left atrium. This lowers the pressure behind the obstructed mitral valve. You have already learned why a low pressure in the left atrium makes a wide 2—OS interval.

14. What effect does standing have on the A_2—P_2 interval? Why?

ANS.: The A_2—P_2 interval either remains the same or narrows [18]. The reason for this is covered on page 195. However, in brief, although there is a decrease in volume to both ventricles, the RV responds to the decrease more than does the LV.

COROLLARY 5: A split second sound that becomes wider on standing has an OS as its second component.

15.   Why should the presence of an OS imply that one should hear a snapping first sound?

ANS.:   The stiffness and doming of the valve that made the OS should also make a snapping S_1. In other words, an OS of the mitral valve usually also has a "closing snap" of the mitral valve.

Note: A loud S_1 may be present even with a completely immobile mitral valve, although it will not probably be snapping or short. Therefore, a loud S_1 does not imply the presence of an OS, but a soft S_1 denies the presence of an OS.

COROLLARY 6: If the S_1 is very soft or only a low-pitched thud, the second component of S_2 is not likely to be an OS.

*16.   How can you separate a 2—OS without changing the A_2—P_2 interval or left atrial pressure?

ANS.:   Raise aortic pressure with a vasopressor agent (either phenylephrine or methoxamine). This has almost no effect on the A_2—P_2 interval except in the presence of an ASD. A slow rate in ASD will widen the A_2—P_2 interval [20].

Summary of Methods of Differentiating an A_2—P_2 from a 2—OS

1.   If the second component of a split S_2 is loudest at the apex, it is an OS.
2.   If the second component of an S_2 is only moderately loud and yet is heard at the second right interspace as well as at the apex, it is an OS in the absence of LBBB.
3.   If the second component increases with expiration in the absence of LBBB, it is an OS.
4.   If the split tends to widen on expiration in the absence of LBBB, it is a 2—OS.
5.   If a triple second sound is present, there is an OS present.
6.   If the split widens on standing, the second component is an OS.
7.   If the S_1 is soft or muffled, the second component of a split S_2 is not a mitral OS.
8.   If a vasopressor agent widens the split in the absence of an ASD, the second component is an OS [20]. (The way to tell an OS from an S_3 is detailed on pp. 237—239.)

*THE TRICUSPID OPENING SNAP

*1.   When will a tricuspid OS be present in the absence of tricuspid stenosis (TS)?

ANS.:   If there is an increased flow through a normal tricuspid valve, e.g.,

a) With an ASD or anomalous pulmonary drainage into the right atrium, partial or complete, the torrential flow may cause a tricuspid OS along the left sternal border, 30—50 msec from the P_2.

Note: The presence of a phonocardiographic tricuspid OS in one study was found only in patients with a pulmonary/systemic flow ratio of 2:1 or more [16].

b) With pulmonary hypertension and tricuspid regurgitation. Whether this is a true tricuspid OS or some other pulmonary artery or RV event has yet to be clarified.

c) With deformed tricuspid valves, as in Ebstein's anomaly, the second component of a widely split S_2 is synchronous with the echocardiographic maximum opening point of the tricuspid valve [6].

*2.   What is the major difference between a mitral and tricuspid OS?

ANS.:   A tricuspid OS becomes louder on inspiration because more blood flows through the tricuspid valve on inspiration. This is important when a tricuspid OS is as loud at the apex area as at the left sternal border due to a huge RV's taking over the usual site of the apex beat.

*3.   Which opens first, the tricuspid or mitral valve?

   ANS.:   The tricuspid valve usually opens first. However, in the presence of MS and TS, the mitral OS usually comes first [10]. This is because when both MS and TS are present, the MS is usually much more severe. Therefore, the mitral OS will occur earlier.

   Note: a) In the presence of mild MS, the tricuspid OS may occur prior to the mitral OS. This is expected in view of the fact that the isovolumic relaxation time of the RV is shorter than that of the LV by about 50–80 msec.

   b) In Ebstein's anomaly, the tricuspid opening snap comes late, presumably because the smaller-than-normal RV is usually a poorly contractile and expansile structure.

*4.   How can you distinguish a tricuspid OS from a widely split A_2–P_2?

   ANS.:   a) Listen for the snare-drum effect of a triple S_2 with the last sound becoming louder on inspiration.

   b) Have the patient stand up and note whether or not the split becomes narrower. An A_2–P_2 may remain the same or become narrower when the patient is standing, but an A_2–tricuspid OS interval either remains the same or becomes wider.

*THE Q–1 AND C–1 INTERVALS

*1.   What is meant by the Q–1 interval?

   ANS.:   It is the time from the onset of the QRS complex to the first major component of the S_1; i.e., it is the Q–M_1 interval. It actually consists of two shorter intervals, namely, the Q–1 and the C–1 intervals. The Q–1 interval is the time between the onset of electrical activity and the onset of mechanical activity of the LV (electro-mechanical interval). This interval varies from 10–70 msec from person to person. In the early literature on the Q_1, the top limit of normal was 50 msec. This was probably because of instrumentation that exaggerated the low frequencies. Thus, the investigators may have been measuring from the Q to the first low-frequency component of the S_1, which would not be considered the M_1 today.

   The C–1 interval is the time between the onset of LV contraction and closure of the mitral valves. This is the preisovolumic contraction period. It is also known as the deformation time.

   Note: a) The C–1 interval is better than the Q–1 interval for assessing MS severity because the C–1 eliminates the unknown factor of the electromechanical interval.

   b) Some factors that control the C–1 interval are

   1) The ability of the LV to contract rapidly and strongly (inotropic state).

   2) The difference between left atrial and LV pressure at the beginning of contraction.

   3) The stiffness or resistance of the mitral valve.

*2.   Why does MS prolong the Q—1 interval?

ANS.:   The stiff mitral valve and the high left atrial to LV pressure gradient forces the LV to rise to a higher pressure before it can close the mitral valve; i.e., the LV has to contract for a longer period of time before it can close the mitral valve.

Note: Some other factors known to prolong the Q—1 are: hypertension; a poorly functioning myocardium; a shunt flow through a VSD or patent ductus arteriosus; and conduction defects, such as right bundle branch block (RBBB), LBBB block, anterior divisional blocks, and Wolff-Parkinson-White preexcitation.

*3.   In MS with atrial fibrillation, how does the Q—1 vary with various diastolic lengths, and how can this variation be used to determine the severity of the MS?

ANS.:   The shorter the previous diastole, the longer the Q—1, because with short diastoles the left atrium cannot empty well through a stenotic valve. This leaves a very high left atrial pressure at the beginning of the next ventricular contraction, and thus the ensuing Q—1 interval will be prolonged. (In patients without MS, atrial fibrillation does not cause significantly different Q—1 intervals.)

If the Q—1 does not become longer after 700-msec cycles, the MS is mild. If the Q—1 requires at least 1-sec cycles to stabilize, it is probably severe.

*The Q—1 Minus the 2—OS Interval

*1.   How can both the Q—1 and the 2—OS intervals be used to make estimation of severity more accurate than either one alone?

ANS.:   Since with increasing severity of MS the Q—1 becomes longer and the 2—OS becomes shorter, the index (Q—1) minus (2—OS) becomes increasingly large as the MS worsens [22]. It has been found that with heart rates between 70 and 80 a (Q—1) minus (2—OS) of at least 20 msec or more always means severe MS [5, 19]. If the index is less than 20 msec, it may or may not be associated with severe MS, because the index may be made invalid by factors that prolong the 2—OS excessively [15].

Another way of using the Q—1 and 2—OS is to correlate the ratio of Q—1 / 2—OS with left atrial mean pressure. One study found the correlation coefficient to be 0.90 [24]. The calculated regression equation was

$$17.8 \ (Q—1)/(2—OS) + 1.33$$

To use the ratio, the systolic blood pressure should not be over 150 mm Hg, and in patients with atrial fibrillation, the heart rate should be between 70 and 90 per minute.

*2.   How can the Q—1 and 2—OS in the presence of atrial fibrillation tell you whether or not the mitral valve is pliable enough to warrant a valvotomy?

ANS.:   If atrial fibrillation is present, patients in whom the Q—1 changes inversely and the 2—OS changes directly with the previous cycle length almost always have a pliable valve. If these intervals are fixed, regardless of cycle length, the valves are likely to be rigid and will require replacement [4].

*THE APEX CARDIOGRAM IN ASSESSING THE
SEVERITY OF MITRAL STENOSIS

*1.   How can you use the C—1, i.e., the C—M_1, interval in helping to diagnose the presence or absence of MS?

ANS.:   C represents the onset of ventricular contraction on the apex cardiogram, and M_1 represents mitral valve closure. Since there is delayed mitral valve closure due to the long time it takes for LV pressure to reach the high left atrial pressure, the C—1 interval should be delayed. If the C—1 interval is less than 30 msec, MS is very unlikely. If, on the other hand, the C—1 interval is over 50 msec in a normotensive patient, MS is likely.

Note: If the patient is hypertensive, the C—1 interval may be as long as 60 msec [13].

*2.   What is the O—F interval? How does MS affect this interval?

ANS.:   The O—F interval is from the O point on the apex cardiogram to the F point. It represents the early rapid filling movement of the LV, and it is shortened by MS. The more severe the MS, the shorter the O—F. If the diameter of the mitral valve is less than 10 mm, the rapid filling wave is absent altogether in two-thirds of patients.

Both the C—1 and the O—F intervals together can be used to assess MS severity. If an index of C—1 minus O—F is used, the higher the number, the more severe the MS. (It is not necessary to correct for heart rate because the C—M_1 is very short, and the O—F is not much affected by heart rate.) A value of —1 or greater suggests severe MS. Even if MR is present, as long as the MS is dominant, a value of —1 suggests that the mitral valve diameter is 1.5 cm or less [14]. It must be realized, however, that the O point is highly dependent on the time constant of the transducer used to record the apex impulse. If the time constant is short, various degrees of differentiation occur. The longer the time constant, the later is the O point after the OS. With an infinite time constant, the O point of the apex cardiogram is simultaneous with the nadir of the LV pressure curve [23]. The above C—1 minus O—F index requires a pulse unit with a time constant of about 1.3 sec.

REFERENCES

1.   Arevalo, F., and Sakamoto, T. On the duration of the isovolumetric relaxation period (IVRP) in dog and man. *Am. Heart J.* 67:651, 1964.

2.   Bayer, O., Loogen, R., and Wolter, H. H. The mitral opening snap in the quantitative diagnosis of mitral stenosis. *Am. Heart J.* 2:234, 1956.

3.   Brandfonbrener, M. Backward masking. *Am. Heart J.* 78:833, 1969.

4.   Cheng, T. O. Phonocardiographic sign for pliability of a stenotic mitral valve. *N. Engl. J. Med.* 286:266, 1972.

5.   Craige, E. Phonocardiographic studies in mitral stenosis. *N. Engl. J. Med.* 257:650, 1957.

6.   Crews, T. L., Pridie, R. B., Benham, R., and Leatham, A. Auscultatory and phonocardiographic findings in Ebstein's anomaly. *Br. Heart J.* 34:681, 1972.

7. Delman, A. J., Gordon, G. M., Stein, E., and Escher, D. J. W. The second sound—mitral opening snap (A_2—OS) interval during exercise in the evaluation of mitral stenosis. *Circulation* 33:399, 1966.
8. Harrison, T. R., Dixon, K., Russel, R. O., Jr., Bidwai, P. S., and Coleman, H. N. The relation of age to the duration of contraction, ejection, and relaxation of the normal human heart. *Am. Heart J.* 67:189, 1964.
9. Luisada, A. A., and Argano, B. Triplication and quadruplication of the second sound. *Chest* 59:316, 1971.
10. Luisada, A. A., Slodki, S. J., and Krol, B. Double (mitral and tricuspid) opening snap in patients with valvular lesions. *Am. J. Cardiol.* 16:800, 1965.
11. Millward, D. K., McLaurin, L. P., and Craige, E. Echocardiographic studies to explain opening snaps in presence of nonstenotic mitral valves. *Am. J. Cardiol.* 31:64, 1973.
12. Nixon, P. G. F., Wooler, G. H., and Radigan, L. R. The opening snap in mitral incompetence. *Br. Heart J.* 22:395, 1960.
13. Oreshkov, V. I. Q—1 or C—1 interval in the diagnosis of mitral stenosis. *Br. Heart J.* 29:778, 1967.
14. Oreshkov, V. I. A new mechanocardiographic index in evaluation of the severity of mitral stenosis: An apexcardiographic study. *Am. Heart J.* 79:789, 1970.
15. Rackley, C. E., Craig, R. J., McIntosh, H. D., and Orgain, E. S. Phonocardiographic discrepancies in the assessment of mitral stenosis. *Arch. Intern. Med.* 121:50, 1968.
16. Rees, A., Farru, O., and Rodriguez, R. Phonocardiographic, radiological, and haemodynamic correlation in atrial septal defect. *Br. Heart J.* 34:781, 1972.
17. Ross, R. S., and Criley, J. M. Cineangiocardiographic studies of the origin of cardiovascular physical signs. *Circulation* 30:255, 1964.
18. Surawicz, B. Effect of respiration and upright position on the interval between the two components of the second sound and between the second sound and opening snap. *Circulation* 16:422, 1957.
19. Surawicz, B., Mercer, C., Chlebus, H., Reeves, J. T., and Spencer, F. C. Role of the phonocardiogram in evaluation of the severity of mitral stenosis and detection of associated valvular lesions. *Circulation* 34:795, 1966.
20. Tavel, M. E., Frazier, W. J., and Fisch, C. Use of phenylephrine in the detection of the opening snap of mitral stenosis. *Am. Heart J.* 77:274, 1969.
21. Uyttenhove, P., VanLoo, A., and Haerens, R. Phonocardiography in mitral stenosis. *Acta Cardiol.* 18:24, 1963.
22. Wells, B. The assessment of mitral stenosis by phonocardiography. *Br. Heart J.* 16:261, 1954. Classic article.
23. Willems, J. L., DeGeest, H., and Kesteloot, H. On the value of apex cardiography for timing intracardiac events. *Am. J. Cardiol.* 28:59, 1971.
24. Yigitbasi, O., Nalbantgil, I., Birand, A., and Terek, A. Q—1/IIA—OS formula for predicting left atrial pressure in mitral stenosis. *Br. Heart J.* 32:547, 1970.

11
The Third Heart Sound

NOMENCLATURE

1. What is the difference between *a* third heart sound and *the* third heart sound?

    ANS.: Any sound after a second sound (S_2) may be *a* third sound, e.g., an opening snap (OS) or a presystolic sound such as the S_4. However, only the specific sound that occurs just after the S_2 near the end of the rapid filling phase of a ventricle (about 120–180 msec [0.12–0.18 sec] after the S_2) should be called *the* third sound. To avoid confusion, we shall call this third sound the S_3.

    Note: 120 msec (0.12 sec) is about the length of time it takes to say "two-three" or "tu-huh" at a leisurely speed.

2. What are other names for the S_3?

    ANS.: A protodiastolic gallop sound, ventricular gallop, early filling gallop sound, and early or rapid filling sound.

3. What is the difference between an S_3 and a ventricular gallop sound?

    ANS.: A gallop cannot be one sound. The word *gallop* must refer to a rhythm or cadence made by at least three sounds in succession. A ventricular gallop is the triple rhythm made by the sequence of the S_1, S_2, and S_3.

4. What is misleading about the word *protodiastolic* in describing the S_3?

    ANS.: a) It was originally coined by Wiggers [16] to represent the time on the aortic pressure pulse between the end of reduced ejection and the closure of the aortic valve. This interval was thought to represent the beginning of ventricular relaxation or diastole. The auscultator defines diastole as the period beginning with aortic valve closure as signaled by the S_2 and not before it.

---

*indicates material that is for electives or fellows in cardiology, or concerns rate phenomena, of interest primarily to cardiologists.

Boldface type indicates that the term is explained in the Glossary.

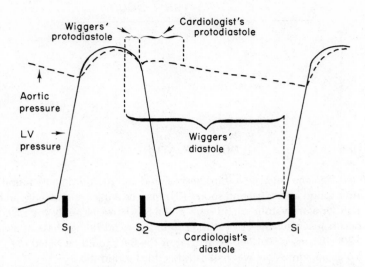

The physiologist considers diastole to begin with the earliest point suggestive of ventricular relaxation or where ejection begins to slacken off. This is not so precise or useful a point as the cardiologist would like, so he considers that diastole begins with the S_2 or the incisura of the arterial pulse.

      b) *Protodiastolic* is used as a synonym for *early diastolic,* yet the prefix *protos* does not mean "early," but means "first." Therefore, the S_4 should be called *hystidiastolic,* from *hystidos* which means "last." Since we do not use such a word for the S_4, it is inconsistent to use Greek nomenclature only for the S_3.

5. What factors besides brevity make the term S_3 preferable to *rapid filling sound*?
   ANS.:   a) The S_4 is also due to rapid filling of the left ventricle (LV) but secondary to atrial contraction.
             b) Only S_3 relates the sound and timing to the S_2.
             c) The pathological S_3 of congestive heart failure may be associated with relatively slow ventricular filling.
             d) The S_3 has been produced in a vigorously contracting dog heart with no blood in it at all [15].

6. How has the meaning of the term *gallop rhythm* changed over the decades?
   ANS.:   It was originally used to describe any rapid series of three or more sounds in the presence of a tachycardia and heart failure. Since this included any extra sounds in systole (systolic gallop) as well as diastole and also eliminated any S_3 with a normal heart rate or without failure, the term *gallop rhythm* has changed its meaning. It now refers to any series of three or more sounds in which the extra sounds occur *only in diastole* and are due to an S_3, or an S_4, or both. Because most physicians cannot tell a gallop from a canter or a trot, some cardiologists prefer *triple* or *quadruple rhythm* to describe a series of sounds with an S_3 or an S_4. The term S_3 or S_4 *gallop,* however, is so universally understood that it may be used without fear of misunderstanding when referring to the rhythm of the usual heart sounds plus a specific extra diastolic sound.

TIMING

1.   Does the ventricle fill most rapidly in early, middle, or late diastole?

     ANS.:   In early diastole. Once the aortic valve closes, the LV expands very rapidly, dur-
             ing which it goes through the stages of **isovolumic relaxation** in about 100 msec
             (0.10 sec) (the time it takes to say "pa-pa" as quickly as possible) and then rapid
             filling. When the mitral valve opens, the ventricle continues its rapid expansion
             phase for about another 60 msec (0.06 sec), until it is suddenly checked by un-
             known forces and the slow expansion phase takes over. The ventricle therefore
             has two rates of expansion: an early quick one and a late slow one.

2.   What percentage of ventricular filling occurs in the early rapid filling phase of diastole in
     comparison with the later slow filling phase of diastole?

     ANS.:   About 80%. After the initial rapid filling, the volume of the ventricle changes
             very little until atrial contraction squeezes the last 20% of blood into the ventricle.

3.   At what point of the rapid filling phase of the LV pressure curve does the S_3 occur?

     ANS.:   At the end of the rapid pressure drop in the LV, i.e., at the point at which the
             rapid expansion changes to the slow expansion phase.

                 Note: There is still some rapid filling occurring after the S_3, presumably due
             to the inertia of the blood mass.

4.   When does isovolumic relaxation begin and end in the LV?

     ANS.:   It begins with aortic valve closure and ends with mitral valve opening. As soon as
             isovolumic relaxation ends and the mitral valve opens, the LV fills rapidly from
             the left atrium.

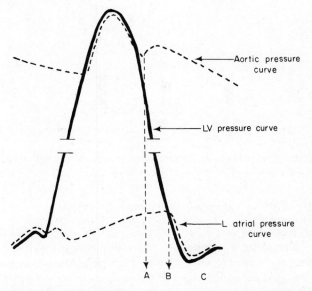

Between point A (aortic valve closure) and point B (mitral valve opening) the volume in the LV
is unchanged. This is therefore the isovolumic relaxation period.

     Note: Normally isovolumic relaxation ranges from about 60—100 msec in
     the LV, and from 30—120 msec in the RV [2].

*5.   What conditions shorten the A_2–S_3 interval?

   ANS.:   Anything that shortens isovolumic relaxation time such as

   a) Constrictive pericarditis.

   b) A sudden increase in venous return to the heart, as when a subject goes from a standing to a recumbent position.

   c) Heart rates over 100 beats per minute.

   Note: The time between the opening of the mitral valve and the S_3 remains relatively constant for all heart rates under 100. Tachycardias shorten the slow filling phase of diastole, but have little effect on the rapid filling phase of ventricular expansion.

6.   In what part of diastole does the S_3 fall, i.e., in the first, middle, or last third?

   ANS.:   In any part, depending on heart rate.

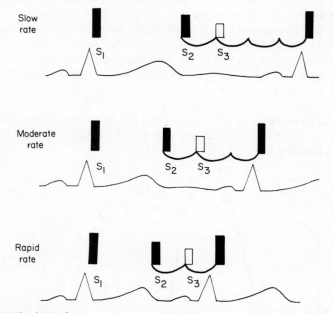

At slow rates (top line) the S_3 is much closer to the S_2 than to the following S_1; i.e., it falls in the first quarter of diastole. At fast rates (bottom line) it may occur in mid-diastole.

MECHANISM OF PRODUCTION

1.   How is the S_3 produced?

   ANS.:   The mechanism is unknown. One useful theory is that it is due to a sudden "pulling short" of the rapidly expanding ventricle by unknown myocardial forces at the end of the rapid expansion phase of the ventricle in early diastole. At the moment of the S_3, the ventricle has stopped rapid expansion, and pressure in the ventricle is no longer falling but becomes relatively stable for about 40 msec (0.04 sec), despite continued rapid filling due to the inertia of the blood mass. Therefore, the S_3 seems to occur at the transition between rapid active and rapid passive ventricular filling [1]. The blood volume in the ventricle at the time of the sudden transition may act as a sudden distending force that causes the sound.

Note: Further proof that the S_3 occurs at the moment of sudden cessation of rapid expansion of the LV is shown by:

    a) A sudden deceleration of the Y descent of the left atrial pressure curve at the time of the S_3 [13].

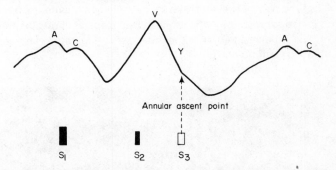

The abrupt change of slope of the Y descent at the time of the S_3 has been called the "annular ascent point" because it was thought to be due to the ascent of the annulus, or atrioventricular valve ring.

    b) Disappearance of the slight pressure gradient between the left atrium and LV at the moment the S_3 occurs. The LV expands faster than it fills during the rapid expansion phase producing this slight pressure gradient, which increases during rapid expansion, to reach a maximum at the time of the S_3. At the moment of the S_3, the gradient is abolished. Only a sudden checking of rapid expansion of the LV could suddenly abolish the pressure gradient.

    c) A sudden change of slope from rapid to slow expansion of the LV at the time of the S_3 has been observed in echocardiograms.

*2. Can a sudden stretch of ventricular muscle or papillary muscle and chordae tendineae produce a heart sound?

ANS.: No sound can be produced if one end of a piece of ventricle is fixed and the other end is suddenly pulled by various amounts of sudden force [4]. This refers to one small piece of muscle. Perhaps this is not true for an entire sphere of ventricular muscle.

A sudden stretch of papillary muscle and chordae can produce a heart sound. This has been shown by the technique just described. It was done under a tank of water with the microphone applied to the tank.

Note: The following is evidence that the S_3 is not caused by a sudden stretch of the papillary muscles and chordae attached to mitral valves.

    a) It can occur with homograft (human cadaver) or heterograft (porcine) replacement of the mitral valves, which necessarily implies that chordae tendineae attachments to the valves are absent [5, 6].

The fact that prosthetic mitral valves (plastic balls or disks) do not usually have S_3s was once used as evidence that chordae tendineae and attachments were necessary to the production of the S_3. However, there is always at least a slight degree of obstruction caused by the prosthetic valve, and the S_3 requires unimpaired flow between atrium and ventricle for its production. When the flow into the LV is increased by a severe paravalvular leak, an S_3 does occur [3].

b) Echocardiography shows that after the mitral valve opens, to initiate the rapid filling phase of ventricular expansion, it flips back into a partially closed position immediately after it has reached its maximum opening probably as a result of eddy currents. (See figure on p. 236.) The S_3 occurs when it is about a fourth of the way between maximum opening and maximum extent of partial closure position, with only a slight change in slope at about the time of the S_3. There is no evidence here that the mitral valve apparatus plays any important role in the production of the S_3.

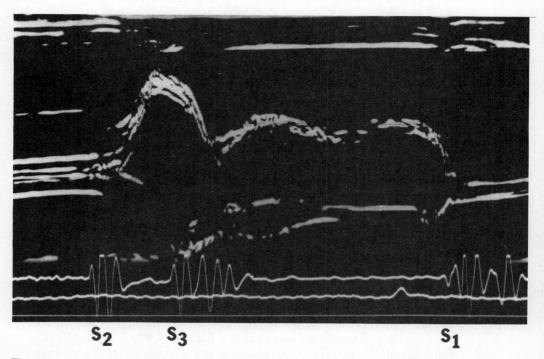

S_2 S_3 S_1

This simultaneous mitral valve echo and low-frequency phonocardiogram was taken at very fast film speed from a 20-year-old man with heart failure and atrial fibrillation due to a severe idiopathic cardiomyopathy. The apical phonocardiogram shows the loud S_3 beginning just before the change of slope in the first closing movement of mitral valve. This man had at times a double S_3 (very rare). However, on the day of this tracing the S_3 was more like a prolonged S_3 or an S_3 followed by a short rumble. (The cause of a split S_3 is unknown.)

*3.   How has it been proved that the S_3 is not produced by either (a) movement of the heart against the chest wall, or (b) a rebound pressure wave reflecting back against the atrioventricular (AV) valves?

ANS.:   a) An S_3 can be heard with direct application of a stethoscope to the heart, even with the chest laid open.

Note: The only time that a sound is produced by the heart striking the chest wall is probably in very rare instances of pericardial effusion, when a systolic thrust of the heart against the chest wall coincides with a loud systolic sound [9].

b) In dogs with empty hearts, an S_3 can be recorded as long as the heart is beating vigorously [15].

4.   What does an apex cardiogram show at the time of the S_3?

ANS.:   A peak of rapid outward movement. (See pp. 124—131 for description of apex cardiogram.)

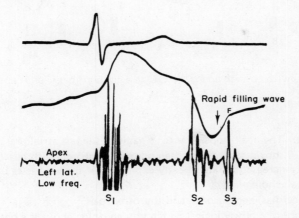

The S_3 occurs at the peak of the rapid filling wave of the apex cardiogram.

THE PHYSIOLOGICAL S_3

1.   Is the physiological S_3 present in all normal subjects?

ANS.:   It is frequently audible in normal subjects under age 30, but it is recordable in most subjects under age 30 on a phonocardiogram near the apex if one can achieve a great enough low-frequency gain (see **frequency**). It is rarely audible or recordable in subjects over age 30. It may persist into the fifth decade in some women.

2.   What cardiovascular conditions tend to produce an audible S_3 in the normal heart?

ANS.:   Anything that increases the velocity of ventricular expansion, such as an increase in flow or sympathetic stimulation.

Note: There is some physiological proof that the more energetic the expansion of the LV, the more likely it is that there will be an S_3.

a) Atrial pressure is normally slightly higher than ventricular pressure at the end of the pre-S_3 part of rapid filling. The S_3 usually occurs only if atrial pressure is *more than slightly* higher than ventricular pressure at this time. The more vigorously the ventricle expands, the greater will be the pressure **gradient** between the left atrium and LV.

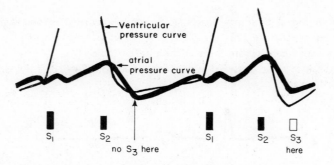

Ventricular pressure curve ←

atrial pressure curve ←

S₁ S₂ S₁ S₂ S₃
        no S₃ here   here

When the LV expands with enough energy to create a gradient between it and the left atrium, an S3 occurs.

   b) The peak slope of V to Y nadir of the left atrial pressure pulse has been shown to be faster than normal in subjects with heart failure and an S3 [14].

3.   What conditions increase the rate of early expansion of the ventricles by means of sympathetic tone or catecholamines?

      ANS.:   Tachycardias, nervousness, and thyrotoxicosis.

4.   Does the presence of a physiological S3 tell you anything about the patient's circulation time?

      ANS.:   Yes, it suggests at least a normal **circulation time.** The same sympathetic tone and catecholamines that are acting on the hearts of these patients to produce the rapid early expansion necessary for the S3 will also increase their cardiac output and thus have an accelerating effect on their circulation time.

5.   What other auscultatory phenomenon is often associated with normal to rapid circulation time?

      ANS.:   A venous hum in the neck is usually present with normal or rapid circulation times, and its presence helps to confirm that the S3 is not associated with heart failure, except in the presence of thyrotoxicosis. The absence of a venous hum has no significance. (See p. 331 for method of eliciting a venous hum.)

6.   When will a tachycardia produce a loud physiological S3 in a patient over age 30 with normal volume flowing through the mitral valve?

      ANS.:   If the rapid filling phase of ventricular expansion is augmented by an atrial contraction. The gallop rhythm that results is then known as a summation gallop. This will occur when the atrial contraction occurs in the early part of diastole, as with marked tachycardias, or with moderate tachycardias plus first-degree atrioventricular (AV) block (long P–R interval).

              Note: It has been calculated that with a P–R of 0.14 sec, a tachycardia of 120 beats per minute may have a summation gallop; with a P–R of 0.16 sec, the summation rate is 115; with a P–R of 0.18, it is 110; and with a P–R of 0.20, it is 105 [8].

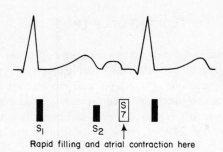

Rapid filling and atrial contraction here

Simultaneous occurrence of atrial contraction and early rapid filling produces a summation sound facetiously called the "S_7" ($S_3 + S_4$). This usually requires a prolonged P–R interval.

7.   How can you tell whether or not a summation gallop is present?

ANS.:   If you can slow the heart rate by carotid sinus pressure, you will lengthen diastole, and the gallop will disappear. This is because slowing the heart rate separates atrial contraction, which is late in diastole, from the rapid filling phase, which is early in diastole.

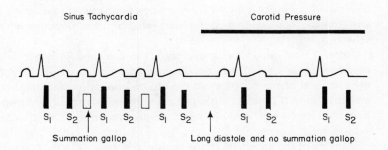

Carotid pressure slows the heart rate and separates the time of atrial contraction from the time of early rapid ventricular filling, thus eliminating a summation gallop. (See also the figure on p. 257.)

8.   Is the summation sound soft or loud?

ANS.:   It is nearly always very loud.

   Note: If a *pathological* S_4 is made louder by occurring during the early rapid filling phase, the rhythm is called an augmented gallop [8]. (See figure on p. 257.) If a physiological or pathological S_3 is made louder by an early atrial contraction, that triple rhythm may also be called an augmented gallop.

LOUDNESS OF THE S₃

1.   What chest piece and degree of stethoscope pressure best bring out the S₃?
     ANS.:   The bell, applied with the lightest possible pressure so that the low frequencies
             will not be damped out. If the S₃ is loud, no amount of pressure will eliminate
             it, since, as a sound becomes louder, it acquires more medium and high frequen-
             cies. If the S₃ is soft, however, even slight pressure with the bell may eliminate
             it. (See Note on p. 249 for the rare exception to the last statement.)

2.   Can an S₃ be made louder by a tachycardia or by bradycardia? Why?
     ANS.:   Tachycardias can make an S₃ louder, because more blood is received by the ven-
             tricle, due to the increased cardiac output that occurs with tachycardias, assuming
             that the rate is not too rapid (a very fast heart rate can actually lower cardiac out-
             put). Also, the catecholamines and sympathetic tone effect on the myocardium
             associated with the tachycardia can cause all myocardial events to be more ener-
             getic.

3.   What increases the loudness of the S₃, inspiration or expiration?
     ANS.:   Either. Expiration can make it louder by
             a) Squeezing blood out of the lungs into the left atrium and ventricle.
             b) Bringing the stethoscope closer to the heart.
             Inspiration can make it louder by increasing sympathetic tone to the heart (**sinus
             arrhythmia**), thus speeding up the heart rate and blood flow through the mitral
             valve.
                 Note: Either inspiration or expiration can make the S₃ louder by causing the
             apex beat to pulsate between the ribs in any particular patient. In some patients,
             the apex beat comes out between the ribs on inspiration, and in others it does so
             on expiration. If it comes out on inspiration one interspace lower than on expira-
             tion, then the S₃ will be louder one interspace lower on inspiration than it is on
             expiration.

4.   Since the proximity of the apex beat to the stethoscope appears to be a factor in intensify-
     ing the S₃, how can you bring the apex beat closer to the chest wall?
     ANS.:   By turning the patient into the **left lateral decubitus position**.

In the left lateral decubitus position
shown, the apex of the heart is brought
as close to the stethoscope as possible.
This is an absolute necessity for hearing
a soft S₃, because it is sensitive to proximity.

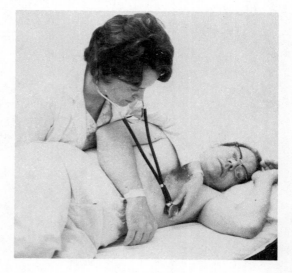

Note: The occasional soft S_3 is heard better with moderate rather than light pressure, usually in chests that make it difficult to place the stethoscope close to the apex beat, due to thick layers of muscle or fat.

5. What proof is there that volume and flow control the audibility of the S_3?

ANS.:   a) All conditions that increase the volume of flow make the S_3 louder; e.g., exercise, having someone hold the subject's legs up, or having the subject in the squatting position.

b) All conditions that decrease flow to the heart cause a decreased audibility of the S_3; e.g., standing up, venous tourniquets, or the water-loss effect of diuretics [10].

Note: One of the characteristics that is most confusing to the beginner when listening to a soft S_3 is its intermittency; i.e., it waxes and wanes in and out of one's hearing threshold. This is probably because the loudness is very sensitive to slight changes in proximity and volume caused by respiration.

THE EXAGGERATED PHYSIOLOGICAL S_3

1. What can exaggerate the physiological S_3?

ANS.:   Any condition that causes an excessive flow through the mitral valve.

Note: The only exception to the rule that excessive flow into the LV exaggerates the physiological S_3 is moderate aortic regurgitation (AR), which does not usually generate an S_3. Chronic, severe AR may or may not produce an S_3. Sudden, severe AR, however, usually does produce an S_3.

2. List the common shunts and the valvular lesion that can cause excessive flow through the mitral valve.

ANS.:   a) Left-to-right shunts, e.g., **ventricular septal defect** (VSD) and **patent ductus arteriosus** (PDA).

b) Incompetent mitral valves, i.e., mitral regurgitation (MR).

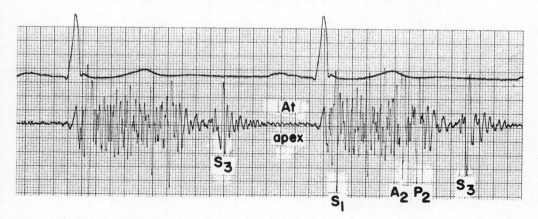

Low-frequency phonocardiogram from a 15-year-old girl with severe rheumatic MR. Besides the loud MR murmur and S_3, note the following: (1) The widely split S_2 (A_2P_2) expected in moderate to severe MR is present. (2) The P_2 is well heard at the apex, and should make you suspect some pulmonary hypertension. The patient's pulmonary artery systolic pressure was 35 mm Hg (upper normal is 25 mm Hg).

3.   Does excessive flow through a tricuspid valve cause a right-sided S_3, i.e., is there a physiological right-sided S_3?

ANS.:   Not usually. The right ventricular S_3 requires not only a large right ventricle (RV) but also a high right atrial pressure. Increased flow alone on the right side is apparently not enough to produce an S_3. For example, in uncomplicated **atrial septal defects** with very large flows through the tricuspid valve, there is usually no S_3. This is probably because the S_3 occurs when there is an abnormal relation between the rate of rapid filling and the ventricle's ability to accommodate its increasing diastolic volume [7]. The normal RV is more compliant than the LV and expands easily to accommodate the increased flow. This presumably eliminates the mechanism for an S_3.

4.   When will a patient with a large VSD or PDA not have an S_3?

ANS.:   If flow is decreased by the development of severe pulmonary hypertension, secondary to a fixed pulmonary artery obstruction, i.e., when an **Eisenmenger reaction** occurs.

5.   When will the pulmonary arterioles react to increased flow by a reflex constriction and so create pulmonary hypertension?

ANS.:   a) If more than three times the normal flow into the lung occurs. This is called "hyperkinetic" pulmonary hypertension.

b) If less than three times the normal flow occurs, but there is a hyperreactive pulmonary vasoconstrictive response to the increased flow.

*6.   How can the detection of an S_3 in the presence of pulmonary hypertension with a VSD or PDA tell you whether the pulmonary hypertension is due to an increased flow (hyperkinetic) or to a fixed irreversible resistance?

ANS.:   The presence of a left-sided S_3 signifies that there is increased flow through the pulmonary valve and that therefore the pulmonary hypertension is hyperkinetic. This means that surgical correction may lower the pulmonary artery pressure to normal [17].

THE PATHOLOGICAL S_3

1.   What are the commonest associated findings in subjects with a pathological S_3?

ANS.:   A high left atrial pressure due to a high V wave, and a large ventricle resulting from a loss of **compliance** or distensibility and a poor **ejection fraction**.

Note: That noncompliance of the ventricle is partly responsible for the occurrence of an S_3 is suggested by its occurrence in a considerable proportion of patients with **hypertrophic subaortic stenosis** (HSS), who have very thick, noncompliant ventricles.

2.   What pathological cardiac condition is generally present when a pathological S_3 occurs in the presence of a high left atrial pressure due to a low ejection fraction?

ANS.:   A **cardiomyopathy**.

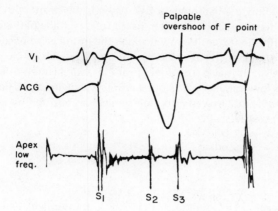

This apex cardiogram and simultaneous apex phonocardiogram is from the same 20-year-old man as in the echocardiogram on p. 228. The pathological S_3 was extremely loud and could be heard anywhere on his chest. It is difficult to say whether it was the overshoot of the rapid filling wave (F point) or the vibrations of the S_3 that was palpable.

THE PHYSIOLOGICAL VERSUS THE PATHOLOGICAL S_3

1. What is the difference in timing and quality between the physiological and pathological S_3?
    ANS.:   None, except that the S_3 found in **constrictive pericarditis** may come earlier than usual.
2. How can you usually tell a physiological from a pathological S_3?
    ANS.:   Only by knowing the circumstances under which it occurs, i.e., by finding the reason for the pathological S_3, such as symptoms and signs of heart failure or of myocardial abnormalities.
    Note: Some patients with a pathological S_3 secondary to a past infarction are relatively asymptomatic, i.e., they do not seem to have the decreased exercise tolerance that is the usual consequence of a high left atrial V wave. The S_3 here may have a different etiology from the usual pathological S_3.
3. Is the physiological S_3 ever as loud as the loudest pathological S_3?
    ANS.:   Almost. Conversely, a pathological S_3 may be very faint.
4. Is the physiological S_3 best heard in areas other than those where pathological sounds are heard?
    ANS.:   No. Both are best heard near the apex area. The rarer RV S_3 is exceptional in that it is best heard more medially unless the RV usurps the usual LV apex area.
5. What is the difference between the physiological and pathological S_3 in their response to pooling of blood in the legs by venous tourniquets or by standing?
    ANS.:   Since it is much more difficult to pool blood in the legs in an edematous patient with a high venous pressure, in the patient in congestive failure, less of an attenuating effect on the S_3 than usual with be shown on standing or when venous tourniquets are applied.

6.   What noise may follow the pathological S$_3$? When is this heard with the physiological S$_3$?
     ANS.:   A short diastolic rumble is often heard following the pathological S$_3$. It is also
             heard with the torrential flow through the mitral valve occurring when the physio-
             logical S$_3$ is exaggerated either by MR or a PDA, which increases flow through the
             mitral valve. It is also sometimes heard in young children following their normal
             S$_3$. This low-frequency diastolic murmur following the S$_3$ occurs while the AV
             valves are rapidly moved into their semiclosed position by eddy currents under
             the mitral leaflets.

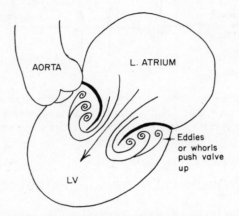

If the flow is fast, eddy currents may push the valve up enough to create a partial obstruction
and so produce turbulent flow and a short diastolic murmur.

             After a pathological S$_3$, the flow under high pressure through a narrowed AV
         valve presumably produces this rumble. Remember that there is still rapid ven-
         tricular filling for a short time after the S$_3$.
             Note: This diastolic murmur following the pathological or physiological S$_3$
         may be mistaken for the murmur of mitral stenosis (MS). (See p. 357 for method
         of distinguishing this murmur from the murmur of mitral stenosis.)

7.   Do high **filling pressures** always mean heart failure?
     ANS.:   No. If it is caused primarily by a high V wave, then the high V wave can be caused
             either by heart failure or by MR. If it is caused primarily by a high A wave, a strong
             left atrial contraction can produce a high A wave at the end of diastole and so
             cause a high filling pressure. Not all high filling pressures mean heart failure, as
             shown by the fact that neither a high V wave due to MS or MR, nor a high A wave
             due to a strong atrial contraction as seen in aortic stenosis, is necessarily associated
             with low ejection fractions.

THE RIGHT VERSUS THE LEFT VENTRICULAR S$_3$

1.   How can you tell a RV from a LV S$_3$?
     ANS.:   a) A RV S$_3$ is louder over the RV area, i.e., near the lower sternal area or epigas-
             trium, unless the ventricle is markedly enlarged, in which case it may be loud
             anywhere on the part of the chest wall that overlies the RV.

b) A RV S_3 is louder on inspiration (more flow into the RV). The LV S_3 may be louder on either inspiration or expiration. (See p. 232 for explanation.)

c) A RV S_3 is associated with a RV heave or rock (see p. 116), a large jugular V wave, and a rapid Y descent.

2. Will increased flow through the tricuspid valve produce a RV S_3?

    ANS.:   No. (See p. 234 for explanation.)

3. List some of the common causes of a RV S_3.

    ANS.:   Right ventricular dilatation and high right atrial pressures, secondary to

    a) Severe tricuspid regurgitation due to pulmonary hypertension.

    b) Sudden RV outflow obstruction, as in massive pulmonary embolism.

    Note: a) Although pulmonary stenosis is also a RV outflow obstruction, it requires severe enough chronic stenosis to produce RV failure before the RV will dilate and cause an S_3 to occur. This is very rare.

    b) A double S_3 can occasionally be heard in patients with severe congestive failure. This is postulated to be due to a combination of a LV and a RV S_3. This is questionable, since both components are often best heard at the site of a LV impulse.

THE S_3 VERSUS THE OPENING SNAP

1. What is the difference between the A_2–OS interval and the A_2–S_3 interval?

    ANS.:   The A_2–OS interval is rarely over 100 msec (0.10 sec), while the smallest A_2–S_3 interval is usually 120 msec (0.12 sec). The difference between 100 and 120 msec is merely the difference between saying "pa-pa" as quickly as possible and saying it at a normal speaking rate.

    Note: There are rare exceptions to both these figures; e.g., the A_2–OS has been seen to be as long as 120 msec, and the S_3 in constrictive pericarditis can come as early as 100 msec after the S_2.

2. How does the quality or pitch of the S_3 help to distinguish it from the OS?

    ANS.:   The S_3 is low in pitch, sounds like a thud or boom, and is best heard with the bell. The OS, on the other hand, is usually a high-frequency, short clicking sound, best recognized with the diaphragm.

    Note: Occasionally, the OS is atypical and deceptively low in pitch. This occurs when the valve is very fibrosed or calcified or if ventricular relaxation is very poor due to severe myocardial damage, resulting in low flow.

3. How does the site of best auscultation help to distinguish the S_3 from an OS?

    ANS.:   An OS is commonly loudest at some point between the apex and the left sternal border, while the S_3 is commonly loudest near the apex.

    Note: Exceptions to this occur when

    a) There is the rare right-sided S_3, which will be loudest along the left sternal border.

    b) There is a large LV. The OS may then be loudest at the apical area.

*4.   Why will pericardial constriction produce an early and loud S_3?

ANS.:   This is the only condition in which, despite normal AV valves, there is a high-pressure V wave in the atrium proximal to a ventricle that is neither dilated nor reduced significantly in function. Since the ventricle is restricted in its extent of expansion, it reaches its maximum rapid expansion state early, and the high filling pressure causes it to expand with more energy and to generate a loud sound. There is also some suggestion from systolic time interval studies that in constrictive pericarditis there is an excessive catecholamine effect on the LV.

Note: On cineangiograms of patients with constrictive pericarditis, this early filling of the LV is seen to be accomplished with exceptional rapidity.

5.   What has the loud S_3 of pericardial constriction been called? Why?

ANS.:   A pericardial knock, because it is very loud.

Note: a) The pericardial knock is not usually present in **tamponade**. However, in patients with the effusive-constrictive type of pericarditis (see p. 63 for explanation), the pericardial knock is usually present.

*b) Although the usual pericardial knock is early, i.e., 100—110 msec after the A_2, the knock may come at the usual S_3 time, i.e., at 120 msec after the A_2, presumably due to a concomitant cardiomyopathy that slows up early ventricular expansion.

6.   How may the quality of the S_1 help to verify whether it is an S_3 or an OS that you hear after the S_2?

ANS.:   An OS is almost always associated with a snapping first sound, i.e., it is short and high-pitched (the closing snap). Therefore, a soft or muffled first sound tends to deny the presence of an OS and confirms that the extra sound is an S_3.

*Note: Unfortunately, constrictive pericarditis is frequently associated with a loud S_1, thus making the early pericardial knock seem even more like an OS [11].

7.   Why may both an OS and an S_3 be present in the same person?

ANS.:   If a healthy, mobile septal (anterior) leaflet is associated with a mural (posterior) leaflet that is thickened, immobile, rolled on itself, and held to the ventricular wall by short, thick chordae, it will allow severe MR and an S_3, while the normal septal leaflet produces an OS [12].

8.   What is the rhythm of an S_1 followed by an S_2, OS, and S_3? Can you make a rhythmic phrase that fits?

ANS.:   Tum   Tu Du Boom   Tum   Tu Du Boom
           1   2   OS   3   1   2   OS   3

*9.   How can an apex cardiogram help to tell an S_3 from an OS?

ANS.:   The OS will fall near the O point, and the S_3 near the peak, of the early filling phase of the apex cardiogram. (See figures on pp. 229 and 345.)

*10.   What is meant by a "tumor plop"?

ANS.:   A left (or right) atrial myxoma attached to a stalk can prolapse through the mitral (or tricuspid) valve in diastole. If it does, it may cause an early diastolic sound that occurs either at the time of an OS or of an S_3. It may be intermittent, vary in loudness, and even vary its time relationship to the second sound [7]. It may differ from an S_3 even if it occurs at the same interval from the A_2 as the usual S_3 by being

a) Louder than expected.

b) More easily heard at the left lower sternal border than expected. (An S_3 is not usually heard at the left lower sternal border unless it is extremely loud.)

Summary of How to Tell an S_3 from an Opening Snap

1. The OS is not usually over 100 msec (0.10 sec) (a rapid "pa-pa") from the S_2. The S_3 is rarely less than 120 msec (0.12 sec) from the S_2 (usually 140 [0.14 sec] msec).
2. The OS is usually a short, sharp click, best heard with the diaphragm; the S_3 is a thud or boom, best heard applying light pressure with the bell.
3. The OS is usually best heard between the apex and the left lower sternal border. The S_3 is almost always best heard at the apex.
4. The OS is always associated with a sharp, loud S_1. The S_3 may or may not have a loud S_1.
*5. An apex cardiogram will show the OS occurring at or near the O point, while the S_3 occurs at or near the peak of the rapid filling wave, or F point.
6. An OS will separate further from the A_2 on standing. An S_3 will not change its distance from the A_2 on standing.

THE S_3 AND MITRAL STENOSIS

1. Why would a left ventricular S_3 not be expected in significant MS?
   ANS.:   Mitral valve obstruction prevents rapid filling of the LV in early diastole, despite a high left atrial pressure. Without rapid early filling, there is usually no S_3.
2. How can you distinguish the S_3 from the occasionally explosive beginning of a diastolic murmur due to MS?
   ANS.:   If the diastolic murmur following the loud sound extends throughout diastole, it is probably a loud beginning to an MS murmur. The length of the diastolic mur- * mur reflects the continuous high gradient, plus a fair flow throughout diastole. The beginning of the murmur is loud presumably because it reflects the high gradient, a good flow, and probably good LV function; i.e., the LV can expand rapidly. This means that if the history and physical examination suggest a low output state, the loud beginning to the murmur is probably due to an S_3. Poor flow is incompatible with a loud beginning to a murmur due to significant MS.

   Note: In the French literature, the loud S_3-like beginning to the diastolic murmur has been called the "initial jerk" of the MS murmur.
3. When may an actual S_3 be heard in MS?
   ANS.:   a) If the right atrial pressure is high and the RV is dilated due to pulmonary hypertension and congestive failure, one may hear a *right* ventricular S_3. If the RV, in its enlargement, usurps the apex area, the S_3 may be heard well in the middle of the left thorax and may be mistaken for a LV S_3.
   b) If the MS is trivial and the dominant condition is MR or perhaps a rheumatic cardiomyopathy.

REFERENCES

1. Arevalo, F., Meyer, E. C., MacCanon, D. M., and Luisada, A. A. Hemodynamic correlates of the third heart sound. *Am. J. Physiol.* 207:319, 1964.
2. Arevalo, F., and Sakamoto, T. On the duration of the isovolumetric relaxation period (IVRP) in dog and man. *Am. Heart J.* 67:651, 1964.
3. Coulshed, N., and Epstein, E. J. Third heart sound after mitral valve replacement. *Br. Heart J.* 34:301, 1972.

4. Dock, W. The forces needed to evoke sounds from cardiac tissues, and the attenuation of heart sounds. *Circulation* 19:376, 1959.

5. El Gamal, M., and Smith, D. R. Occurrence of a left ventricular third heart sound in incompetent mitral heterografts. *Br. Heart J.* 32:497, 1970.

6. Gianelly, R. E., Popp, R. L., and Hultgren, H. N. Heart sounds in patients with homograft replacement of mitral valve. *Circulation* 42:309, 1970.

7. Goldschlager, A., Popper, R., Goldschlager, N., Gerbode, F., and Prozan, G. Right atrial myxoma with right to left shunt and polycythemia presenting as congenital heart disease. *Am. J. Cardiol.* 30:82, 1972.

8. Grayzel, J. Gallop rhythm of the heart. *Circulation* 20:1053, 1959.

9. Kay, C. F., Joyner, C. R., Helwig, J., Jr., and Raymond, T. F. The "late systolic heartbeat" of pericardial effusion. *Am. Heart J.* 72:7, 1966.

10. Leonard, J. J., Weissler, A. M., and Warren, J. V. Modification of ventricular gallop rhythm induced by pooling of blood in the extremities. *Br. Heart J.* 20:502, 1958.

11. Moreyra, E., Knibbe, P., and Segal, B. L. Constrictive pericarditis masquerading as mitral stenosis. *Chest* 57:245, 1970.

12. Nixon, P. G. F., Wooler, G. H., and Radigan, L. R. Mitral incompetence caused by disease of the mural cusp. *Circulation* 19:839, 1959.

13. Radner, S. Left atrial pressure curve: Significance of annular ascent wing. *Acta Med. Scand.* 159:219, 1957.

14. Shah, P. M., and Yu, P. N. Gallop rhythm hemodynamic and clinical correlation. *Am. Heart J.* 78:823, 1969.

15. Smith, J. R. Observations on the mechanism of the physiologic third heart sound. *Am. Heart J.* 28:661, 1944.

16. Wiggers, C. J. Studies on the consecutive phases of the cardiac cycle. *Am. J. Physiol.* 56:415, 1921.

17. Wood, P. The Eisenmenger syndrome or pulmonary hypertension with reversed central shunt. *Br. Med. J.* 2:701, 755, 1958. Classic article.

12
The Fourth Heart Sound

NOMENCLATURE

1. What are some of the names given for the triple rhythm produced by the sequence of fourth heart sound (S_4), the S_1, and S_2?

    ANS.:   An atrial gallop, a presystolic gallop, or an S_4 gallop.

2. What is misleading about the term *atrial gallop*?

    ANS.:   It implies that the atrium itself is the source of the extra sound. The contraction of the atrium itself is actually not audible with the stethoscope.

3. What is misleading about the term *presystolic gallop*?

    ANS.:   A gallop produced by a third heart sound (S_3) can be "presystolic" during a tachycardia, because with rapid rates the first sound follows very shortly after the S_3.

4. What is the advantage of the term *S_4 gallop*?

    ANS.:   It specifies exactly which extra sound is thought to be producing the triple rhythm, regardless of any vagaries of diastolic length and without reference to exact mechanisms. It also separates it best from the S_3 gallop and suggests where the extra sound ought to be found in relation to the first heart sound (S_1), the second heart sound (S_2), and the third heart sound (S_3). It also enables you to refer to the single sound of S_4 without the necessity of always using the term *gallop,* which requires that you mean at least three sounds.

*THE INAUDIBLE S_4 COMPONENT

*1. Does atrial muscle itself produce vibrations as it contracts?

    ANS.:   Yes, but they are inaudible, because they are too low in frequency and amplitude. They can be picked up by special phonocardiographic techniques, e.g., by placing a phonocatheter inside the atrium and in the esophagus.

     Note: The interval from the onset of the P to the onset of the audible S_4 (henceforth simply called the S_4) averages 160 msec (120—200 msec). It therefore occurs about 40 msec after the inaudible component, which occurs at an average of 120 msec after the onset of the P (80—120 msec range).

---

* indicates material that is for electives or fellows in cardiology, or concerns rare phenomena, of interest primarily to cardiologists.

Boldface type indicates that the term is explained in the Glossary.

*2.   In what condition may each contraction of an atrium by itself cause an audible sound?

ANS.:   a) In complete atrioventricular (AV) block or junctional rhythm. Atrial vibrations can sometimes be recorded during systole as the atrium contracts against closed AV valves.

b) In some cases of atrial flutter, clicking sounds, maximal at the base of the heart, occur just after each F wave [10]. They can be heard during both systole and diastole and may become increasingly louder during diastole. These sounds tend to become inaudible with the treatment of congestive heart failure.

Since the only chamber in which such sounds can be recorded by intracardiac phonocatheter is in the atrium, they would appear to represent some effect of atrial contraction itself [29]. They have even been heard during flutter-fibrillation, and it has been postulated in this instance that coarse atrial fibrillation occurred in one atrium and activated the other atrium in a slow, almost regular manner [30].

THE AUDIBLE S_4

Mode of Production

1.   Where is the audible S_4 best recorded by an intracardiac phonocatheter, in the atrium or in the ventricle?

ANS.:   In the ventricle.

2.   What does the apex cardiogram show at the time of the S_4?

ANS.:   A hump just before the systolic outward impulse. This presystolic hump is often large enough to be palpable and is called an A wave, or atrial hump. Since the designation of A wave is used for a jugular wave, we shall henceforth use the term *atrial hump* when referring to this hump on the apex cardiogram.

Note: a) The peak of the atrial hump coincides with the largest vibrations of the S_4.

b) An S_4 or atrial hump never occurs in the presence of atrial fibrillation.

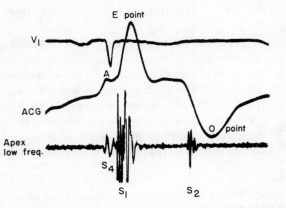

Apex cardiogram and phonocardiogram from a 50-year-old man with a previous infarction. The S_4 is simultaneous with a large palpable atrial hump (A wave) on the apex cardiogram.

Note: The A wave is 15% of the total apex pulse amplitude, or vertical E to 0 distance. Atrial humps of 15% or more of the E—0 amplitude are usually palpable.

3.   What causes this atrial hump or end-diastolic outward movement on the apex cardiogram?

ANS.:   It is the effect of left atrial contraction, causing a slight increase in the volume of the left ventricle (LV) at the end of diastole. This slight increase in volume before the ventricle contracts can be seen on a cineangiogram with contrast material in the LV, even in normal subjects.

Note: The atrial hump grows at the expense of the systolic ejection bulge. An atrial hump of over 12% of the total apex cardiogram movement is probably abnormal, and if it is 14% or more, it will probably be palpable [12]. (See figures on pp. 242 and 252.)

*4.   Is the pressure in the atrium at the time of the atrial contraction higher or lower than in the ventricle at the time of the simultaneous atrial hump producing the S_4?

ANS.:   The atrial A wave pressure is higher than LV atrial hump pressure at the time of the S_4 [26].

Note: a)   An atrial hump may be palpable even when the S_4 may be too low in frequency to be audible. On the other hand, a pathological S_4 may be heard in the absence of a palpable atrial hump. This is obvious when you realize that only a chest that allows an apex beat to be easily palpated will allow you to palpate the atrial hump, yet the S_4 sound may still be heard. There are many cardiologists who believe that you should never call an S_4 pathological unless you can find a palpable atrial hump with it [36]. If you follow this teaching, you will misinterpret every pathological S_4 in which the apex beat is difficult to palpate.

b)   Although the S_4 and peak of the atrial hump on the usual apex cardiogram are simultaneous, they both occur on the upslope of the atrial hump of the simultaneous LV pressure curve. The greater the loss of compliance of the LV, the lower does the S_4 occur on the atrial hump of the LV pressure curve [31]. This may be due to different time constants of the transducers used for apex cardiograms and for LV pressure curves [39].

5.   Can an audible S_4 be produced by an atrium contracting against a stenotic atrioventricular (AV) valve as in mitral stenosis (MS)?

ANS.:   No.

Note: The atrium must be able to transmit its pressure freely to the LV, or else only a presystolic murmur will be heard.

6.   How can atrial contraction prevent the AV valves from moving into the ventricles?

ANS.:   By the flow through the valves, causing eddy currents that curl around the underside of the valves and push them upward (see figure on p. 236). Thus, although atrial contraction can open the valves, eddy currents limit the extent to which the valves can be pushed into the downward position, and they even tend to cause valve closure.

Note: Echocardiograms show that after atrial contraction opens the valves, they rise immediately to a semiclosed position presumably due to eddy currents.

7.   What theory could account for the production of the audible S_4 if it (a) occurs at the peak of atrial contraction, (b) causes such an increase in LV end-diastolic volume that it produces a recordable and often palpable systolic outward movement, (c) occurs when atrial pressure is higher than ventricular pressure, (d) sounds the same as an S_3, (e) cannot occur if the AV valves are closed or stenotic?

ANS.:   Atrial contraction, by causing eddy currents on the undersurface of the AV valves, tends to hold them upward. However, since atrial contraction also raises the volume in the ventricle, there is stretching of the chordae tendineae and papillary muscles at exactly the same time that the AV valves are being pulled or held in the opposite direction. If it has enough energy, this tug on the chordae and papillary muscles could account for the sound.

AIDS TO RECOGNIZING THE RHYTHM OF THE S_4 GALLOP

If you remember that the P wave indirectly produces the S_4, and the QRS produces the S_1, then if you know that the S_2 occurs at the end of the T, the rhythm of S_4, S_1, and S_2 is the same as P, QRS, and end of T.

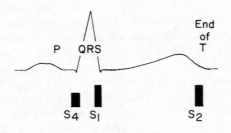

If you realize that the T wave is a *systolic* event, it will be easy to remember that the S_2 comes at the end of the T wave. Thus, the rhythm of an S_4 gallop is the rhythm symbolized by P, R ――― T, where R represents the QRS complex and T represents the end of the T.

Since the P is closer to the QRS than the QRS is to the end of the T, the rhythm or cadence is a pair of sounds close together followed by a pause, then the second sound. Therefore, the rhythm of two cycles would be: 4―1――――2   4―1――――2.

Vocal imitation of the heart sounds can help you in perceiving the actual phenomena. Since the S_4 is low-pitched, you should practice imitating the S_4―S_1 ――――S_2 by saying "huh-one――――two." Place the "huh" as closely as possible to the "one," so that they are practically one word, "Huh-one." Also, say the "huh" as softly as possible, because the S_4 is often just within the realm of audibility and in fact like the S_3, tends to disappear in and out of consciousness from beat to beat when it is soft.

THE PHYSIOLOGICAL S_4

1.   Can an S_4 be heard in normal subjects?

ANS.:   It can occasionally be heard in some normal subjects in all age groups. However, it is so rarely normal that unless it is heard in a young person with a concomitant physiological S_3, or in an athlete with physiological hypertrophy, you should suspect that it is an abnormal finding.

Note: Almost all tall athletes (e.g., basketball professionals) have a physiological S_4. It can be recorded in almost two-thirds of young boys with a high-gain, low-frequency phonocardiogram [5]. It can be recorded in 35–70% of apparently normal subjects over age 40 [2, 33]. This may only mean that different equipment has different recording capabilities for low frequencies and does not necessarily mean that these vibrations are audible. Since in a third of patients in one series of asymptomatic patients over age 40 with a recorded S_4 the maximal treadmill test results were positive, it is questionable how often a physiological S_4 is heard in perfectly normal hearts in persons over age 40 [2].

2.   Why is the physiological S_4 so rarely heard?

ANS.:   a) It is usually too soft and too low in frequency of vibrations.

b) It is often too close to the S_1 to be separated from it by ear. It is then called the atrial component of the S_1 and it will be seen on a simultaneous phonocardiogram and ECG to begin with or after the QRS.

*3.   What is the mechanism of the physiological S_4?

ANS.:   It seems at first to be the same as the pathological S_4, because both occur at about the same time. The normal atrium, however, may contract in a peristaltic fashion toward the ventricle. Therefore, by the time atrial contraction has caused the ventricle to reach its peak pressure, most of the atrium is relaxed and has a low pressure. This reversal of pressure at the AV valves will tend to close them, pull on the chordae tendineae, and so produce a sound [19]. This peristaltic atrial movement is probably not present in a hypertrophied, strongly contracting atrium and cannot yet be considered to cause the pathological S_4.

Note: A first-degree AV block often produces an S_4 in the absence of apparent heart disease, probably by the method suggested above; i.e., by raising pressure in the LV enough to reverse the pressure gradient across the mitral valve, producing a sudden upward movement of the valve and a tug on chordae tendineae and papillary muscles [17]. (See pp. 247 and 248.)

THE PATHOLOGICAL S_4

Causes and Associated Conditions

1.   After what age is an S_4 gallop most likely to be pathological?

ANS.:   After age 20. You should, however, consider any S_4 possibly pathological, even in a young subject, until proved otherwise. This means that before you call it physiological in the younger age group, you should probably hear a physiological S_3 and a physiologically split S_2, feel a normal apex beat, perhaps hear a venous hum in the neck without having to elicit it by marked head turning (see p. 331), and obtain normal ECG and chest x-ray findings.

2.   What kind of atrial contraction is necessary for the production of an audible S_4?

ANS.:   A strong atrial contraction is the most important requirement for an audible S_4.

3.   What condition generates a strong atrial contraction?

ANS.:   Any condition in which the ventricle is "stiffer" than normal, i.e., in which the ventricle has decreased distensibility or **compliance**.

4.   How could loss of distensibility of a ventricle cause a strong atrial contraction, i.e., how does the atrium "know" that it must contract more strongly when the ventricle has lost compliance?

ANS.:   The left atrium and ventricle are one chamber in diastole, i.e., while the mitral valve is open. Therefore, whatever pressure changes occur in one chamber during diastole also occur in the other chamber. It may be called an "atrioventricle" during diastole. If the LV is poorly distensible, as with left ventricular hypertrophy (LVH), the pressure rise due to filling of the atrioventricle from the pulmonary veins is steep. By the time the P wave and its subsequent atrial contraction occur, the atrial pressure is so high that it has a strong **Starling effect**, and the atrium will contract with greater energy than normal. (See figure on p. 111.)

5.   What conditions cause a decreased compliance of the ventricle?

ANS.:   Those in which the ventricle is
   a) Thickened by LVH, as when it is laboring under a chronic **pressure load**.
   b) Stiffened by replacement of myocardium by fibrous tissue or infiltrate, e.g., amyloid heart disease or an old myocardial infarction.
   c) Stiffened by **ischemia** due to angina or acute infarction.

6.   What is the commonest cause of LVH in which an S_4 is heard?

ANS.:   Hypertension.

7.   How can a strong atrial contraction at the end of diastole cause a stronger contraction in a poorly compliant ventricle?

ANS.:   By forcing blood into the ventricle just before the ventricle contracts. This causes an extra stretch of the ventricular myocardium, and Starling's law tells us that such an extra stretch will give a stronger contraction; i.e., increase in end-diastolic volume will increase the energy of the subsequent contraction.

*8.   Why will a patient whose filling pressure is elevated by a strong atrial contraction be less dyspneic than the patient who has the same high filling pressure due to a high V wave?

ANS.:   A high A wave starting from a low left atrial pressure and trough will result in a lower mean left atrial pressure than will a high V wave falling to a high Y trough.

   Note: This implies that a patient with an S_4 is less likely to be dyspneic than one with an S_3.

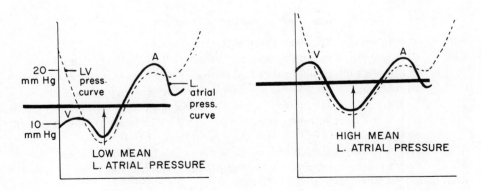

A low V wave and a disproportionately high A wave are seen on the left. These give a lower mean left atrial pressure and therefore less dyspnea than do both a high V wave and a relatively poor atrial contraction, as seen on the right.

9.   What can prevent the effect of even a strong left or right atrial contraction from being transmitted to their respective ventricle?

ANS.:   Mitral or tricuspid stenosis.

Note: If the mitral obstruction is due to a left atrial myxoma, an S_4 can occur. This is presumably either because the sound is due to some effect of atrial contraction on the tumor, or because the atrial contraction can transmit its pressure to the LV via the atrial tumor.

10.   What makes an atrium in sinus rhythm too weak to help out a ventricle?

ANS.:   a) If it is too large, as in chronic severe rheumatic mitral regurgitation (MR), the atrium may be overstretched and therefore contract less efficiently. This can also occur when the left atrium is severely damaged by myocarditis, infarction, or infiltrate. It may be the damage rather than the enlargement that prevents an efficient contraction under these circumstances.

b) If there is excess vagal stimulation [18].

c) If there is too little blood in the atrium, i.e., decreased venous return due to either diuresis or standing the patient up.

*11.   How can you distinguish clinically and by phonocardiogram between the physiological and the pathological S_4 that is very close to the S_1?

ANS.:   a) Pressure on the carotid sinus does not change the intensity or position of the physiological S_4, but will cause the pathological S_4 to fade or disappear into the S_1.

b) If the S_4 is over 70 msec from the S_1, it is likely to be a pathological S_4 [5].

12.   How can the S_4 assist in the diagnosis of **constrictive pericarditis** or **tamponade**? Explain.

ANS.:   An S_4 is not heard in constriction or tamponade. This seems surprising at first, since in tamponade the pressure rises high quickly in the "atrioventricle" during diastole, and you would think that the stretch of the atrium would stimulate it to contract strongly. On the other hand,

a) The inability of the ventricle to expand at the end of diastole due to the constriction could account for the loss of the forces necessary for an S_4.

b) The LV pressure rises so high at the end of diastole that the left atrium may not be able to open the mitral valve well.

c) The atrium may be tethered with the constriction, so that it cannot contract well.

*THE DOUBLE S_4

*1.   What mechanism can approximate the AV valves during atrial relaxation?

ANS.:   When the atrium relaxes after its systole, the pressure inside the atrium decreases. At this time, however, the ventricle is not relaxing, and there is a momentary reversal of pressure gradient; i.e., the pressure in the ventricle is momentarily higher than that in the atrium. This naturally causes the AV valves to come closer together and perhaps even to close if there is enough time in diastole before ventricular contraction. This closure movement may produce a sound.

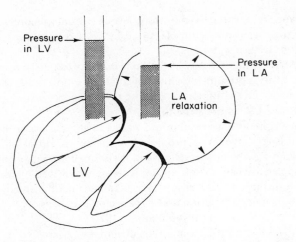

The higher pressure in the LV relative to that in the left atrium (LA) caused by atrial relaxation can "push" the mitral valves upward and may produce a sound.

*2.   When is this valve closure sound audible?
      ANS.:   a) If first-degree AV block is present, i.e., when there is a long P—R interval.
              b) If second-degree or complete AV block is present, i.e., when there is no QRS
                 at all after some P waves [6].
                 Note: This second method of AV valve closure is probably a different mechanism than that for the pathological S_4 as suggested by
              a) The atrial pressure is higher than ventricular pressure at the time of the usual
                 pathological S_4, but lower than ventricular pressure at the time of the second
                 S_4 component in complete AV block in both animals and man. (See figure.)
              b) In complete AV block with heart damage, split S_4 sounds are frequently audible,
                 with the first component at the usual distance of an S_4 and the second one
                 200 msec or more from the P wave.
              c) The P—S_4 interval of the pathological S_4 is rarely more than 180 msec. The
                 P—S_4 interval in complete AV block is usually about 200 msec or more.
                 (P—S_4 intervals have a range of 120—200 msec.)

The S_4 in Myocardial Infarction and Angina

1.   What proportion of patients with acute myocardial infarction have an S_4?
      ANS.:   Almost all will have a phonocardiographic S_4 unless they have MS, or atrial infarction, or faint sounds due to impending death. It is heard by auscultation in about
              a half of patients during the first few days following infarction [35]. Although
              this hyperacute S_4 may disappear, it will rarely ever do so if present beyond the
              first few days.
2.   How could you explain the frequent S_4 heard in the first few days of myocardial infarction?
      ANS.:   The infarcted area, whether dyskinetic (bulges out like an **aneurysm** in systole)
              or akinetic (no movement during systole) should not cause a loss of compliance
              of the LV, although one study claims that it does [20]. Therefore, we must assume
              that in the first few days of infarction, the ischemia, or the excess catecholamines, or
              both together can cause a loss of compliance of the LV [9].

3.   Why may angina patients have an S_4 only during an attack of angina?
      ANS.:   There is a marked increase in stiffness of the LV during angina, both at the
                beginning and end of diastole [3].

The S_4 in Volume Overloads

1.   When is ventricular enlargement usually associated with a normally compliant ventricle
      and therefore with an absent S_4?
      ANS.:   When there are chronic volume overloads due to regurgitant or shunt flows, e.g.,
                in **ventricular septal defect** (VSD), **patent ductus arteriosus**, chronic aortic
                regurgitation (AR), and chronic MR secondary to disease of the valve itself.
                      Note: An S_4 can, however, occur with a volume overload if there is a *relative*
                loss of compliance of the LV in situations in which there is increased flow to the
                LV not due to a shunt or regurgitant flow. This occurs in hyperthyroidism,
                thyrotoxicosis, or severe anemia [1]. Here, the loss of compliance may be due
                to the effect of catecholamines on a volume-overloaded LV. Excessive catechol-
                amines are not found in ventricles overloaded by uncomplicated chronic shunts
                or regurgitation.
2.   When in MR will there be an S_4?
      ANS.:   When the MR is
                a) Secondary to papillary muscle dysfunction or dilatation due to fibrosis or
                    ischemia.
                b) Sudden and severe due to a ruptured chorda in an otherwise normal heart, so
                    that the atrium enlarges only moderately.
                      Note: In rheumatic, chronic MR uncomplicated by chordae rupture, there is
                almost never a left-sided S_4.

LOUDNESS AND AUDIBILITY OF THE S_4

1.   Where is the LV S_4 usually best heard?
      ANS.:   At the apex, in the **left lateral decubitus position**.
                      Note: The LV S_4 is occasionally better heard at the left lower sternal border
                than at the apex. The reason for this is unknown, but it occurs mostly in patients
                with angina or a past history of infarction [37].
2.   Why should you usually use a bell to bring out the S_4?
      ANS.:   Most of the energy of the S_4 (as with the S_3) is in the low-frequency range. The
                diaphragm is designed to dampen low frequencies.
                      Note: An S_3 or S_4 may occasionally best be heard with a diaphragm type of
                chest piece or with firm bell pressure. This happens because
                a) When the S_3 or S_4 is loud, high frequencies develop, and attenuating the low
                    frequencies by firm bell pressure can sharpen the perception of the extra
                    sounds by helping to separate them from the S_1 or S_2, especially during
                    tachycardias [28].
                b) When the S_4 is soft and a thick or obese chest hides the apical movements,
                    pressure may cause them to strike the bell of the stethoscope and will bring
                    out an almost inaudible S_3 or S_4.

3.   What are the pitfalls of using held expiration to bring the stethoscope closer to the heart in order to help hear the S_4?
     ANS.:   After a few beats the venous return will decrease. The soft S_4 is very sensitive to venous return. Remember that the lungs act like a pump and help to speed up the circulation time.

4.   How can S_4 gallops be made louder?
     ANS.:   a) By increasing the flow to the atrium.
             b) By increasing the need for a stronger atrial contraction.
             c) By bringing ventricular movements closer to the stethoscope.

5.   How can you increase the flow to the atrium besides having the patient exercise?
     ANS.:   a) By holding the patient's legs up or having him flex his knees. Unfortunately, the supine position for these maneuvers will attenuate the S_4 by causing the heart to fall away from the chest wall.
             b) By a post-**Valsalva** increase in flow.
             c) By having the patient cough. This is really another form of exercise, as well as a Valsalva maneuver.
             d) By having the patient squat. This increases cardiac output for a few beats.
             e) By isometric contraction via handgrip. This increases cardiac output, as well as blood pressure.
             f) By having the patient take four or five deep, rapid breaths. This activates the lung pump and thus increases flow to the heart.

6.   How can you artificially increase the need for a stronger atrial contraction, so that the S_4 is made louder?
     ANS.:   a) Increase the blood pressure with vasopressors (methoxamine or ephedrine), by having the patient squat, or by a handgrip for one minute.
             b) Decrease the coronary flow and increase blood pressure by having the patient smoke a cigarette.

7.   How can you bring ventricular movements closer to the stethoscope?
     ANS.:   Turn the patient into the left lateral decubitus position. If one listens immediately, the effects of exertion will also be operative for a few beats.
             Note: When all these maneuvers fail to produce an S_4 that is suspected, have the patient go from the standing to the left lateral decubitus position. This often produces an S_4 for a few beats.

HANDGRIP AND THE S_4

1.   When does isometric handgrip contraction bring out an S_4?
     ANS.:   Only if it raises pressure at the end of diastole in the LV. This occurs only if
             a) There is abnormal LV function. (This does not occur in all subjects with abnormal LV function.)
             b) There is normal LV function but severe MR or AR is present, probably because isometric contraction increases the regurgitation by increasing blood pressure.

2.   When and how does handgrip increase blood pressure?
     ANS.:   In most subjects, by increasing cardiac output through an augmentation of heart rate and contractility [16, 25]. In hypertensive patients, in patients with a reduction in cardiac reserve, and in patients with a significant obstructive lesion, as in MS, it also increases peripheral resistance [22].

Note: Handgrip has been widely recommended to bring out an S_3 and an S_4. It does not always help, probably because the increased contractility of the LV reduces the need for both an S_4 and the high left atrial pressure necessary for the S_3. If, however, the patient has angina or a pressure-loaded LV as in aortic stenosis or elevated blood pressure, the end-diastolic pressure will usually be elevated by handgrip, and an S_4 will be brought out, especially if the heart is small [8, 25].

3.   Does the strength of the handgrip control the peak heart rate and blood pressure rise?

ANS.:   No, as long as equal degrees of fatigue are produced. The strength of the hand-grip only controls the rate of development of the peak heart rate and blood pressure. For example, a 75% maximum voluntary contraction for 1 minute achieves about the same effect as a 25% effort for 5 minutes.

DIFFERENTIATION FROM THE S_3

1.   How does the quality or the pitch of the S_4 differ from that of the S_3?

ANS.:   They do not differ. They may both be described as a low-pitched thud or a boom. Often, they feel more like a physical movement of the eardrum than like a sound.

2.   When is it difficult to tell an S_3 from an S_4 gallop?

ANS.:   During tachycardia.

3.   How can you tell without a phonocardiogram or pulse tracing whether an S_3 or S_4 is present with a tachycardia?

ANS.:   a) If you can slow the rate with carotid sinus pressure, you may be able to detect that the extra sound keeps a constant relationship with the S_1, in which case it is an S_4. If it maintains a constant relationship with the S_2 and moves away from the S_1, it is an S_3.

b) Wait for a postpremature beat pause. An S_4 will obviously precede the next S_1 after the pause.

Note: The long diastole after a premature ventricular contraction does not always bring out an S_4. This is unfortunate, because if it did, it would always separate an S_3 from an S_4 or from a summation gallop. Often, the S_4 disappears at the end of a long diastole. The reason is unclear.

4.   How can you tell by phonocardiogram whether an extra sound is an S_3 or an S_4?

ANS.:   a) Since the longest distance between an S_2 and an S_3 is 200 msec, any interval longer than this suggests that the extra sound is an S_4.

b) Since the shortest distance between a P wave and an S_4 is 60 msec, any interval less than this suggests that the extra sound is an S_3.

c) A phonocardiogram plus apex cardiogram will show the S_3 at the peak of the early rapid filling wave, while an S_4 occurs at the peak of the atrial hump or A wave. (See figure on p. 252.)

5.   What is the rhythm called if both an S_3 and S_4 are present?

ANS.:   Quadruple rhythm, train-wheel rhythm, or double gallop.

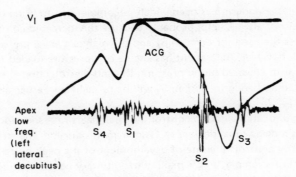

Apex cardiogram and phonocardiogram from a 55-year-old male with two previous infarctions. Surprisingly, despite his S_3 and S_4, or double gallop, he was almost asymptomatic without treatment. His atrial hump was easily palpable.

DIFFERENTIATION OF AN S_4–S_1 FROM A SPLIT S_1 (M_1–A_1 OR M_1–T_1)

1.   When is an S_4–S_1 difficult to distinguish from a split S_1 due to an M_1–A_1 or M_1–T_1?
     ANS.:   When the S_4 is very close to the S_1.
     Note: Even experienced auscultators can mistake a split S_1 for an S_4–S_1 as shown by the study in which they were asked to record whether or not an S_4 was heard in 200 consecutive patients over age 50. Among 34 patients without an S_4 on phonocardiogram, there were 56% false-positives [33] .

2.   How can you make an S_4 occur farther from the S_1 and so exaggerate the gallop rhythm?
     ANS.:   a) By increasing venous return, e.g., by having the patient raise his legs, exercise, or squat, or by the post-Valsalva effect.
             b) By causing more coronary insufficiency, e.g., by having the patient smoke a cigarette or exercise, or by giving handgrip exercise to a patient with coronary insufficiency.
             c) By increasing the work of the LV, e.g., by raising peripheral resistance with drugs, squatting, smoking, or handgrip. (See p. 306 for type of patient in whom handgrip will raise resistance.)

3.   What is the difference in quality between an S_4 and an S_1?
     ANS.:   When loud, the S_4 is a booming thud; the S_1 is sharper, shorter, and crisper. When the S_4 is loud, it is difficult to tell the difference in quality between an S_4 and an S_1; but when soft, the S_4 has fewer high frequencies, so that it is often inaudible with the diaphragm pressed hard against the chest. The S_1 is usually heard almost as well with the diaphragm and firm pressure as with the bell, regardless of whether it is loud or soft.

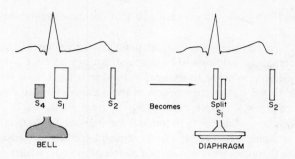

Pressure with the bell or the use of a diaphragm will eliminate most soft S_{4s} and may bring out the narrow, sharp, clicking physiological split of S_1.

*4.   How can you distinguish between an S_4-S_1 and M_1—ejection sound by phonocardiogram and pulse tracings?

ANS.:   a) By taking a phonocardiogram simultaneously with an ECG. You may see a sound that starts before the QRS. Although an S_1 can never do this, an S_4 may, and usually does.

b) By taking a phonocardiogram simultaneously with an apex cardiogram. The S_4 is always simultaneous with the peak of the atrial hump of the apex cardiogram; the S_1 always appears after this atrial hump. The A_1, or aortic ejection sound, tends to occur at or near the peak of the upstroke of the apex cardiogram.

5.   How can the site of auscultation tell you whether you are listening to an S_4-S_1 rather than to a split M_1-A_1 or M_1-T_1?

ANS.:   Since the S_4 tends to disappear anywhere away from the apex beat, a split S_1 that sounds the same at the left sternal border as at the apex probably does not contain an S_4.

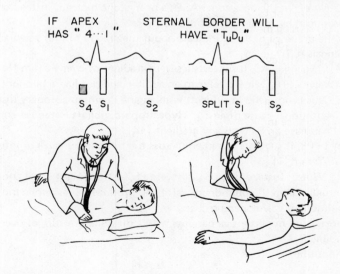

An S_4 is rarely heard at the left lower sternal border, but the two sharp sounds of the normally split S_1 are commonly heard there as well as at the apex. Therefore, if you hear the same split in both places, it is not likely due to an S_4.

6. How do changes from cycle to cycle tell you that the patient probably has an S_4 instead of an $M_1 - A_1$?

    ANS.: A soft S_4 tends to disappear from perception from beat to beat; an M_1 does not characteristically do this. The change from beat to beat is due to the fact that the S_4 is very sensitive to changes in volume in the LV, as well as to proximity of the LV to the stethoscope. Both of these parameters are affected by respiration.

7. How can postural changes differentiate an $S_4 - S_1$ from an $M_1 - A_1$?

    ANS.: The S_4 is very sensitive to blood-volume changes, so that standing will generally make it disappear. The $M_1 - A_1$ may even become more apparent on standing, because this represents **isovolumic contraction** time, which can be prolonged by standing.

SEVERITY OF CARDIAC DYSFUNCTION AND PRESENCE OF AN S_4

1. When does an S_4 occur with the pressure overloads caused by mild pulmonary or aortic stenosis, or *mild* pulmonary or systemic hypertension?

    ANS.: When enough myocardial damage has resulted from coronary disease (in the older age groups), then an S_4 may occur even with mild systemic hypertension or mild aortic stenosis (AS).

*2. When is a right-sided S_4 not expected despite severe pulmonary hypertension?

    ANS.: When the contraction of the right atrium can decompress itself through a large atrial septal defect (ASD) or VSD. When the right atrium contracts at the end of diastole, it usually cannot transmit its pressure entirely to the RV if there is an ASD or VSD present. It will instead transmit a portion of its pressure to the left atrium or LV through the abnormal connection.

    Note: In the occasional ASD, a presystolic murmur instead of an S_4 may be produced by atrial contraction.

3. What does the presence of an S_4 indicate about the gradient in (a) valvular AS and (b) pulmonary stenosis (PS)?

    ANS.: a) In valvular AS, it suggests a severe gradient of over 70 mm Hg across the aortic valve. (This should refer to an audible and not just a phonocardiographic S_4.) This is not valid in subjects with angina in whom coronary disease may be an additional cause of an S_4. **Hypertrophic subaortic stenosis** subjects, however, can have an S_4 with any gradient [14].

    b) In PS, it suggests a gradient across the pulmonary valve or **infundibulum** of over 70 mm Hg [38].

    Note: Instead of an S_4 in severe PS, a strong right atrial contraction may actually open the pulmonary valve and produce a presystolic murmur or even a pulmonary valve opening click.

4. What proportion of hypertensive patients with a diastolic pressure of over 100 mm Hg will have an audible S_4?

    ANS.: About half.

5.   What is a more serious sign of heart disease, the pathological S_3 or the S_4?

ANS.:   In the absence of increased AV valve flow, an S_3 is more serious, because it means an increased left atrial pressure, which is a sign of decompensation at rest. An S_4, on the other hand, merely means that a poorly compliant ventricle is "calling on the atrium for help." The help it receives may be enough to keep the output adequate, even with moderate exercise.

6.   What happens to the S_4 when failure becomes severe and an S_3 develops?

ANS.:   After a stage in which both an S_3 and an S_4 may be present, the S_4 tends to soften and then disappear, and the patient with severe failure may be left with only an S_3 [4].

*7.   When is an S_4 heard in the neck? Why?

ANS.:   a) When there is a strong right atrial contraction (as in PS or pulmonary hypertension), the strong jugular A wave strikes the stethoscope chest piece to produce a sound with the timing of an S_4. It is not surprising that the effect of a strong right atrial contraction can be heard in the neck, because sudden tensing of strips of various tissues has shown that the superior vena cava gives the loudest sounds of all cardiac tissues that have been tested, e.g., pulmonary artery, aorta, mitral, tricuspid valves, and the walls of the atria and ventricles [9a].

b) When the LV S_4 is moderately loud, however, it is often audible in the right supraclavicular area. The reason is unknown. It is surprising in view of the fact that the S_3 is rarely heard there, even if moderately loud.

Note: Right-sided S_{4s} are heard under the same circumstances for the right side of the heart as are left-sided S_{4s} for the left side. Therefore, they are heard in the presence of RV overloads that cause loss of compliance of the RV, such as severe PS and pulmonary hypertension. They are also heard in sudden, severe tricuspid regurgitation due to ruptured chordae or endocarditis (right-sided endocarditis is usually seen only in heroin addicts). An S_4 usually is heard at rest in PS only when the PS is severe, i.e., when the RV pressure is 120 mm Hg or more.

SEVERITY OF THE CARDIAC DYSFUNCTION AND TIMING AND AMPLITUDE OF THE S_4

1.   What is the relation between the $P-S_4$ interval and the severity of the pathological condition that causes the S_4 gallop?

ANS.:   The shorter the $P-S_4$ interval, the more severe the pathological condition [11]. It follows then that if the $P-S_4$ interval is short, the S_4-S_1 interval will be long.

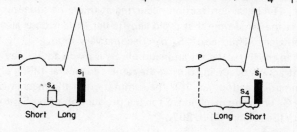

SEVERE STIFFNESS   SLIGHT STIFFNESS

The longer the S_4-S_1 interval, the greater is the loss of compliance of the LV (provided the $P-R$ interval is not prolonged) and usually the louder is the S_4.

2.   What will happen to the S_4–S_1 interval in a patient who is hypertensive and is either given an antihypertensive agent or in whom the flow to the heart is decreased by having him stand up?

ANS.:   Both of these maneuvers will make a narrow S_4–S_1 interval; i.e., the S_4 moves toward the S_1 and may join with it, to become indistinguishable [21]. This could explain why an S_4–S_1 interval may be narrow despite severe hypertension or AS if the flow is decreased due to diuretics or heart failure.

3.   What happens to the loudness of the S_4 if it comes early rather than late, i.e., if the P–S_4 interval is short and the S_4–S_1 interval long? Why?

ANS.:   The S_4 becomes louder. By pacing the atria of dogs electrically, it has been shown that the earlier in diastole the atrium is made to contract, the more powerfully it contracts. It has also been shown that long S_4–S_1 intervals result in a more energetic ventricular contraction than do short S_4–S_1 intervals.

*4.   What happens to the loudness of the S_1 if the S_4 moves farther from it? Why?

ANS.:   The S_1 becomes softer [21, 27]. If the atrium reaches its peak pressure early, it may allow left atrial relaxation to reach low levels early, and left atrial pressure will be relatively low when the ventricle starts to contract. Therefore, the LV will close the mitral valve at the slowest part of its acceleration curve. (See figure on p. 165.)

*5.   Why would the S_4–S_1 interval in hypertensive patients be well separated even if the P–S_4 interval were not shortened?

ANS.:   In LVH patients, the Q–M_1 interval is prolonged because the electromechanical interval is prolonged [4].

*6.   Why will acute myocardial infarction tend to narrow the S_4–S_1 interval, even if the P–S_4 is shortened?

ANS.:   Catecholamines, which reach a high level in acute infarction, tend to shorten the Q–M_1 interval. This may make the S_4 difficult to appreciate.

SUMMATION AND AUGMENTED GALLOPS

1.   Why can a first-degree AV block augment the effect of an atrial contraction?

ANS.:   A first-degree AV block, i.e., with the P wave coming very early in diastole, may cause the atrium to contract early enough to coincide with the time of rapid ventricular filling. Unless the P–R interval is extremely prolonged, this contraction of the atrium at the time of rapid ventricular filling will only occur with a tachycardia. The atrial contraction occurring at this time squeezes blood into the ventricle at the same time that rapid ventricular expansion is also drawing blood into the ventricle. Thus, a soft S_4 can become very loud.

2.   What is the gallop rhythm called if an inaudible S_3 is made audible by the augmented flow of an atrial contraction occurring during the rapid ventricular filling phase?

ANS.:   A summation gallop, i.e., it is the summation of the mechanism for the production of the S_3 with the mechanism for the production of an S_4, to make an audible sound. (See figure on p. 257.)

*3. When are summation gallops pathological?

ANS.: When a pathological S_3 is augmented by atrial contraction occurring very early in diastole. Similarly, a pathological S_4 may be augmented by occurring during the early rapid filling phase. These are called "augmented gallops" [15]. This implies that an S_3 or S_4 was augmented by the fortuitous assistance of a marked tachycardia or prolonged P—R interval. Thus, an augmented gallop may be a pathological type of summation gallop. If a physiological S_4 is augmented by a long P—R interval plus tachycardia, the summation gallop is physiological.

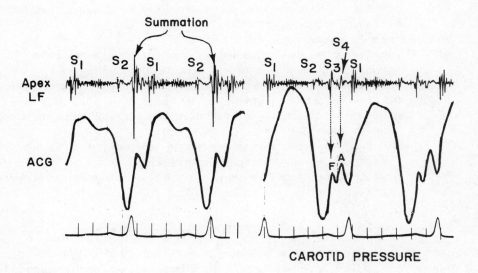

In this patient with heart failure and AS, a tachycardia of 115 with a P—R of 150 msec (0.15 sec) causes a summation gallop. When the rate is slowed by carotid pressure, both an S_3 and an S_4 appear. Therefore, this is an *augmented* type of summation gallop.

4. What may you hear if the heart rate of a patient with a summation gallop is slowed by carotid sinus pressure?

ANS.: Either nothing or a pathological S_3, a pathological S_4, a physiological S_3, or both a pathological S_3 and S_4, i.e., a double gallop.

5. How long a P—R interval is necessary for a summation gallop to occur?

ANS.: It depends on the length of diastole, i.e., on the heart rate. With very fast rates, only a slightly long P—R will produce summation. With normal rates, a very long P—R is necessary. (See p. 230 for actual P—R intervals that will produce summation for various heart rates.)

*6. How can a summation or augmented gallop be differentiated from an S_3 or S_4 if you cannot slow the heart rate?

ANS.: A simultaneous phonocardiogram and apex precordiogram will show that the peak of the early filling wave and atrial hump are fused, and the single peak will occur simultaneously with the summation sound.

*THE PACEMAKER S₄-LIKE CLICK

*1.   When can an electronic pacemaker produce an extra sound? When does the extra sound occur?

  ANS.:   When it causes intercostal skeletal muscle contraction, it can produce a high-pitched, clicking, inspiration-accentuated sound just preceding the M_1, so that it sounds like a right-sided S_4 click [23, 24]. It occurs about 6 msec after the pacing stimulus [7].

  Perforation of the myocardium of the RV by a transvenous pacing electrode should be suspected when the pacemaker-induced sound occurs. This, however, is not a necessary concomitant.

*2.   Where on the chest are pacemaker sounds best heard?

  ANS.:   Sometimes at the apex and sometimes at the left lower sternal border. They are occasionally only audible in the left lateral decubitus position.

*3.   Where has the pacemaker been situated when it produced a click plus diaphragmatic contraction with each click, without perforation of the heart?

  ANS.:   a) In the coronary sinus, where it stimulated the left hemidiaphragm, according to one report [34].

  b) In the RV posteroinferior apical region in close proximity to the left hemidiaphragm, according to another report [32].

  c) At the apex of the RV anteriorly, where it caused diaphragmatic stimulation that was distressing to the patient [13].

REFERENCES

1.   Argano, B. J. Phonocardiographic findings in anemia. *Chest* 60:599, 1971.
2.   Aronow, W. S., Cassidy, J., and Uyeyama, R. R. Effect of position on the resting and post-exercise phonocardiogram. *Chest* 61:439, 1972.
3.   Barry, W. H., Brooker, J. Z., Alderman, E. L., and Harrison, D. C. Changes in diastolic stiffness and tone of the left ventricle during angina pectoris. *Circulation* 49:255, 1974.
4.   Bethell, H. J. N., and Nixon, P. G. F. Understanding the atrial sound. *Br. Heart J.* 35:229, 1973.
5.   Bridgman, E. W. Notes on a presystolic sound. *Arch. Intern. Med.* 14:474, 1914.
6.   Brockman, S. K. Dynamic function of atrial contraction in regulation of cardiac performance. *Am. J. Physiol.* 204:597, 1963.
7.   Cheng, T. O., Ertem, G., and Vera, Z. Heart sounds in patients with cardiac pacemakers. *Chest* 62:64, 1972.
8.   Cohn, P. F., Thompson, P., Strauss, W., Todd, J., and Gorlin, R. Diastolic heart sounds during static (handgrip) exercise in patients with chest pain. *Circulation* 47:1217, 1973.
9.   Diamond, G., and Forrester, J. S. Effect of coronary artery disease and acute myocardial infarction on left ventricular compliance in man. *Circulation* 45:11, 1972.
9a.   Dock, W. The genesis of diastolic heart sounds. *Am. J. Med.* 50:178, 1971.
10.   Dolara, A., and Tardini, B. Atrial flutter sounds: Report of a case. *Am. Heart J.* 78:369, 1969.
11.   Duchosal, P. A study of gallop rhythm by a combination of phonocardiographic and electrocardiographic methods. *Am. Heart J.* 7:613, 1932.

12. Epstein, E. J., Coulshed, N., Brown, A. K., and Doukas, N. G. The "A" wave of the apex cardiogram in aortic valve disease and cardiomyopathy. *Br. Heart J.* 30:591, 1968.

13. Gaidula, J. J., and Barold, S. S. Diaphragmatic origin of the pacemaker sound. *Chest* 61:195, 1972.

14. Goldblatt, A., Aygen, M. M., and Braunwald, E. Hemodynamic-phonocardiographic correlations of the fourth heart sound in aortic stenosis. *Circulation* 26:92, 1962.

15. Grayzel, J. Gallop rhythm of the heart. *Circulation* 20:1053, 1959.

16. Grossman, W., McLaurin, L. P., Saltz, S. B., Paraskos, J. A., Dalen, J. E., and Dexter, L. Changes in the inotropic state of the left ventricle during isometric exercise. *Br. Heart J.* 35:697, 1973.

17. Hamby, R. I., Aintablian, A., and Wisoff, B. G. Mechanism of closure of the mitral prosthetic valve and the role of atrial systole. *Am. J. Cardiol.* 31:616, 1973.

18. Harris, W. S., Robin, P., and Tabatznik, B. Modification of the atrial sound by the cold pressor test, carotid sinus massage, and the Valsalva maneuver. *Circulation* 28:1128, 1963.

19. Herbert, W. H. Basis for effects of atrial dynamics on ventricular function. *N. Y. State J. Med.* 67:675, 1967.

20. Hood, W. B., Jr., Bianco, J. A., Kumar, R., and Whiting, R. B. Experimental myocardial infarction, reduction of left ventricular compliance in healing phase. *J. Clin. Invest.* 49:1316, 1970.

21. Kincaid-Smith, P., and Barlow, J. The atrial sound in hypertension and ischaemic heart disease. *Br. Heart J.* 21:479, 1959.

22. Kivowitz, C., Parmley, W. W., Donoso, R., Marcus, H., Ganz, W., and Swan, H. J. C. Effects of isometric exercise on cardiac performance. *Circulation* 44:994, 1971.

23. Kluge, W. F. Pacemaker sound and its origin. *Am. J. Cardiol.* 25:362, 1970.

24. Kramer, D. H., Moss, A. J., and Shah, P. M. Mechanisms and significance of pacemaker-induced extracardiac sound. *Am. J. Cardiol.* 25:367, 1970.

25. Krayenbuehl, H. P., Rutishauser, W., Shoenbeck, M., and Amende, I. Evaluation of left ventricular function from isovolumic pressure measurements during isometric exercise. *Am. J. Cardiol.* 29:323, 1972.

26. Kuo, P. T., Schnabel, T. G., Jr., Blakemore, W. S., and Whereat, A. F. Diastolic gallop sounds: The mechanism of production. *J. Clin. Invest.* 36:1035, 1957.

27. Leonard, J. J., Weissler, A. M., and Warren, J. V. Observations on the mechanism of atrial gallop rhythm. *Circulation* 42:1007, 1958.

28. Luisada, A. A., and Bartolo, G. High frequency phonocardiography. *Am. J. Cardiol.* 8:51, 1961.

29. Massumi, R. A., Hernandez, T., Just, G., and Tawakkol, A. A. The audible sound of atrial tachyarrhythmia (flutter?). *Circulation* 33:607, 1966.

30. Neporent, L. M., and DaSilva, J. A. Heart sounds in atrial flutter-fibrillation. *Am. J. Cardiol.* 19:301, 1967.

31. O'Rourke, R. A. The atrial sound. Factors regulating its occurrence and timing. *Am. Heart J.* 80:715, 1970.

32. Pupillo, G. A., Talley, R. C., and Linhart, J. W. "Pacemaker heart sound" caused by diaphragmatic contractions. *Am. Heart J.* 82:711, 1971.

33. Rectra, E. H., Khan, A. H., Pigott, V. M., and Spodick, D. H. Audibility of the fourth heart sound, a prospective, "blind" auscultatory and polygraphic investigation. *J. A. M. A.* 221:36, 1972.

34.   Schluger, J., and Wolf, R. E. Sound caused by diaphragmatic contraction resulting from transvenous cardiac pacemaker. *Chest* 61:693, 1972.

35.   Stock, E. Auscultation and phonocardiography in acute myocardial infarction. *Med. J. Aust.* 1:1060, 1966.

36.   Tavel, M. E. The fourth heart sound — A premature requiem? *Circulation* 49:4, 1974.

37.   Turner, P. P., and Hunter, J. The atrial sound in ischaemic heart disease. *Br. Heart J.* 35:657, 1973.

38.   Vogelpoel, L., and Schrire, V. Auscultatory and phonocardiographic assessment of pulmonary stenosis with intact ventricular septum. *Circulation* 22:55, 1960.

39.   Willems, J. L., DeGeest, H., and Kesteloot, H. On the value of apex cardiography for timing intracardiac events. *Am. J. Cardiol.* 28:59, 1971.

13

Ejection Murmurs

PHYSICAL CAUSES

1. What is the cause of murmurs?
   ANS.: Turbulent flow in the cardiovascular system.

2. What anatomical situations tend to produce turbulence?
   ANS.: a) Obstruction to blood flow, either by circumferential narrowing or by a local protrusion into the stream.
   b) Flow into a distal chamber of larger diameter than the proximal one.

3. What happens to the velocity of flow at an orifice?
   ANS.: It increases, just as when you narrow the nozzle of a hose.

4. How does the area of an orifice affect both the flow across it and the loudness of the murmur?
   ANS.: The smaller the orifice area with the same volume of flow, the greater the velocity at the orifice and the greater the turbulence of murmur.
   *Note: Turbulence is also affected by the following:
   a) Viscosity. The greater the viscosity, the less the turbulence. It is to be expected, then, that the high hematocrit in patients with cyanotic congenital heart disease can increase viscosity to attenuate murmurs.
   b) The irregularity of the shape of the orifice. The greater the irregularity, the louder the murmur.
   c) The smoothness or sharpness of the orifice edges. The greater the sharpness, the louder the murmur.

*5. What is a Reynolds number, and how does it apply to murmurs in man?
   ANS.: Turbulence in a tube is calculated by a formula known as the Reynolds number. It includes diameter, viscosity, and velocity of flow. The greater the Reynolds number, the greater the turbulence. The trouble with the turbulence theory as a cause of murmurs is as follows:
   a) The Reynolds number in man is rarely great enough to produce a murmur [7].
   b) Turbulence implies wave fronts in all directions, and they should cancel each other out and produce no sound at all.

*6. What is the vortex or eddy theory of the cause of murmurs?
   ANS.: Turbulence sets up vortices or eddies, and these can strike the walls of the vascular system to produce vibrations that have frequencies and amplitudes compatible with actual murmurs.
   Note: A good analogy for eddies is that they are like smoke rings. (See figure on p. 236.)

---

* indicates material that is for electives or fellows in cardiology, or concerns rare phenomena, of interest primarily to cardiologists.

Boldface type indicates that the term is explained in the Glossary.

7.   How does the **frequency** or pitch of a murmur relate to the **gradient**?
     ANS.:   The greater the gradient, the higher the frequencies produced.
8.   What happens to the frequency and pitch of a murmur as the flow is increased?
     ANS.:   The greater the flow across an orifice, the more low and medium frequencies are
             produced.

CHARACTERISTICS OF THE EJECTION MURMUR

1.   What cardiac event is implied by an ejection murmur?
     ANS.:   The term implies that the murmur is produced by blood flowing forward through
             a **semilunar valve** during systole.
2.   What is characteristic of ejection murmurs on a phonocardiogram?
     ANS.:   They start with the final component of the first heart sound (S_1), are crescendo-
             decrescendo, and finish before the second sound of the side of the heart from
             which the murmur originates. This means that a left-sided murmur will finish
             before the A_2, and a right-sided murmur will finish before the P_2.

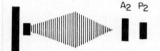

This murmur could be either pulmonary or aortic, since it ends before both components of the
second sound.

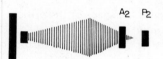

This murmur can be a pulmonary ejection murmur, since although it extends beyond the A_2, it
finishes before the P_2.

3.   Why must an ejection murmur be crescendo-decrescendo?
     ANS.:   The loudness of a murmur across a valve is controlled by the gradient. This
             gradient is controlled by the velocity and acceleration of flow; i.e., the greater
             the velocity and acceleration of flow, the greater the gradient and the louder the
             murmur.
                 The shape of the murmur across an obstruction reflects the shape of the gradient.
             For example, in aortic stenosis (AS), as the pressure in the left ventricle (LV) rises
             to just above diastolic pressure in the aorta, it takes a short time to overcome the
             inertia of the aortic blood and walls. Therefore, the initial gradient across the
             aortic orifice is slight, and the murmur starts softly. The pressure gradient then
             increases toward midsystole, as does the murmur. As soon as the ventricle begins
             to reach the stage of reduced ejection, just past the middle of systole, the flow
             decreases, the gradient decreases, and the murmur decreases.

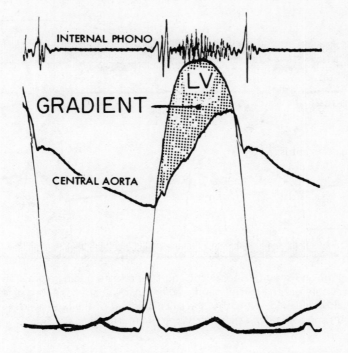

A simultaneous aortic and LV pressure tracing (taken with a catheter tip micromanometer to eliminate time delays through tubes) in a subject with valvular AS. The shape of the murmur follows the shape of the gradient (shaded area).

4. Why does the aortic or pulmonary ejection murmur end before the semilunar valve closure sound of its side?

  ANS.: Just before the valve closes, the velocity of forward flow has so decreased that even if the murmur does go to the second sound, the ear cannot hear the very end of this faint decrescendo part of the murmur.

5. What happens to the loudness of an ejection murmur after a long diastole, as in the long pauses after premature ventricular contraction or after the long diastoles of atrial fibrillation? Why?

  ANS.: It becomes louder, because the long period of diastole allows a larger volume to collect in the LV, and this increased volume is ejected during the next systole.

  Note: a) The **postextrasystolic potentiation** caused by an early depolarization of a ventricle, as with a premature ectopic beat, produces a positive inotropic effect on the ventricle for the next contraction and contributes to the loudness of the ejection murmur after a long diastole.

  b) Since the gradient across a stenotic valve increases as the square of the increase in flow, a slight increase in flow can cause a great increase in gradient and therefore a great increase in the murmur.

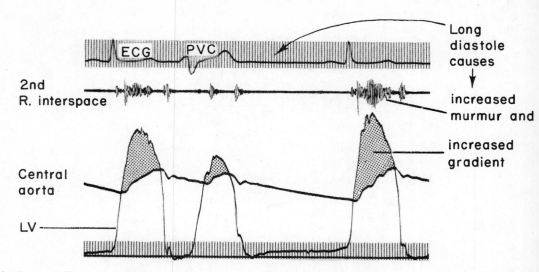

A phonocardiogram and simultaneous aortic and LV pressure tracing from a 16-year-old boy with valvular AS. Not only did the murmur and gradient increase after the long diastole, but the ejection sound also increased. Note that the small gradient of the premature ventricular contraction (PVC) itself produced only a short early systolic murmur.

6. What happens to the pitch or frequency characteristics of an ejection murmur when the murmur is soft? Why?

ANS.: It retains the low and medium frequencies. (This is important, since regurgitant murmurs do not do this.) This is because the greater the flow, the greater are the number of low frequencies in a murmur. Ejection murmurs are produced by the entire stroke volume passing through the aortic or pulmonary valve with each systole, even when the obstruction or gradient across the valve is trivial.

7. What was the original meaning of the term *ejection murmur*? Why is this definition misleading?

ANS.: A midsystolic murmur that was crescendo-decrescendo and ended before the second sound of its side [29]. It ignores the following:
a) On phonocardiograms, most ejection murmurs can usually be seen to start without any pause after the S_1.
b) Regurgitant murmurs may also be crescendo-decrescendo.

8. How can you best define an ejection murmur?

ANS.: It is best defined as an "ejection murmur complex"; i.e., it is a murmur that begins with the end of the S_1 or with an ejection sound, is crescendo-decrescendo, ends before the second sound of its side, usually becomes louder after long diastoles, and, when soft, retains low and medium frequencies.

9.   How can you tell by auscultation alone that a crescendo-decrescendo (diamond or rhomboid shape on a phonocardiogram) is present in a murmur?

   ANS.:   The S_1 plus the peak of the crescendo plus the S_2 makes a rhythmic cadence of:

duh - huh - duh

peak

S_1 of S_2

diamond

   Note: a) Remember that this rhythm is not all that you hear. This should be thought of only as the background effect to the systolic noise that contains the S_1 and S_2. If an S_2 is missing, "duh - huh" tells you that the murmur is crescendo-decrescendo. If the S_1 is missing, the rhythm of "huh - duh" tells you that the murmur is crescendo-decrescendo.

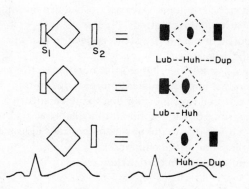

If you imagine the string section of an orchestra playing a long note during systole and the drums playing a rhythm of two or three notes, you will have the impression given by the peak of an ejection murmur plus either an S_1, an S_2, or both.

         *b) Since the pitch of an ejection murmur is also often crescendo-decrescendo, the higher frequencies being in midsystole, the shape of some ejection murmurs is sometimes best appreciated with the diaphragm or with the high-frequency band of a phonocardiogram [33].

10. How can you tell by the loudness of an ejection murmur whether or not there is a significant gradient across a valve?

   ANS.:   A very soft murmur, i.e., grade 2 or less, is likely to occur with an unimportant gradient, provided artifactual reasons for the softness, such as obesity, are ruled out. If the murmur is very loud, i.e., grade 4 or more, the gradient is likely to be significant, but spurious causes of excessive loudness must be ruled out.

11. List the commonest spurious cause of softening of systolic murmurs besides the obvious ones of obesity or an increased anteroposterior diameter that keeps the stethoscope too far from the heart.

   ANS.:   Congestive heart failure.

12.   List some factors that spuriously increase the loudness of systolic ejection murmurs, i.e., without reflecting the degree of the gradient.

 ANS.:   a) The systolic expansion of a markedly dilated pulmonary artery or aorta creating artifactual crackles or crunches by pressure against the surrounding lung tissue.

 b) A very thin chest wall, forcing a tortuous aorta close against the anterior chest wall.

 c) Any cause for increased flow, such as exercise, thyrotoxicosis, arteriovenous fistulas, anemia, shunts, or increased diastolic filling as in bradycardias or aortic regurgitation.

TYPES OF EJECTION MURMURS

1.   List the three types of thoracic ejection murmurs.

 ANS.:   1) The systolic semilunar valve nonobstructive murmur with normal or increased flow (systolic flow murmur).

 2) The aortic or pulmonary stenosis ejection murmur.

 3) The thoracic arterial murmur.

2.   List the five types of systolic semilunar valve nonobstructive murmurs.

 ANS.:   1) The normal impulse gradient murmur due to thin chest or quiet room.

 2) The increased flow murmur due to increased stroke volume or rate of ejection.

 3) The murmur due to ejection into a dilated artery.

 4) The murmur due to unknown anatomical causes of turbulence: namely, the humming murmur of childhood.

 5) The murmur due to **aortic sclerosis**.

SYSTOLIC FLOW MURMURS

The Normal Impulse Gradient Murmur and the Increased Flow Murmur

1.   How can a systolic murmur be produced across a normal semilunar valve?

 ANS.:   There is always a forward pressure gradient across a semilunar valve, as there must be in any pipe with a forward flow.

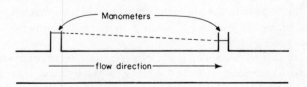

The gradient between the upstream and downstream manometers may not be measurable by the usual cardiac catheter techniques. If, however, the gradient is increased enough by obstruction to flow, a semilunar valve, or even a local protuberance from one wall, enough turbulence may occur to produce a murmur.

2.   What is the relationship between the gradient across a semilunar valve and the shape of
     the murmur?
     ANS.:   a) The greater the gradient, the louder and longer the murmur and the later the
             peak of the crescendo-decrescendo.
             b) The shape of the gradient is responsible for the shape of the murmur across
                a stenotic valve. Across a normal valve, however, the shape of the murmur is
                controlled by the velocity of flow, which is crescendo-decrescendo with an
                early peak to the crescendo; i.e., it is mainly an early ejection murmur.
                Note: In the absence of AS, the normal peak gradient across an aortic valve
             (known as the impulse gradient) is very early, because gradient is related to acceler-
             ation of flow, and acceleration peaks early in the absence of stenosis. Murmurs,
             on the other hand, are related to velocity of flow, which has a slightly later peak
             than does acceleration. Therefore, the peak of the normal flow murmur across a
             semilunar valve is later than the peak gradients.

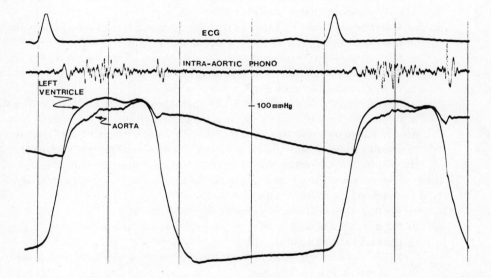

Aortic and LV pressure tracings together with a phonocardiogram from a 40-year-old man with
an innocent aortic ejection murmur. Note the early systolic gradient between the LV and aorta,
which is the normal impulse gradient found not only in normal left-sided chambers but also
normally seen between the right ventricle and pulmonary artery. This tracing is taken by a single
catheter with two end holes, in order to obtain absolutely accurate timing and pressure differences
across the aortic valve.

3.   In what percentage of normal subjects is an ejection murmur heard?
     ANS.:   In 100%, depending on:
             a) Soundproofing of the room. All normal subjects have an ejection murmur in a
                soundproof room [22].
             b) The number of times the subject is examined for murmurs.
             c) The physical or emotional state of the subject; exercise may be required to
                bring out the murmur.

d) The degree to which the shape and thickness of the chest separate the stethoscope from the heart.

e) The age of the subject. About 96% of healthy children up to age 14 have ejection murmurs on ordinary clinical examination in a quiet but not sound-proof room [31]. These murmurs are usually maximal at the left sternal border.

4. Why are young patients most likely to have an easily audible flow murmur?

ANS.: Because of their more rapid **circulation time** and their relatively thin chests.

5. What terms are used for an easily audible ejection murmur across a valve that is produced by an increase in flow rather than by valve narrowing?

ANS.: a) *Systolic flow murmur* is the preferred term.

b) *Systolic murmur of relative stenosis* (see question 6).

c) *Functional murmur.* This implies only the kind of change of function that causes an increase in flow. However, this is not as clear a term as *flow murmur.* It is often wrongly applied to ejection murmurs of unknown etiology that are not necessarily due to increased flow.

d) *Innocent murmur.* This implies that the prognosis is definitely known and therefore cannot refer to all flow murmurs.

e) *Benign murmur.* This implies that flow murmurs are malignant if they are associated with any abnormality such as anemia or a shunt.

*6. Does the term *relative stenosis* aptly explain the flow murmur?

ANS.: Almost, although not exactly. It is true that increased flow across an orifice such as a normal valve does cause a fall in pressure beyond the valve just as in pulmonary or aortic stenosis. But since the murmur shape across a normal valve is related to velocity changes more than to gradient, the flow murmur is different from a stenosis murmur, in which the gradient and murmur have the same shape.

7. List the commonest causes of a flow murmur across a pulmonary or aortic valve, besides the rapid circulation of a young person.

ANS.: a) An excessively narrow anteroposterior chest diameter.

b) Flow into a suddenly dilated vessel beyond a semilunar valve.

c) Increased stroke volumes due to

1) Shunt flows, e.g., central shunt flows of an atrial septal defect and ventricular septal defect.

2) Regurgitant leaks such as aortic and pulmonary regurgitation.

3) Marked bradycardia, as in complete atrioventricular (AV) block.

4) Increased cardiac outputs, such as in thyrotoxicosis, anemia, exercise, pregnancy, and systemic arteriovenous fistulas.

Note: a) Cardiac output is not significantly increased in anemia until the hemoglobin and hematocrit drop to about 50% of normal.

b) About 95% of pregnant women have ejection murmurs [21].

5) A bicuspid aortic valve.

Note: A bicuspid aortic valve, probably by becoming slightly thickened, may create an ejection murmur that is loudest at the second right interspace. An ejection murmur that is loudest at the second right interspace is probably always due to some abnormality.

8.   What is meant by a "hemic" murmur?

ANS.:   Any murmur that is present in the anemic state and disappears when the anemia is corrected. This includes:

a) Pathological murmurs, especially mitral regurgitation (MR), that are heard only with the increased heart size, increased blood volume, and increased need for coronary flow caused by the severe anemia [12].

b) Ejection flow murmurs produced by increased blood volume caused by the severe anemia.

Note: The so-called aortic regurgitation murmurs heard only during severe anemias are probably the diastolic high-frequency components of a venous hum transmitted down to the second right interspace.

9.   When is a *decreased* velocity of flow responsible for an ejection murmur in the absence of valvular obstruction to account for it?

ANS.:   Flow that suddenly enters a dilated chamber; i.e., a dilated pulmonary artery or aorta can produce turbulence that results in a murmur. The flow into the dilated vessel will suddenly *decrease in velocity,* just as flow from a river decreases in velocity when it enters a lake. The two major examples of this are idiopathic dilatation of the pulmonary artery and dilatation of the ascending aorta, as in **aneurysm** or pulmonary atresia.

Note: It is possible that some of these murmurs are artifactually produced by adhesions between a dilated ascending aorta or main pulmonary artery and the surrounding pleura. (See p. 270, question 4.)

Atrial Septal Defect Systolic Flow Murmurs

1.   What causes the systolic murmur in patients with an uncomplicated ASD?

ANS.:   Increased flow through a dilated pulmonary artery.

2.   Why is there no murmur through the defect in the atrial septum?

ANS.:   Because there is almost no gradient across the defect. If the defect is large, the two atria act as a single chamber, so that the pressures on each side of the defect are almost equal. Even if the defect is small, the gradient between left and right atrium is never more than a few millimeters of mercury and therefore will still not produce a murmur.

Note: a) A murmur through an ASD may be inaudible even if one occurred at that site, because an acoustic signal produced artificially by a mechanical sound generator in the right atrium is almost completely dissipated before it reaches the chest wall [17].

b) A murmur may be produced across an ASD in the presence of a small defect plus MR or rheumatic mitral stenosis (MS), which raises the pressure in the left atrium higher than in the right atrium. An ASD plus MS is called Lutembacher's syndrome. A continuous murmur may be heard under these circumstances.

3. Where is the ASD systolic ejection murmur best heard? What is surprising about its radiation?

ANS.: The ejection murmur is best heard at the second or third left interspace. There is frequent transmission to the apex, even when the murmur is soft [30]. This is probably due to the greatly dilated right ventricle (RV), which transmits all RV and pulmonary artery events to the apex.

4. What suggests that part of the pulmonary murmur of ASD is extracardiac, i.e., probably due to adhesions between the dilated pulmonary artery and pleura?

ANS.: a) It is often crackly, crunchy, or scratchy [30].

b) It is often louder and longer than a mere flow murmur should be despite the absence of PS.

c) Other causes of marked pulmonary artery dilatation sometimes produce this crackling or crunchy type of murmur (e.g., idiopathic dilatation of the pulmonary artery).

d) In some ASDs there is almost no murmur at all, despite a normal pulmonary artery pressure. (See p. 286 for the effect of respiration on the ASD ejection murmur.)

5. What skeletal deformities suggest that an ejection murmur is due to an ASD?

ANS.: a) Any Marfan deformity (see p. 29) suggests not only pulmonary artery or aortic dilatation, but also an ASD.

b) A prominent left precordium suggests not only that the RV was dilated during childhood but also that it was working against a high pressure. This suggests that the ejection murmur is due to an ASD with pulmonary hypertension.

c) A thumb deformity such as a finger-like thumb (three phalanges) or an extra-short thumb.

d) An ulnar-radial deformity that prevents good forearm supination or pronation. These and the thumb abnormalities with an ASD have been called the Holt-Oram syndrome [32].

The Straight Back Syndrome Ejection Murmur

1. What is meant by the straight back syndrome?

ANS.: Compression of the heart due to loss of normal dorsal curvature of the spine [38]. This results in a pulmonary ejection murmur in almost all cases. This murmur is usually mistaken for that of either pulmonary stenosis (PS) or ASD.

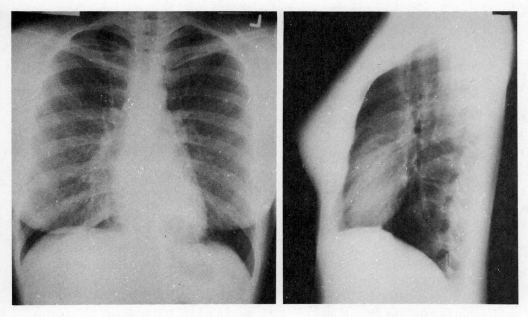

In this patient with the loss of dorsal curvature the anteroposterior diameter is one-third of the transverse diameter. The "straight front," plus the slight anterior bowing of the lower thoracic spine, probably contributed to the compression effect on the heart. (Courtesy of Dr. Antonio C. deLeon, Jr.)

2. What other palpatory and auscultatory findings in the straight back syndrome mimic ASDs?
    ANS.:   a) An exaggerated left parasternal movement may be present.
            b) The split of S_2 may be wide.
            c) The second component of S_1 may be accentuated [14].
            d) The systolic murmur is often scratchy or crunchy.
3. How loud is the ejection murmur of the straight back syndrome?
    ANS.:   It may be from grade 1/6 to grade 4/6. Even without a **pectus excavatum**, a markedly narrowed anteroposterior diameter can occasionally cause a murmur loud enough to have a thrill [10].
            Note: a) The murmur has occasionally been noted to change markedly in intensity from grade 2 to grade 4 with stethoscope pressure.
                    b) A short, early, grade 1/6, scratchy diastolic murmur that increases with inspiration is present in many patients with the straight back syndrome.

*4. Why will loss of the normally gentle dorsal kyphosis cause a pulmonary ejection murmur?

ANS.: The upper mediastinal structures may be compressed against the sternum and so create murmurs. In a small percentage of such patients, there is actually a gradient of 5—15 mm Hg in the pulmonary outflow tract, apparently created by this compression.

Note: a) An anteroposterior chest diameter of one-third or less of the transverse diameter (measured at just above the right dome of the diaphragm) is almost diagnostic of the straight back syndrome [10].

b) The objection to the term *straight back syndrome* is the fact that many subjects with straight backs have an anteriorly bowed sternum that gives ample space for the heart and thus have no pseudocardiac disease [11].

c) Scoliosis and pectus excavatum are commonly found with the straight back syndrome.

The Humming Systolic Ejection Murmur

1. What adjectives have been used to describe the quality, or timbre, of the humming (innocent) ejection murmur found in children? What eponym has been used for it?

ANS.: It has been described as a buzzing, vibratory, twanging, moaning, or groaning murmur. It has been called Still's murmur after the British author of a pediatric textbook published in 1918, who described it as "twanging."

The regular vibrations on this phonocardiogram of a humming systolic murmur (SM) tell you that the murmur has a musical quality. The peak of the crescendo occurring in the first third of systole tells you that the gradient across the semilunar valve is probably trivial.

2. What does the humming or twanging character of an ejection murmur in childhood tell you about the gradient across the semilunar valve?

ANS.: It means that there is only a slight gradient across the valve producing the murmur. It also suggests strongly that the murmur is innocent and will either disappear when puberty is complete or sound the same 15 years later [15].

3.   What two theories have been proposed to account for the humming murmur?

ANS.:   a) It has been proposed that a taut pulmonary valve fibrous ring structure or "trigonoidization" can cause vibrations as blood passes through it. Against this theory is the fact that pulmonary hypertension or pulmonary artery dilatation from any cause that also would tense the valve ring does not cause a humming murmur.

b) It has also been thought to be caused by a flow murmur through the aortic valve.

4.   What evidence suggests that this murmur does not come from the pulmonary area?

ANS.:   a) Intracardiac phonocardiograms from the pulmonary artery in patients with this murmur show only the same ejection murmur as picked up in most normal persons; i.e., it is not vibratory either by paper recordings or when heard through a loudspeaker [46].

b) After a **Valsalva** maneuver, the murmur does not return immediately. (See p. 286 for explanation of effect of the Valsalva maneuver on murmurs.)

c) A fine **thrill** can be recorded on the carotid tracings of some children with this murmur.

5.   Where is the humming or twanging murmur usually best heard?

ANS.:   Between the apex and the left sternal border, but it may also be heard anywhere along the left sternal border. It is a little surprising how widespread and difficult it is to localize this innocent murmur.

6.   What suggests that it is a form of "flow" ejection murmur?

ANS.:   a) It becomes louder with the subject supine and often disappears with the subject in the upright position.

b) The murmur is never louder than grade 3/6.

c) The murmur is usually short, reaching its peak early.

d) Children with this murmur tend to have shorter preejection periods than those without it [15]. (See p. 387 for explanation of preejection period.)

e) It consists of low and medium frequencies, i.e., between 75 and 160 cycles per second. A murmur that is relatively low in pitch suggests that it is mostly due to flow with very little gradient.

Note: These humming murmurs may become as long as an important murmur in the presence of increased flow, such as occurs with high fevers or severe anemias.

7.   Why is the term *innocent murmur* better than *functional* or *benign* to describe to the family a murmur that is not associated with any known cardiological abnormality?

ANS.:   *Innocent* conveys an immediate impression of unimportance without implying a lesion. *Benign,* on the contrary, implies that an abnormality is present but is not malignant. *Functional* may have no meaning to a layman, although to a physician it has a specific meaning of "due to increased flow."

The Aortic Ejection Murmur in the Elderly

1.   What percentage of patients over age 50 have an easily audible aortic ejection murmur without valvular stenosis?

ANS.:   About 50%. Therefore, we have called this the "50 over 50" (50/50) murmur. Actually, the incidence rises with age from about 30% at age 50, to about 70% at age 90 [8].

2.   What is the cause of this aortic ejection murmur?
      ANS.:   There are several theories:
                a) It is due to the fibrotic, thickened aortic valves, often with some calcification,
                   which do not fully open because of stiffness (aortic valve sclerosis) and are
                   seen at autopsy in about 70% of elderly patients with unimportant aortic ejec-
                   tion murmurs.
                b) It is due to calcific spurs in the aortic ring, which may protrude into the stream
                   when calcium is laid down at the roots of the cusps.
                c) It is due to atherosclerotic plaques in the ascending aorta, which may cause
                   turbulence as the aortic stream strikes the roughened endocardium.
                   Note: The general condition alluded to by these theories is called aortic sclerosis.

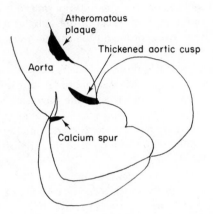

A slight but abrupt protuberance (e.g., a calcium spur) is capable of producing a murmur of considerable intensity.

3.   What factors in the elderly are known to increase the incidence of the 50/50 murmur?
      ANS.:   a) Hypertension. The higher the blood pressure, the more likely is the murmur.
                   Note: In one series of severely hypertensive patients, every one had an ejection
                   murmur [24].
                b) Sex. The incidence of this murmur is almost twice as high in women as in men.
4.   How loud can a murmur be that is due to aortic sclerosis?
      ANS.:   Up to grade 4. A grade 4 murmur, however, is rare, and constitutes only about 2%
              of such murmurs.
5.   What is the most important method of distinguishing a loud murmur of aortic sclerosis
      from that of AS?
      ANS.:   Palpation of the carotid will generally differentiate between the slow rise of AS
              and the normal rate of rise of aortic sclerosis. (See p. 38 for the use of ejection
              times in differentiating these two lesions.)

AORTIC STENOSIS EJECTION MURMURS

Valvular Aortic Stenosis Murmurs

Murmur Shape, Duration, and Quality

1. How can you tell the severity of an aortic gradient by the shape and length of the murmur?

   ANS.:   In general, the later the peak of the crescendo and the longer the murmur, the more severe the gradient.

   Note: Even though the peak of the crescendo in valvular AS goes only very slightly beyond midsystole no matter how severe the stenosis, a rough correlation can be found between the Q—peak interval and the presence of either mild or severe AS. If the Q—peak interval is less than 200 msec, severe stenosis (valve area less than 0.75 cm) is very unlikely. If the Q—peak interval is over 240 msec, severe stenosis is likely [4].

2. What may happen to the pitch and quality of the aortic murmur that is heard at the apex? Why is this confusing? What is this phenomenon called?

   ANS.:   The high-frequency components tend to radiate to the apex and may even sound musical at this site. Therefore, a murmur of MR is suggested. This is called the Gallavardin phenomenon.

   Note: In the elderly patient, the murmur at the apex is often musical or cooing. This is probably due to the commonly absent commissural fusion seen in the tricuspid stenotic valves of elderly patients. These nonfused cusps may vibrate, and produce pure frequencies [39].

3. What is characteristic of the quality of the loud murmur of significant AS?

   ANS.:   It tends to be harsh, rasping, grunting, and coarse, sounding like a person clearing his throat. This murmur can be imitated by placing your palm on the diaphragm of a stethoscope and listening through the earpieces while you scratch the dorsal surface of the hand with your fingernail.

Loudness and Site

1. Where is the aortic systolic murmur of valvular AS heard loudest?

   ANS.:   Anywhere in a straight line from the second right interspace to the apex. If, however, the patient is obese or has emphysema, the murmur may be loudest above the clavicle.

2. Where is the classic *aortic area*? What is wrong with this term?

   ANS.:   In the second right interspace. All aortic valvular events are best heard anywhere in the "sash" or "shoulder harness" area from the second right interspace to the apex.

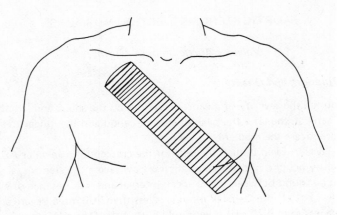

AORTIC AREA

Since aortic ejection murmurs and clicks are often best heard at the apex area, and aortic regurgitation murmurs are usually best heard along the left lower sternal border or midsternum, it should no longer be taught that the "aortic area" is the second right interspace.

3.   What term should be substituted for *aortic area*?

  ANS.:   The *second right interspace.* It is confusing to a student to be told that aortic murmurs and ejection sounds are often best heard at the left sternal border or apex and then to hear the second right interspace called the "aortic area."

4.   What is characteristic of the upward radiation of an aortic murmur?

  ANS.:   It tends to radiate into the neck bilaterally, but often radiates well along the innominate vein, to make the murmur slightly louder on the left, contrary to earlier impressions reported in the literature.

  Note: If it radiates better to the right, you should suspect supravalvular AS. (See p. 280 for description of supravalvular AS.)

5.   Is a loud ejection murmur (at least grade 4/6) ever associated with mild AS?

  ANS.:   Although a loud murmur usually signifies severe AS, a small percentage occur in moderate AS and even mild AS [1].

  Note: a) A loud murmur, together with an absent or very soft A_2, almost always means severe AS [1].

  b) The mere transmission of an aortic systolic murmur to the neck does not tell you the degree of AS.

6.   If a murmur of AS is grade 6, i.e., can be heard with the stethoscope off the chest, how soft can the murmur become if heart failure with resultant reduced stroke volume develops?

  ANS.:   It may almost disappear because of the poor myocardial contraction.

  Note: Concomitant mitral stenosis (MS) will also decrease the loudness of the AS murmur, but unless the MS is very severe, the AS murmur will dominate the picture and even cause the MS murmur to be absent [42].

*7.   Why will a low flow due to a cardiomyopathy or mitral obstruction produce almost no murmur across a moderately obstructed aortic valve?

     ANS.:   The physiological cross-sectional area of the aortic valve is always smaller than the anatomical area, and the lower the flow, the smaller the physiological cross-sectional area used by the forward stream. It has been shown that if the flow is low, the anatomical cross section of the aortic valve could be narrowed by nearly 60% without impinging on the functional cross-sectional area [41].

8.   Why may there be a soft murmur in the absence of heart failure in severe AS in the elderly?

     ANS.:   a) There is commonly an increased anteroposterior chest diameter in the elderly, especially at the base.

           b) The lack of commissural fusion of the three cusps seen commonly in the stenotic aortic valves of elderly persons may cause the ejected blood to come out in the form of a "spray" rather than a jet. This may modify the murmur and make it not only more musical but also less loud and harsh than when there is a fixed orifice due to commissural fusion and the production of a high velocity jet, as from the narrow nozzle of a hose [39].

Summary of Auscultatory Clues to the Diagnosis of Severe Valvular Aortic Stenosis

The AS is probably severe, i.e., the gradient is over 70 mm Hg, or, in the presence of congestive heart failure, over 50 mm Hg, if:

1.   An S_4 is present in a patient under age 40 [9].
2.   The murmur is long, is accompanied by a thrill, and the A_2 is soft or absent.
3.   The murmur is long and only grade 3/6, but the patient has a large, thick chest, heart failure or significant MS, and the A_2 is very soft or absent.

Hypertrophic Subaortic Stenosis Murmurs

1.   When in systole does the obstruction begin in **hypertrophic subaortic stenosis (HSS)**?

     ANS.:   Midsystole.

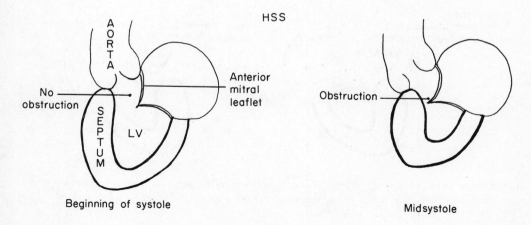

The asymmetric hypertrophy of the LV (sometimes shortened to ASH) causes no obstruction until the disproportionately hypertrophied septum meets the anterior mitral leaflet in midsystole.

2.   When does the ejection murmur begin in HSS?

ANS.:   If the obstruction is moderate or severe the murmur will begin at the same time as in valvular stenosis, i.e., in early systole, contrary to many statements in the literature that are probably based either on mild cases or on phonocardiograms that are too well filtered or too hastily examined. The reason the murmur so often begins early in HSS, even though the obstruction occurs late, is because tremendously rapid early ejection is characteristic of HSS. Normally, only 50% of ventricular volume is ejected during the first half of systole, but in HSS, 80% or more is ejected during this period [37]. This rapid flow even through a normal valve can produce a murmur in early systole. Then the obstruction to outflow occurs and produces the rest of the murmur. However, if the obstruction is mild, there may not be an early flow murmur and only the delayed murmur due to the midsystolic obstruction may be present.

Note: Occasionally, a low-amplitude ejection sound can be seen on a phonocardiogram preceding the murmur. The rapid ejection in early systole can set up the necessary conditions for sudden expansion of the aorta and the production of a root sound.

3.   How can raising the blood pressure by a vasopressor agent or by having the patient squat help to differentiate between the ejection murmur of valvular AS from HSS?

ANS.:   In valvular AS, raising the blood pressure has no effect unless an inotropic vasopressor, such as metaraminol, stimulates contraction and thus increases the gradient. If the vasopressor agent produces a bradycardia by the vagal effect of suddenly raising blood pressure, there may be more time for diastolic filling, and the greater stroke volume may increase the loudness of the murmur.

In patients with HSS, on the other hand, a pure vasopressor, such as methoxamine which has no inotropic effects, will decrease the murmur. The increased resistance to outflow probably tends to hold the **outflow tract** open by pushing down on the anterior mitral leaflet.

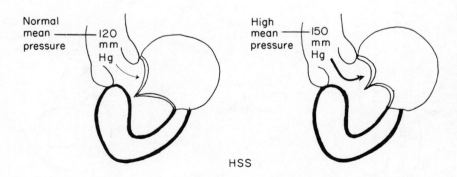

Normal mean pressure ——— 120 mm Hg

High mean pressure ——— 150 mm Hg

HSS

A high blood pressure during ejection pushes up on the mitral valve and spreads apart the LV outflow tract, which is made up of the septum and the anterior mitral leaflet.

4.   What tends to make an HSS obstruction worse, making the cavity smaller, or making it larger? Why?

ANS.:   Making it smaller, because the hypertrophied septum obliterates the cavity space faster if it is a smaller cavity at the beginning of systole.

5.   How can a **Valsalva maneuver** help differentiate the ejection murmur of valvular AS from HSS?

ANS.:   During the Valsalva maneuver, the venous return is decreased. Thus, the stroke volume is decreased, and the ejection murmur of valvular AS is decreased. However, in a patient with HSS, the decreased venous return produces a smaller LV and therefore more obstruction and a louder murmur.

Note: This may not always work, because the Valsalva maneuver may produce such a rise in systemic resistance and aortic pressure that it overcomes the effect on heart size.

6.   How can amyl nitrite inhalation differentiate the ejection murmur of valvular AS from that of HSS?

ANS.:   The blood pressure will drop immediately with amyl nitrite inhalation, but the flow does not increase until the tachycardia and increased cardiac output occur about 20 sec later. Therefore, the murmur of valvular AS, which is dependent on flow, will not begin to increase for about 20 sec. The murmur of HSS, on the other hand, will become louder within a few beats after inhalation, because as soon as the blood pressure drops (which is almost immediately), the loss of resistance to outflow causes a loss of support for the anterior leaflet of the mitral valve as the ventricle contracts. (See p. 307 for hemodynamic effects of amyl nitrite.)

7.   What can cause both an increased peripheral resistance and increased venous return? What effect will this have on the murmurs of HSS and of valvular AS?

ANS.:   Squatting, especially for the first few beats, will diminish the murmur of HSS and tend to increase the murmur of valvular AS, because it causes both an increased venous return for a few beats and then a persistent increase in peripheral resistance [35].

*8.   What is peculiar about the site of greatest loudness of the HSS murmur?

ANS.:   It is usually loudest near the apex but occasionally it is loudest at the left lower sternal border. However, when septal hypertrophy is so great that it produces RV as well as LV outflow obstruction, the infundibular obstruction may cause the murmur to be louder at the base than at the apex or left lower sternal border.

Note: "Asymmetric septal hypertrophy of the heart" describes well the heart in HSS, because the septum is so disproportionately hypertrophied that it can cause both outflow and inflow obstruction of the LV and RV, i.e., it can cause not only AS but also PS and even occasionally some mitral or tricuspid gradients or both. The dominant obstruction, however, is almost always AS.

9.   Why is the HSS murmur often mistaken for an MR murmur?

ANS.:   a) Because the HSS murmur often tends to be loudest at the apex.

b) Some MR is usually present. It is thought that either the hypertrophied septum distorts the direction in which the papillary muscles pull on the valve cusps, or a **Bernoulli effect** pulls the anterior leaflet toward the septum. Echocardiograms show an abnormal anterior movement of the anterior mitral leaflet during systole.

*In one series there was a 75% incidence of ballooning of the mitral valve associated with HSS [25]. This may be due to the reduced end-systolic volume's narrowing the distance between the papillary muscle and the anterior mitral leaflet, permitting the latter to project excessively into the left atrium.

*Note: The MR murmur associated with HSS should change in the same way as the ejection murmur with any maneuvers or pharmacological agents. If it does not or is pansystolic (the MR murmur of HSS is either delayed in onset or ends before the A_2), primary MR is probably present and will not disappear after corrective surgery for the HSS.

10.   How can the presence of aortic regurgitation (AR) help distinguish valvular AS from HSS?

ANS.:   An AR murmur is not expected with HSS, but it is very common to have at least some AR with valvular AS.

Note: Since valvular AS may coexist accidentally with HSS, the presence of AR does not rule out HSS.

Supravalvular and Subvalvular Discrete Aortic Stenosis Murmurs

1.   Where in the aorta is the stenosis of supravalvular AS?

ANS.:   Above the **sinuses of Valsalva.**

*Note: It may be focal (hourglass), discrete membranous, or diffusely hypoplastic in type.

2.   At what unusual site might the murmur be loudest in supravalvular AS? Does this help differentiate it from valvular AS?

ANS.:   In the suprasternal notch or first right intercostal space [3]. (However, it may also be loudest in the second intercostal space, which is not an unusual best site for the valvular AS murmur.)

Note: Radiation of the murmur to the right carotid louder than to the left carotid may also suggest that it is supravalvular rather than valvular AS. (See p. 38 for explanation.)

*3.   What other murmurs are often found in patients with supravalvular AS?

ANS.:   a) Those due to branch stenosis of the pulmonary arteries.

b) A murmur due to AR.

*4.   Where may the obstructive ridge in subvalvular discrete AS be located, and of what may it consist?

ANS.:   a) Just below the aortic valve, and consisting of a thin membrane on the ventricular septum.

b) About 1 cm below the aortic valve, consisting of a fibrous ring and associated with muscular hypertrophy that narrows the outflow tract.

*5.   What other murmur is common in patients with discrete subaortic stenosis?

ANS.:   Aortic regurgitation may occur in as many as one-third of such patients [28].

Note: If the murmur is preceded by an ejection click, it is not likely to be due to discrete subvalvular AS, unless it happens to be associated with a bicuspid aortic valve.

Summary of Clinical Findings in Supravalvular Aortic Stenosis

1. Peculiar "elfin" facies in nonfamilial type. (See p. 30 for facies of supravalvular AS.)
2. Pulse volume greater and murmur louder in the right than in the left carotid.
3. Blood pressure higher in the right arm.
4. No ejection sound.
5. Slight AR murmur.

PULMONARY STENOSIS EJECTION MURMURS

1. Where is the classic "pulmonary area," and what is wrong with this term?
    ANS.:   The second left interspace. Pulmonary events may be best heard anywhere along the left sternal border (or even in the epigastrium in patients with chronic obstructive pulmonary disease).
2. Where is the murmur of (a) valvular PS and (b) infundibular PS usually best heard?
    ANS.:   a) At the second left interspace.
             b) At the third or fourth left interspace.
             Note: The third left interspace parasternally has often been called Erb's point. This name seems unnecessary and confusing, first, because some authors include the fourth left interspace, and, second, because medical dictionaries do not often give a definition of Erb's point on the chest, but describe one on the neck over the brachial plexus.
3. What is the relation between the peak of the crescendo of the PS murmur and the severity of the obstruction?
    ANS.:   The later the peak, the more severe the obstruction. It may be as late as 80% of the way through RV systole [44].
             Note: In about 50% of adults with coarctation, PS may be imitated by the auscultatory complex of an ejection click being followed by a murmur with a late peak [6]. In coarctation, the murmur may begin with a gap after the ejection click. This gap is never present in PS. The murmur in coarctation is heard best along the left sternal border and is probably due to flow through intercostal collaterals or possibly through the coarcted segment.
4. Why is it that in AS the murmur rarely peaks much beyond midsystole, yet in PS it may easily go beyond midsystole?
    ANS.:   The RV is shaped like a teapot, with a main body, namely, the inflow tract, and an exceptionally thick, high spout, which is the outflow tract, or **infundibulum**.

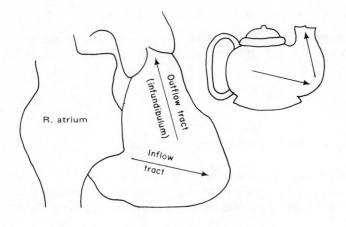

The outflow tract of the RV is a tubular structure made up mostly of muscle, called the crista supraventricularis, which separates the tricuspid from the pulmonary valves.

The worse the obstruction at the valve, the more do the muscles of the RV outflow tract hypertrophy, and the later it contracts relative to the inflow tract. It may be late contraction of this RV outflow tract that produces the late peak of the crescendo.

Note: Intracardiac phonocardiograms have shown that above a severely stenotic pulmonary valve, there is a loud pansystolic murmur reaching its peak late in systole, but just below the valve, only the late component of the murmur is present [19].

The LV, on the other hand, has only a partially complete muscular outflow tract, because the anterior mitral valve and its chordae and papillary muscles form the posterolateral wall of a merely functional outflow tract, which is probably seldom anatomically independent enough to contract more than slightly later on the left side.

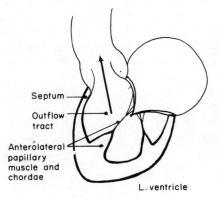

There is no infundibulum in the LV because the mitral and aortic valves are in direct continuity.

*5. How can you be sure by stethoscope alone that the murmur has an early peak, as in mild PS?

ANS.:   If the first (aortic) component of the second sound is clearly audible despite listening where the murmur is heard loudest, the chances are that the murmur has both an early peak and an early ending. This is both because the P_2 is delayed, usually coming long after the A_2 in PS, and because the murmur of mild PS (RV pressure less than 50 mm Hg) is rarely louder than grade 3/6.

*6.   How does infundibular PS affect the length of the murmur? Why?
    ANS.:   If the infundibular stenosis is due to a congenital diaphragm somewhere in the
        RV outflow tract, there is no unexpected effect on the length of the murmur.
        If, however, the infundibular stenosis is due to hypertrophy of the outflow tract,
        the murmur tends to be slightly longer than in valvular stenosis of similar sever-
        ity [44]. In this "contractile" type of stenosis, the infundibulum starts to con-
        tract later than does the main RV and reaches its maximum during the early
        relaxation phase of the body of the RV. Therefore, the infundibulum (and pul-
        monary artery) pressures are higher than pressure in the body of the RV for about
        100 msec before the pulmonary valve closes [26]. This causes a wide splitting of
        the A_2–P_2 interval, whether the stenosis is mild, moderate, or severe.
            Note: Infundibular stenosis can be imitated by a RV anomalous muscle bundle
        that traverses the RV cavity below the infundibulum, extending from its anterior
        wall to the low crista supraventricularis area. This can obstruct blood flow, pro-
        ducing a high-pressure inflow chamber and a distal low-pressure chamber. Apart
        from a loud ejection murmur, the clinical findings in this condition have not been
        well studied, because it is rare as a solitary lesion, most commonly being found
        together with a VSD.

7.   How can the analysis of a phonocardiogram suggest the severity of the gradient across the
    pulmonary valve in PS with an intact septum?
    ANS.:   By the length of the murmur, the site of the peak of the crescendo, the presence
        or absence of an ejection click, and the width of the split of the S_2 [44].

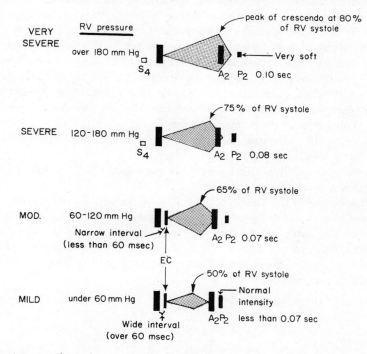

As the gradient across the pulmonary valve increases, the murmur peaks later and lasts longer, and
the P_2 becomes further separated from the A_2 and softer. The ejection click (EC) may be absent
above 60 mm of pressure in the RV, but may reappear on sitting or standing.

*8.   When may an acquired PS murmur occur?
       ANS.:   If a large pulmonary embolus produces a partial pulmonary artery obstruction.

*9.   What kind of facies suggest PS?
       ANS.:   Highly colored moon facies, as in Cushing's syndrome [47]. This facies is found
                in about a third of patients with severe PS. **Hypertelorism** is often found in PS
                with ASD.

Murmurs in Pulmonary Stenosis with Intact Ventricular Septum Versus Tetralogy of Fallot

1.   Besides in severe heart failure, when will PS be severe but the murmur still very short?
       ANS.:   If a VSD with an overriding aorta (**tetralogy of Fallot**) is present, the more severe
                the PS, the shorter the murmur. This is because the greater the obstruction at the
                pulmonary valve, the more the right-to-left shunt increases, and so less blood goes
                through the pulmonary valve. This will make sense only if you know that the
                murmur of a tetralogy of Fallot with **cyanosis** is solely due to the PS. *Right-to-left
                shunts do not usually produce murmurs.*
                   Note: This introduces the concept of two outlets for systole, which is impor-
                tant to the understanding of murmur changes with maneuvers and drugs. If a
                ventricle has two outlets for systole, increased resistance to flow through one of
                the outlets will cause more blood to go through the other outlet. If, on the other
                hand, resistance is decreased beyond an outlet, more blood will move through that
                outlet and less through the other. In tetralogy, the RV has the two outlets of the
                pulmonary artery and the aorta that overrides the VSD. In tetralogy you should
                think of the RV as pumping directly into the aorta and not into the LV first.

*2.   Why will the degree of cyanosis tend to correlate with the softness of the murmur?
       ANS.:   a) Increased cyanosis means increased polycythemia, which in turn means increased
                   blood viscosity. The greater the viscosity, the less the turbulence across an
                   obstruction and so the softer murmur [20]. (See Reynolds number on p. 261.)
                b) The greater the right-to-left shunt, the softer the murmur, because less blood is
                   going through the pulmonary valve.
                   Note: In a very severe tetralogy, the systolic murmur is usually no louder than
                grade 2/6 [43].

*3.   How can amyl nitrite differentiate between the murmur of PS in tetralogy and that occur-
       ring when the ventricular septum is intact?
       ANS.:   The immediate decrease in peripheral resistance with no effect on pulmonary
                resistance causes an increased right-to-left shunt through the septal defect into the
                overriding aorta, and thus there is decreased flow through the stenotic pulmonary
                valve, resulting in a softer murmur. If, on the other hand, there is an intact ven-
                tricular septum, the increase in flow after about 20 sec causes the PS murmur to
                become louder.

Note: The murmur of severe PS with a "muscle-bound" RV well may diminish with amyl nitrite. Therefore, amyl nitrite cannot be used to distinguish *severe* PS from tetralogy [45]. It can still be used, however, to distinguish mild or moderate PS (which are never "muscle-bound") from tetralogy. A "muscle-bound" RV is one with an excessive degree of outflow tract hypertrophy, with resultant failure of the RV systolic pressure to fall to less than 100 mm Hg immediately after valvotomy. It can be suspected by the paradoxical effect of amyl nitrite and by the jugular tracing, which shows a very slow and shallow Y descent (or no Y descent at all) in the absence of tachycardia.

4. How can vasopressor agents such as metaraminol or methoxamine help to differentiate between the murmur of PS with an intact ventricular septum and that of tetralogy?

ANS.:   In PS with an intact ventricular septum, metaraminol may make the murmur louder because of its positive inotropic effect [5]. Methoxamine, however, is a pure vasopressor agent and will produce little significant change in a PS murmur if the septum is intact. However, in tetralogy of Fallot, the PS murmur is increased because the increase in peripheral resistance decreases the right-to-left shunt into the aorta and therefore increases pulmonary flow. If an inotropic vasopressor such as metaraminol is used in tetralogy, variable effects are produced.

*5. How does the effect of a long diastole following a premature beat help to distinguish pure PS from tetralogy of Fallot?

ANS.:   If the postextrasystolic beat has a significantly louder murmur than the normal beats, the septum is probably intact. This reflects the fact that in pure PS, the postextrasystolic pressure in the RV usually rises over 15 mm Hg above its regular pressure, while in tetralogy of Fallot, the pressure rises only slightly above control levels [23].

*6. How can the phonocardiogram of the murmur suggest the rare kind of VSD with PS in which the pressure in the RV is higher than in the LV? (In the usual tetralogy of Fallot, the pressures in the RV and LV are equal.)

ANS.:   The peak of the murmur may be early in systole, and the murmur may end before the S_2, despite signs of severe PS, such as a widely split S_2. This may be because the infundibular stenosis (commonly present in this kind of PS) may be associated with so much outflow hypertrophy that the VSD may be squeezed closed by the hypertrophied muscle around it.

Note: This will produce, in effect, the same acoustic findings as in PS with an intact septum plus the contractile type of infundibular stenosis.

THE EFFECT OF RESPIRATION ON EJECTION MURMURS

1. What phase of respiration can increase a gradient across (a) a pulmonary valve and (b) an aortic valve? How should this affect their murmurs?

ANS.:   a) Inspiration increases the flow across the pulmonary valve. Therefore, it increases the gradient and the loudness of the murmur.

b) Conversely, it decreases the flow into the LV and across the aortic valve and therefore decreases both the gradient and murmur.

2.   Will a pulmonary flow murmur, such as in an ASD, with only a slight gradient across the pulmonary valve, become louder on inspiration? Why?

ANS.:   Only slightly or not at all, because even though the slight increases in velocity of flow due to inspiration should make the murmur louder, this is overcome by the increase in distance from the stethoscope caused by chest expansion. Even by intracardiac phonocardiograms, only two-thirds of ASDs show an increased amplitude of murmurs in the pulmonary artery on inspiration [18].

3.   Why may a PS ejection murmur increase on inspiration?

ANS.:   Because the gradient already present on expiration tends to increase by the square of the increased flow caused by inspiration.

4.   Why may a PS ejection murmur not always increase during inspiration?

ANS.:   a) Inspiration may place too much lung between the stethoscope and the heart. This occurs especially in the upper half of the chest (the basal areas of the heart). Therefore, listen low on the chest or even posteriorly. Do not listen merely where the murmur is loudest.

b) Sinus arrhythmia may cause shorter diastoles during inspiration. This will decrease stroke volume during inspiration and tend to soften the murmur.

5.   Why does standing help exaggerate the increase in a PS murmur caused by inspiration?

ANS.:   a) The increase in pulmonary flow caused by inspiration is about 15 ml, whether the subject is lying down or standing. The stroke volume, however, is decreased on standing, so that the same 15-ml increase in stroke volume on inspiration makes a proportionately larger amount of stroke volume ejected.

For example, the increase is 15% if the stroke volume supine is 100 ml, and the increase on inspiration is 15 ml. If the stroke volume on standing (which can be decreased by 25%) is 75 ml, the 15-ml increase on inspiration is now a 20% increase. Therefore, on standing, there is a proportionately greater increase in gradient across the pulmonary valve. Even though the murmur while standing will be softer on *both* inspiration and expiration, the *difference* will be more marked.

b) The increased sympathetic tone caused by standing may decrease the degree of sinus arrhythmia.

*6.   What is the effect of a Valsalva maneuver on an ejection murmur during and after the straining? Why?

ANS.:   During the straining, all ejection murmurs (with the rare exception of the HSS murmur) decrease, due to decreased venous return.

When the Valsalva strain is released, the maximum loudness of the pulmonary ejection murmur will return immediately, i.e., within two or three beats. The maximum loudness of the aortic murmur will, however, be delayed for about six to ten beats due to the time that it takes for the dammed-up venous blood to pass through the lungs to the LV and aorta [2].

Summary of How to Tell a Pulmonary from an
Aortic Stenosis Murmur by Auscultation

1. The AS murmur increases on expiration, while the PS murmur increases on inspiration, especially on standing and if you listen low on the chest posteriorly.
2. An AS murmur may be maximal in the second right intercostal space or at the apex. The PS murmur will only be maximal somewhere along the left sternal border.
3. The post-Valsalva effect causes an immediate return of loudness of the PS murmur and a delay of the return of the AS murmur loudness.
4. If an ejection click is present, it will decrease or disappear on inspiration only with PS.
5. A wide, normally moving split following the murmur usually indicates a murmur of PS and not of AS.
6. A right-sided S_4 gallop, i.e., one that increases on inspiration, is due to PS, while a gallop heard only at the apex that increases only on expiration suggests that the murmur is due to AS.

THORACIC ARTERY FLOW MURMURS

1. What is the difference between a bruit and a murmur?
    ANS.:   The word *bruit* (pronounced "brooee") is French for "noise" or "sound." In France, the first and second heart sounds are the first and second *bruits*. Our S_1 and S_2 are their B_1 and B_2. We tend to misuse the word to mean an arterial murmur. Since arterial murmurs sound the same as murmurs heard elsewhere, there seems to be no need for a change of terminology, especially since the word has even been used by some for a heart murmur [16].
2. What flow murmur may cause an ejection murmur at the second right or left interspaces even though the excess flow is not through the semilunar valves?
    ANS.:   Rapid flow through the proximal branches of the aorta in young people. This is often mistaken for an aortic ejection murmur.
    Note: A carotid murmur is present in about 80% of children up to 4 years, but in only 10% of those in older age groups.
3. How can you test for the presence of a supraclavicular arterial murmur?
    ANS.:   a) Inch gradually toward the supraclavicular area with your stethoscope. You will note that the murmur becomes loudest in that area and will be heard only in the first third of systole.
    b) If the hand on that side is exercised, the arm flow will be increased, and the murmur may become louder. A valvular murmur will not become louder.
    c) Have the patient stretch his arm downward and backward, and listen to the murmur gradually diminish as the subclavian artery is compressed.
    d) Compress the subclavian artery with your finger, and note how the murmur decreases. If only partial occlusion is obtained, the murmur may increase as the obstruction increases.
    Note: Listen also for a venous hum and an S_3 to confirm the presence of a hyperkinetic circulation [40]. (See p. 331 for a method of eliciting a venous hum.)

4.   What kind of arterial murmur is heard in **coarctation**?

ANS.:   A systolic delayed murmur continuing beyond the S_2 can be heard over the large collateral vessels of the back. This murmur may become softer or disappear if the arteries are compressed.

Note: If the systolic delayed murmur is heard between the left scapula and spine, it is questionable whether it is caused by flow through the coarctation itself or through the collaterals. It has been heard there with complete occlusion of the coarcted segment. It has generally been taught that the more severe the coarctation, the longer the murmur over the coarcted site. Thus, if the narrowed segment is less than 2 mm in diameter, the murmur will start in early systole, have a crescendo in late systole, and go into diastole (continuous murmur). A mild coarctation is said to have a short, early murmur.

*Aorta—Coronary Artery Bypass Surgery Flow Murmurs

*1.   Where are the systolic murmurs due to aorta—coronary artery bypass surgery best heard?

ANS.:   Usually, they are localized to the second and third left interspace parasternally [27].

*2.   What is the timing and intensity of the bypass murmur? How is it brought out?

ANS.:   It is a short, early ejection murmur, not much over grade 2/6 in loudness. It is best heard with the patient sitting up and leaning forward with held expiration.

*3.   What suggests that the systolic ejection murmur heard after coronary bypass surgery is indeed due to the bypass?

ANS.:   a) It was often noted to develop in patients who did not have the murmur prior to surgery.

b) When it disappeared, the bypass was often found occluded.

c) In one study, when the murmur was present, the bypass was invariably found patent [27].

d) It has been heard only when the anterior descending artery was bypassed.

*4.   What suggests that the systolic ejection murmur after bypass surgery is generated at the distal anastomotic site between the vein and artery?

ANS.:   a) It does not occur with a right coronary artery bypass.

b) It has not been heard on or around the aorta with a stethoscope at open heart surgery.

*5.   Why would the bypass graft murmur be expected to be louder in systole than in diastole, even though we know that coronary flow is greater in diastole?

ANS.:   a) The bypass graft has no aortic valve overriding it during systole as does the normal coronary ostium.

b) The murmur may be due to retrograde flow across the native coronary artery stenosis that engendered the operation in the first place. In support of this is the fact that in no patient with a completely occluded native stenosis has the murmur developed, and if the native stenosis was later found completely occluded, the murmur had disappeared.

*6.   What is the significance of (a) a disappearing and (b) a persistent bypass murmur?

ANS.:   a) A disappearing murmur has no meaning, because many become softer after a few months, and by one year, almost all are either softer or disappear.

b) A persistent murmur strongly suggests that the bypass graft is open.

Note: The murmur develops in only about half the patients with a bypass to the anterior descending artery.

Pulmonary Artery Branch Stenosis Murmurs

*1.   What types of pulmonary arterial stenosis are there?
      ANS.:   a) Multiple peripheral stenosis with or without stenosis of the right or left main
                 branch.
              b) Stenosis of the pulmonary trunk or its bifurcations.
              Note: a) There is commonly another congenital lesion present, such as pulmonary
                         valve stenosis or supravalvular AS.
                      b) Pulmonary artery branch stenosis is commonly seen with the rubella
                         syndrome, other features of which may be the cataracts, deafness, mental
                         retardation, or poor growth curves.

*2.   Does peripheral pulmonary branch stenosis produce a pulmonary ejection murmur?
      ANS.:   If the stenosis is unilateral, an ejection murmur may be present. If it is bilateral,
              however, a continuous murmur may or may not be produced [13]. Pulmonary
              hypertension must usually be present to maintain a gradient across the obstruction
              during diastole. It requires bilateral pulmonary branch stenosis or some other
              cause of pulmonary hypertension to produce a continuous gradient and murmur.
                 However, a pulmonary artery branch may be stenosed and produce no murmur
              at all if the distal segment is supplied by enough bronchial collaterals to prevent
              much forward flow [34].

*3.   Where are the murmurs of unilateral pulmonary branch stenosis heard? What can mimic this?
      ANS.:   Anywhere on the chest. Wide radiation with equal loudness throughout, i.e., to
              the axillae and back, is the hallmark of pulmonary artery branch stenosis murmurs.
              It can be imitated in some patients with an ASD by a pulmonary artery flow mur-
              mur that can also be heard anywhere on the chest wall and that disappears with
              closure of the ASD [36].
                 Note: A partially obstructing pulmonary embolus can produce a similar murmur.

*4.   What is characteristic of the timing and loudness of peripheral pulmonary artery stenosis
      murmurs that distinguishes them from valve stenosis or flow murmur?
      ANS.:   They begin, peak, and end later in systole than a proximal stenosis or flow mur-
              mur. They are rarely louder than grade 3/6.

REFERENCES

1. Bergeron, J., Abelmann, W. H., Vazquez-Milan, H., and Ellis, L. B. Aortic stenosis — Clinical
   manifestations and course of the disease. *Arch. Intern. Med.* 94:911, 1954.
2. Bertrand, C. A., Milne, I. G., and Hornick, R. A study of heart sounds and murmurs by
   direct heart recordings. *Circulation* 13:49, 1956.
3. Beuren, A. J., Apitz, J., and Harmjanz, D. Supravalvular aortic stenosis in association with
   mental retardation and a certain facial appearance. *Circulation* 26:1235, 1962.
4. Bonner, A. J., Sacks, H. N., and Tavel, M. E. Assessing the severity of aortic stenosis by
   phonocardiography and external carotid pulse recordings. *Circulation* 48:247, 1973.
5. Bousvaros, G. A. Effect of norepinephrine on the phonocardiographic, auscultatory and
   hemodynamic features of congenital and acquired heart disease. *Am. J. Cardiol.* 8:328, 1961.
6. Bousvaros, G. A. Diagnostic auscultatory complex in coarctation of the aorta. *Br. Heart J.*
   29:443, 1967.

7. Bruns, D. L. A general theory of the causes of murmurs in the cardiovascular system. *Am. J. Med.* 27:360, 1959. Classic article.

8. Bruns, D. L., and VanDer Hauwaert, L. G. The aortic systolic murmur developing with increasing age. *Br. Heart J.* 20:370, 1958.

9. Caulfield, W. H., deLeon, A. C., Jr., Perloff, J. K., and Steelman, R. B. The clinical significance of the fourth heart sound in aortic stenosis. *Am. J. Cardiol.* 28:179, 1971.

10. Datey, K. K., Deshmukh, M. M., Engineer, S. D., and Dalvi, C. P. Straight back syndrome. *Br. Heart J.* 26:614, 1964.

11. Daves, M. L. Cardiovascular anachronisms. *J. A. M. A.* 224:879, 1973.

12. Dawson, A. A., and Palmer, K. N. V. The significance of cardiac murmurs in anemia. *Am. J. Med. Sci.* 25:554, 1966.

13. D'Cruz, I. A., Agustsson, M. H., Bicoff, J. P., Weinberg, M., Jr., and Arcilla, R. A. Stenotic lesions of the pulmonary arteries. *Am. J. Cardiol.* 13:441, 1964.

14. DeLeon, A. C., Jr., Perloff, J. K., Twigg, H., and Majd, M. The straight back syndrome. *Circulation* 32:193, 1965.

15. de Monchy, C., van der Hoeven, G. M. A., and Beneken, J. E. W. Studies on innocent praecordial vibratory murmurs in children. *Br. Heart J.* 35:685, 1973.

16. Dock, W. Examination of the chest: Advantages of conducting and reporting it in English. *Bull. N.Y. Acad. Med.* 49:576, 1973.

17. Feruglio, G. A. An intracardiac sound generator for the study of the transmission of heart murmurs in man. *Am. Heart J.* 63:232, 1962.

18. Feruglio, G. A., and Steenivasan, A. Intracardiac phonocardiogram in thirty cases of atrial septal defect. *Circulation* 20:1087, 1959.

19. Gamboa, R., and Willis, K. The systolic murmur of combined pulmonary stenosis and infundibular stenosis. *Am. J. Cardiol.* 19:880, 1967.

20. Garb, S. The relationship of blood viscosity to the intensity of heart murmurs. *Am. Heart J.* 25:568, 1944.

21. Goldberg, L. M., and Unland, H. Heart murmurs in pregnancy. *Dis. Chest* 52:381, 1967.

22. Groom, D., Chapman, W., Francis, W. W., Bass, A., and Sihvonen, Y. T. The normal systolic murmur. *Ann. Intern. Med.* 52:134, 1960.

23. Hoffman, J. I. E., Rudolph, A. M., Nadas, A. S., and Paul, M. H. Physiologic differentiation of pulmonic stenosis with and without an intact ventricular septum. *Circulation* 22:385, 1960.

24. Humerfelt, S. Bj. An epidemiological study of high blood pressure. *Acta Med. Scand.* (Suppl. 406) 173:64, 1963.

25. Jeresaty, R. M. Mitral ballooning — A possible mechanism for mitral insufficiency in diseases associated with reduced end-systolic volume of the left ventricle. *Chest* 60:114, 1971.

26. Johnson, A. M. Functional infundibular stenosis, its differentiation from structural stenosis and its importance in atrial septal defect. *Guys Hosp. Rep.* 108:373, 1959.

27. Karpman, L. The murmur of aortocoronary bypass. *Am. Heart J.* 83:179, 1972.

28. Kelly, D. T., Wulfberg, E., and Rowe, R. D. Discrete subaortic stenosis. *Circulation* 46:309, 1972.

29. Leatham, A. Systolic murmurs. *Circulation* 17:601, 1958.

30. Leatham, A., and Gray, I. Auscultatory and phonocardiographic signs of atrial septal defect. *Br. Heart J.* 18:193, 1956.

31. Lessof, M., and Brigden, W. Systolic murmurs in healthy children and in children with rheumatic fever. *Lancet* 2:673, 1967.

32. Lewis, K. B., Bruce, R. A., Baum, D., and Motulsky, A. G. The upper limb-cardiovascular syndrome. *J. A. M. A.* 193:98, 1965.

33. Luisada, A. A., and DiBartolo, G. High frequency phonocardiography. *Am. J. Cardiol.* 8:51, 1961.

34. Massumi, R., Just, G., Tawakkol, A., and Hernandez, T. Acoustically silent stenosis of branch of pulmonary artery. *Am. J. Med.* 40:773, 1966.

35. Nellen, M., Gotsman, M. S., Vogelpoel, L., Beck, W., and Schrire, V. Effects of prompt squatting on the systolic murmur in idiopathic hypertrophic obstructive cardiomyopathy. *Br. Med. J.* 3:140, 1967.

36. Perloff, J. K., Caulfield, W. H., and deLeon, A. C., Jr. Peripheral pulmonary artery murmur of atrial septal defect. *Br. Heart J.* 29:411, 1967.

37. Pierce, G. E., Morrow, A. G., and Braunwald, E. Idiopathic hypertrophic subaortic stenosis. *Circulation* (Suppl. 4) 30:152, 1964.

38. Rawlings, M. S. The "straight back" syndrome. *Am. J. Cardiol.* 5:333, 1960.

39. Roberts, W. C., Perloff, J. K., and Costantino, T. Severe valvular aortic stenosis in patients over 65 years of age. *Am. J. Cardiol.* 27:497, 1971.

40. Stapleton, J. F., and El-Hajj, M. M. Heart murmurs simulated by arterial bruits in the neck. *Am. Heart J.* 61:178, 1961.

41. Stein, P. D., and Munter, W. A. New functional concept of valvular mechanics in normal and diseased aortic valves. *Circulation* 44:101, 1971.

42. Uricchio, J. F., Goldberg, H., Sinah, K. P., and Likoff, W. Combined mitral and aortic stenosis. *Am. J. Cardiol.* 4:479, 1959.

43. Vogelpoel, L., and Schrire, V. Auscultatory and phonocardiographic assessment of pulmonary stenosis with intact ventricular septum. *Circulation* 22:55, 1960.

44. Vogelpoel, L., and Schrire, V. Auscultatory and phonocardiographic assessment of Fallot's tetralogy. *Circulation* 22:73, 1960.

45. Vogelpoel, L., Schrire, V., Beck, W., and Nellen, M. The pre-operative recognition of the "muscle-bound" right ventricle in pulmonary stenosis with intact ventricular septum. *Br. Heart J.* 26:380, 1964.

46. Wennevold, A. The origin of the innocent "vibratory" murmur studied with intracardiac phonocardiography. *Acta Med. Scand.* 181:1, 1967.

47. Wood, P. *Diseases of the Heart and Circulation* (2nd ed.). Philadelphia: Lippincott, 1956. P. 411.

14
Systolic Regurgitant Murmurs

1. What is meant by a systolic regurgitant murmur?
   ANS.: A murmur produced by retrograde flow from a high pressure area of the heart through some abnormal opening into an area of lower pressure.

2. List the four usual abnormal openings that allow systolic regurgitation.
   ANS.: a) A **ventricular septal defect** (VSD). (High-pressure area left ventricle [LV] to low-pressure area right ventricle [RV].)
   b) An incompetent mitral valve. (High-pressure area LV to low-pressure area left atrium.)
   c) An incompetent tricuspid valve. (High-pressure area RV to low-pressure area right atrium.)
   d) An arteriovenous communication such as **patent ductus arteriosus** (PDA). (High-pressure area aorta to low-pressure area pulmonary artery.)

3. What characteristics are common to all systolic regurgitant murmurs?
   ANS.: a) If there are early components, they start at the first heart sound (S_1). If there are late systolic components, they always go to or beyond the second heart sound (S_2) of the same side.
   b) When soft, they are predominantly high-pitched and blowing, because the opening is probably very small, and there is a high **gradient** between a ventricle and any chamber into which retrograde flow occurs.
   c) They tend to remain the same after long diastoles. (For rare exceptions to this rule, see p. 294.)

4. How can you imitate various kinds of high-pitched, blowing murmurs?
   ANS.: a) Whisper a drawn-out "haaaa" or "hoo."
   b) Say a drawn-out "shsh."
   c) Hold the diaphragm of the stethoscope against the palm of your hand and listen through the earpieces while you run the pads of your fingers across the back of your hand.

5. What are regurgitant murmurs called if they stretch from S_1 to or beyond S_2?
   ANS.: Pansystolic or holosystolic.

---

*indicates material that is for electives or fellows in cardiology, or concerns rare phenomena, of interest primarily to cardiologists.

Boldface type indicates that the term is explained in the Glossary.

6. What are the advantages and disadvantages of each of these terms?

ANS.: *Holos* is a Greek word meaning "wholly," "complete," "entire," or "all." *Pan* is a Greek word meaning "each" and "every," as well as "all." Therefore, it seems that holosystolic has only one meaning, and it fits the timing of "from S_1 to S_2" well. However, *pan* is such a universally used prefix, with such a well-understood meaning, "all," that there is no point in teaching an unfamiliar prefix such as *holo* for the sake of pedantic purism. *Holo* has probably become popular in English-speaking countries because it means the same as "wholly" which sounds enough like *holo* to be easily remembered.

7. If the regurgitant murmur goes far beyond the S_2, what is it called?

ANS.: A continuous murmur.

THE EFFECT OF A LONG DIASTOLE ON LEFT-SIDED REGURGITANT MURMURS

1. What will happen to the loudness of a left-sided regurgitant murmur, such as in mitral regurgitation (MR) or ventricular septal defect (VSD), after a sudden long diastole?

ANS.: The loudness usually remains about the same (except under special circumstances).

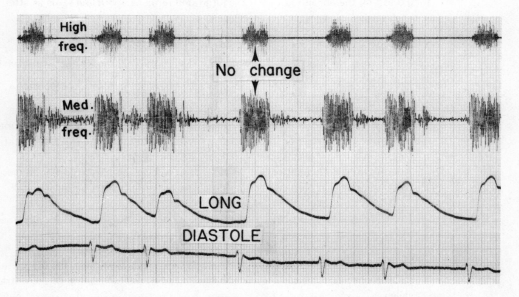

A high- and medium-frequency phonocardiogram taken at the apex together with an external carotid tracing from a 45-year-old woman with moderately severe, chronic, rheumatic MR, with few symptoms on digitalis alone. Because of atrial fibrillation, short and long diastoles are present which demonstrate that the murmur does not grow louder after long diastoles than after short or average diastoles.

Note: a) This is one of the best ways to differentiate an ejection from a regurgitant murmur. If the murmur is accentuated after a long pause at the **base of the heart**, but not at the apex, there is probably both an ejection and a regurgitant murmur present.

b) If the pause is caused by a premature ventricular contraction (PVC), do not compare the postextrasystolic beat with the PVC but with the normal cycle following the postextrasystolic beat. A PVC may be so premature that there is no time for any significant ventricular filling. Therefore, the loudness of a murmur produced by the PVC itself is of no significance.

2.   Since there is a larger volume in the ventricle after a long diastole, why does the left-sided regurgitant murmur not usually become louder?

ANS.:   In MR, VSD, or PDA, the LV has two outlets during systole. The amount ejected through each outlet depends on the relative resistance beyond each outlet. During the PVC, the aortic pressure is less than normal because of the small stroke volume. During the long diastole after the PVC, the pressure beyond the aortic outlet falls still more, due to continued long runoff into the periphery. Thus, by the time of the next systole, the resistance at the aortic valve has dropped so low that blood is preferentially ejected into the aorta, and relatively less is regurgitated through the other orifice. However, since there is more volume in the LV at the end of a long diastole, the absolute quantity regurgitated remains about the same as after short diastoles.

Note: The quantity of retrograde flow in MR and in a VSD actually does increase *during isovolumic contraction* in the beat after the long pause; but this does not affect the loudness of the murmur during the major part of systole, when the amount regurgitated is not increased [44].

*3.   When may a left-sided regurgitant murmur become *louder* after a long diastole?

ANS.:   a) When a larger LV produces more regurgitation, as when MR results from the types of papillary dysfunction in which the papillary muscle is either abnormally short, due to scarring, or displaced downward and laterally, due to LV dilatation.

b) When the outflow resistance is fixed, as in aortic stenosis (AS).

c) When there is a high peripheral resistance, as in severe hypertension or congestive failure, which permits little fall in aortic pressure despite a long diastole.

4.   When may the MR murmur become softer after a long diastole?

ANS.:   a) In the ballooned or prolapsed mitral valve syndrome. (See p. 308 for explanation.)

b) In murmurs due to papillary muscle dysfunction, this often happens. The cause is unknown, but it may possibly occur because these murmurs may result from much the same mechanism involved in the ballooning of the mitral valve.

MITRAL REGURGITATION MURMURS

Terminology

Why may it be preferable to use the term *mitral regurgitation* rather than *mitral incompetence* or *mitral insufficiency,* even though cardiologists are about equally divided as to the preferred usage?

ANS.:   The abbreviation for mitral incompetence or insufficiency is MI, which is also used as an abbreviation for myocardial infarction. There is no confusion when MR is used.

Note: Regurgitation describes the direction of flow, while *incompetence* or *insufficiency* describes the condition of the valve. For the sake of consistency, we shall use *aortic, pulmonary, and tricuspid regurgitation, instead of incompetence or insufficiency.*

Causes

1.   List the four commonest causes of MR murmurs in the adult.

ANS.:   Rheumatic valve damage, papillary muscle dysfunction, ruptured chordae tendineae, and myxomatous degeneration of the mitral valve, causing ballooning or prolapse of the mitral leaflet into the left atrium.

*2.   List some rare causes of MR in the adult.

ANS.:   Left atrial myxoma and endocardial cushion defects with a cleft anterior leaflet. (The former may present as pure MR.)

Note: A cleft mitral valve can also occur with a secundum ASD, but this is rare [34, 75].

*3.   What are the likely causes of a MR murmur at the apex in an infant?

ANS.:   a) Papillary muscle dysfunction, secondary to either an anomalous left coronary artery arising from the pulmonary artery or to endocardial fibroelastosis.

b) Acute myocarditis.

c) Endocardial cushion defect with cleft mitral valve.

d) Myxomatous degeneration of the mitral valve with or without Marfan's syndrome.

Note: About 50% of patients with Marfan's syndrome have MR [67].

e) Ebstein's anomaly of the left atrioventricular (AV) valve (actually a tricuspid valve) in corrected transposition of the great vessels.

4.   What suggests that mitral annular dilatation is in itself a rare cause of MR?

ANS.:   a) Many patients with grossly dilated hearts due to such conditions as aortic regurgitation (AR) or **cardiomyopathies** have no MR.

b) The surface area of the billowing mitral leaflets is more than twice the area of the mitral orifice.

c) Severe LV dilatation may occur without any dilatation of the annulus; i.e., the midportion between the apex and the base expands most.

d) The fibromuscular portion of the annulus contracts during systole and produces a sphincter-like action.

Note: An idiopathic calcification of the mitral annulus can increase the degree of regurgitation in a mitral valve, in which there is another cause of MR, presumably because if the fibro-muscular portion of the annulus is thick or calcified, it cannot act as a sphincter, i.e., it cannot decrease the size of the mitral orifice during systole.

*5.   When will corrected transposition have a murmur that mimics MR?

ANS.:   A corrected transposition means that both the great vessels and the ventricles are transposed. Therefore, an anatomical RV on the left side of the heart feeds the aorta, but receives blood through a tricuspid valve. (It should be easy to remember that the valves stay with the appropriate ventricle rather than atrium because the chordae tendineae and papillary muscles are attached to the valves.) If the tricuspid valve becomes regurgitant, as with an Ebstein's anomaly (downward displacement of a deformed tricuspid valve), it will *seem* to be MR. There is a high incidence of left AV valve (tricuspid) regurgitation in patients with corrected transposition [72]. Anomalous insertion of chordae into the left AV valve has been found to be the cause when no Ebstein's deformity was present.

6.   What are the usual causes of papillary muscle dysfunction murmurs?

ANS.:   a) Myocardial infarction, recent or old, with or without a ventricular **aneurysm** and with or without papillary muscle fibrosis. Infarction of the ventricle at the base of the papillary muscles or the ischemia of that area of the ventricle that may occur with an attack of angina pectoris can cause marked MR even with a normal papillary muscle. An anomalous coronary artery arising from the pulmonary artery can cause MR, probably due to infarction of both the papillary muscle and of the ventricle at the base of the papillary muscle.

   Note: Mitral regurgitation due to papillary muscle dysfunction is most severe when associated with infarction of the ventricular muscle at the base of a papillary muscle. Many patients with papillary muscle fibrosis do not have MR at all. In experiments with dogs, it has not been possible to produce MR by causing papillary muscle ischemia unless it is combined with infarction of the LV at the base of the papillary muscle [59].

   *b) Congenital MR can occur when a poorly developed small papillary muscle arises at a higher-than-normal point on the LV wall.

   c) **Hypertrophic subaortic stenosis** (HSS) can cause MR because the anterior leaflet may be pulled down in systole toward the septum and away from the posterior leaflet. This movement of the leaflet toward the septum is due either to the abnormal angle at which the anterolateral papillary muscle is attached to the grossly hypertrophied septum or to the **Bernoulli effect** of the high-velocity stream being ejected past the anterior mitral leaflet.

7.   When acute infarction results in the murmur of MR due to papillary muscle dysfunction, what happens to the murmur during the course of the acute infarction?

ANS.:   About 10% of papillary muscle dysfunction murmurs due to acute infarction will disappear before the patient leaves the hospital [38].

Loudness, Sites, and Radiation of Mitral Regurgitation Murmurs

1.   Where are MR murmurs loudest?

ANS.:   At the apex area.

Note: There is at least one report of a MR murmur loudest at the second right interspace. This patient had only moderate MR, probably from some unusual cause [79]. Another article reports on 2 patients with probable rheumatic MR with the murmur just as loud at the second right interspace as at the apex area [88]. These patients also had only mild to moderate MR. The jet in these unusual cases probably was directed anteriorly against the aortic root, which lies against the anterior atrial wall. (See p. 303 for diagram.)

2.   When may an MR murmur *seem* to be louder at the left sternal border than at the apex area?

ANS.:   In very long chests in which the apex area is very medially placed; i.e., where the LV impulse is actually near the left sternal border. You must try to shift the apex laterally either by turning the patient to the **left lateral decubitus position** or having him sit up, with his legs on the bed. (Standing the patient up will move the apex area even more medially.)

3.   Where is the best radiation zone of the usual MR murmur?

ANS.:   It usually radiates best to the axilla and the left posterior intrascapular area of the chest. However, if loud enough, it will radiate to the right, but to a lesser degree.

Note: When the murmur is due to ruptured chordae, it may have unusual radiation (see p. 303).

*4.   What kind of conduction abnormality has made an MR murmur louder?

ANS.:   Wolff-Parkinson-White (W-P-W) preexcitation, type B, in which RV contraction precedes LV contraction. The reason for the increased loudness is unknown [7].

Note: W-P-W preexcitation, type B, has also brought out a tricuspid regurgitation and an innocent ejection murmur [7].

5.   Besides an obese or emphysematous chest, what can cause silent, severe MR?

ANS.:   a) Concomitant mitral stenosis (MS) can apparently direct the MR stream in such a way as to make the murmur inaudible [2].

b) Prosthetic mitral valve MR due to a suture breakdown.

c) Slight MR may be silent due to a large RV or a large, thick chest that hides the ventricle from the stethoscope. The MR may become severe and the murmur audible only intermittently when myocardial ischemia develops due to an attack of angina. During these ischemic episodes the MR may become so severe that the patient may even develop pulmonary edema [54a].

Note: Almost all the adults with silent MR who have been reported on had severe regurgitation, and most had paroxysmal nocturnal dyspnea or were in atrial fibrillation [80]. A widely split S_2 in the presence of a large LV and unexpectedly large left atrium were the only clues.

Shape, Pitch, and Duration of Mitral Regurgitation Murmurs

1.   What are all the possible shapes of a MR murmur?
     ANS.:

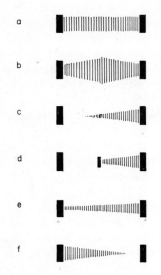

a

b

c

d

e

f

Note that when the MR murmurs begin late, they always go to the second sound, and when they begin early, they always start with the first sound.

2.   What shape are the loudest MR murmurs?
     ANS.:   Pansystolic, crescendo-decrescendo murmurs are usually the loudest. The crescendo-decrescendo in these patients is very slight and is better described as spindle-shaped on a phonocardiogram.
3.   How does the pitch of a murmur correlate with gradient and flow?
     ANS.:   High gradients and little flow produce high-pitched murmurs. High flow and little gradients produce low-pitched murmurs. Combined high flow and high gradients produce murmurs with mixed frequencies.
4.   Which MR murmurs are always associated with almost purely high frequencies, i.e., only a blowing sound?
     ANS.:   All the soft ones with small flows and high gradients, i.e., those due to trivial MR.
             Note: The gradient between a left atrium and LV usually reaches over 100 mm Hg during the peak of systole.
5.   Why does the MR murmur go slightly beyond the S_2?
     ANS.:   Because the LV pressure is higher than the left atrial pressure, even after the aortic valve closes.

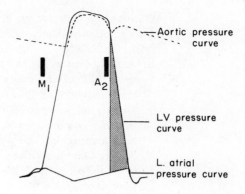

Note that the LV pressure is above left atrial pressure even after the A_2.

6. Is a MR murmur louder on inspiration or expiration?

   ANS.:   It is usually louder on expiration, because that is when blood is pushed into the LV from the lungs.

   Note: Unusual rotations caused by inspiration may bring the heart closer to the stethoscope and make the murmur paradoxically louder on inspiration. This can often be counteracted by placing the stethoscope lateral to the apex beat. If the heart sounds also become louder on inspiration, this suggests that rotation is the cause. Unusual cardiac rotations with respiration are common after cardiac surgery.

7. How can different kinds of papillary muscle dysfunction produce MR murmurs of different shapes?

   ANS.:   If one papillary muscle is unable to contract or is attached to infarcted muscle at its base, its muscle plus chordae will be longer than the opposite contracting papillary muscle plus chordae. The contracting normal papillary muscle will therefore pull down the mitral leaflets on its side during systole [8].

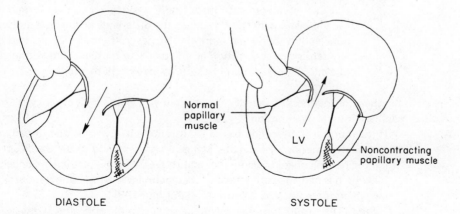

DIASTOLE   SYSTOLE

Normal papillary muscle

LV

Noncontracting papillary muscle

A noncontracting papillary muscle may make its chordae plus papillary muscle relatively longer as the ventricle becomes smaller. This is most likely to produce a murmur that becomes progressively louder as systole proceeds (crescendo murmur to the S_2).

During the progress of systole there are two possibilities, keeping in mind that each group of papillary muscles supply chordae to one half of both anterior and posterior leaflets:

a) As the pressure rises and the LV cavity decreases in size, the portion of the mitral leaflets with the relatively long papillary muscle-plus-chordae projects more and more into the left atrium, to produce a crescendo murmur to the S_2. That is, the noncontracting papillary muscle fails to keep its side of the mitral leaflets down in apposition with the counterpart attached to the opposite papillary muscle. This is probably the commonest type of papillary muscle dysfunction murmur.

b) If, on the other hand, the heart contracts very well, it may become so small at the end of systole that there may be no disparity between the two sides, i.e., the relative length of the chordae plus the papillary muscles is not crucial to maintain apposition to the billowing valves. Thus, even a decrescendo or crescendo-decrescendo murmur can occur.

A papillary muscle plus chordae may, on the other hand, be very short, due to complete scarring. This shortened muscle will pull down on its side of the valve leaflets throughout systole; i.e., it can produce a "bound-down" leaflet, so that the opposite side will tend to overshoot in late systole and produce a crescendo murmur. However, depending on how small the ventricle becomes as the pressure rises, and how well the good papillary muscle contracts, a crescendo, a plateau, a decrescendo, or a crescendo-decrescendo murmur will be produced.

Note: a) If a piece of mitral valve attached to the normal muscle loses support in midsystole due to too short a papillary muscle to the opposite leaflet, it may suddenly flip upward to produce a midsystolic nonejection click or late systolic murmur.

b) The papillary muscles are subendocardial structures and receive their innervation early. Therefore, they usually begin to contract early in systole [39]. Any difference in papillary muscle and chordae length will then usually manifest itself early in systole; i.e., the murmur will usually begin with the M_1, unless the difference produces a midsystolic nonejection sound and murmur. However, it has been suggested that late tensing or contraction of one papillary muscle could be the cause of a sound or click in midsystole in patients with papillary muscle dysfunction.

8.   How can the shape or loudness of the MR murmur tell you whether its etiology is rheumatic or papillary muscle dysfunction?

ANS.: a) If the murmur is crescendo to the S_2, it is more likely to be due to papillary muscle dysfunction. Rheumatic MR is rarely crescendo to the S_2 except during the healing phase of acute rheumatic fever, usually in a patient under age 20, who has had an acute attack of rheumatic fever within a few months, during which there was also a pansystolic murmur [93].

Note: The papillary muscle dysfunction due to the HSS almost always produces a decrescendo murmur, so that if a pansystolic murmur is heard at the apex in a patient with HSS, coincidental rheumatic MR should be suspected, and the murmur will probably become louder with squatting and persist after surgery for the HSS [52].

b) If the murmur becomes louder as the heart becomes smaller when the patient compensates for failure, this is suggestive of fixed rheumatic MR. Papillary muscle dysfunction murmurs tend to become softer as the heart becomes smaller with improving failure.

c) If an S_4 is present, it strongly suggests papillary muscle dysfunction, secondary to a cardiomyopathy. Rheumatic MR rarely is associated with an S_4.

d) Papillary muscle dysfunction murmurs often become softer after long diastoles [14]. Rheumatic MR murmurs remain about the same.

MITRAL REGURGITATION DUE TO RUPTURED CHORDAE

1. How many chordae are capable of rupturing?

   ANS.: There are about 120 attached to both mitral leaflets. There are about 12 chordae attached to each of about six heads of each papillary muscle, and these chordae divide about three times before they attach to their valves [71].

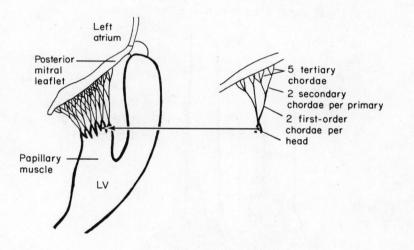

   Note: Spontaneous ruptures usually occur in one of the 25 major chordae closer to the papillary muscles than to the leaflets, thus involving at least four or five small terminal branches [68a]. Only if infective endocarditis has caused the rupture may only a few terminal branches tear off.

2. How can you tell if a MR murmur is due to papillary muscle dysfunction rather than to ruptured chordae?

   ANS.: a) Ruptured chordae superimposed on rheumatic heart disease produce a sudden onset of severe MR and failure (a loud S_3, a grade 3/6 or more murmur, and an increase in symptoms). The usual papillary muscle dysfunction produces signs only of mild to moderate MR, with a murmur that is rarely more than grade 3/6. Exceptionally, however, papillary muscle dysfunction due to a large infarcted area at the base of the papillary muscle can produce severe MR. Also, rupture of only a few unimportant posterior chordae superimposed on a normal heart may produce few symptoms.

Note: The majority of the chordae that insert into the leaflets are inserted into the distal rough zone of the leaflets and are called rough zone chordae. Rough zone chordal rupture of the posterior leaflet may cause only moderate MR. Two rough zone chordae, larger and thicker than the rest, insert into the anterior leaflets. Rupture of one of these two so-called strut chordae often results in severe MR and a flail anterior leaflet [68a].

b) If the murmur is soft or only crescendo to the S_2, it is not likely to be due to ruptured chordae.

c) A decrescendo mixed frequency murmur associated with symptoms of high left atrial pressure (orthopnea or paroxysmal nocturnal dyspnea) suggests ruptured chordae of recent onset. This is because the left atrium does not enlarge much with MR. This poor left atrial compliance may raise the V wave pressure to a very high peak in systole. This late rise in left atrial pressure decreases the regurgitation and the murmur toward the end of systole.

Note: a) Left atrial pressures as high as 70 mm Hg have been recorded toward the end of systole.

b) If a leaflet projects markedly into the left atrium because of ruptured chordae, it is often called a "flail" leaflet.

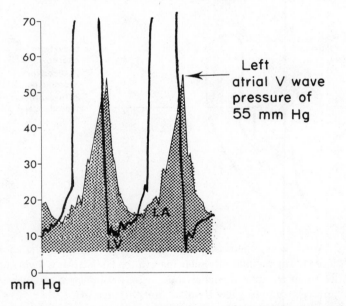

This is a LV and left atrial (wedge) pressure tracing from a 23-year-old woman with ruptured mitral chordae. The shaded area is under the left atrial (wedge) pressure curve. The slight delay in the peak wedge pressure is due to the fact that wedge pressures (taken by a catheter wedged into the distal pulmonary arterial branches) always show a delay in comparison with direct left atrial pressure tracings. The rapid increase in V wave pressure during systole rapidly decreases the gradient across the mitral valve and will tend to cause both a decrescendo gradient and a murmur. The decompressing effect on the LV of the massive loss of blood into the left atrium causes a late systolic fall in LV pressure. This end-systolic decrease in LV pressure further decreases the gradient across the mitral valve toward the end of systole.

3.   Why may ruptured chordae imitate aortic stenosis (AS)?

ANS.:   If the posterior chordae rupture, producing a flail posterior cusp, the stream of regurgitation may strike the atrial septum in such a way as to produce murmurs with the shape and radiation into the carotids typical of that seen with AS murmurs [76]. To further confuse the picture, the murmur at the second right interspace may even be shorter than the one at the apex. About half of the posterior rupture murmurs will radiate into the neck [76].

Note: a) Radiation of the posterior rupture murmur may sometimes be better into the lower back than into the neck. The reason is unknown.

b) Despite good radiation into the second right interspace and neck, the murmur of posterior chordae rupture is still usually loudest at the apex [40a].

4.   How does the murmur caused by a rupture of anterior chordae radiate?

ANS.:   If it causes a flail anterior leaflet, it will not only create an apical murmur but the murmur may also radiate loudly along the midthoracic spine and even to the top of the head [31, 58].

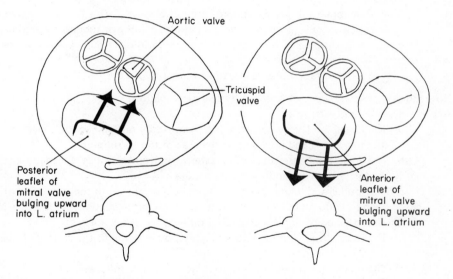

These views of the valve rings from above show how posterior ruptured chordae (on left) can direct the regurgitant stream against the aorta and cause the murmur to be transmitted like an aortic ejection murmur. On the right is shown how ruptured anterior chordae can direct the regurgitant stream posteriorly against the spine.

Note: There have been rare reports of patients with *anterior* chordal rupture who had murmurs that imitated AS [82]. The reason is unknown, but they may have mixed findings, such as the good transmission to the back characteristic of an anterior flail leaflet as well.

5.   How do diastolic sounds tell you that a loud MR murmur is due to ruptured chordae rather than to rheumatic heart disease?

ANS.:   The resistant healthy atrial wall in patients with ruptured chordae responds with a **Starling effect** to the massive regurgitant stream and, by contracting strongly, often produces an S_4. An S_4 is rare in rheumatic MR.

6.   What is the commonest cause of ruptured chordae? What is the next most common cause?

ANS.:   The commonest cause is **infective endocarditis** on an abnormal valve such as found in rheumatic heart disease or in myxomatous transformation. The next most common cause is idiopathic [76].

Note: Myxomatous degeneration of a valve or a chorda can make these structures prone to endocarditis. The endocarditis may then be blamed for the rupture that is really due to myxomatous degeneration. A cleft in the posterior cusp, with billowing, voluminous leaflets, has sometimes been found associated with idiopathic ruptures, suggesting that an unusual strain is placed on at least one chorda [54]. There are reports of patients with the ballooned valve syndrome (see p. 308 for explanation) having chordal rupture [33].

7.   What can imitate the auscultatory findings of ruptured chordae?

ANS.:   Severe myxomatous degeneration of the mitral valves. This is often known as "the floppy valve syndrome." Only a definite history of sudden development of severe MR can rule out the more chronic and insidious floppy valve syndrome.

Quantitating the Degree of Mitral Regurgitation

1.   How can you tell the degree of MR by physical examination?

ANS.:   The MR is greater
   a) The larger the LV by palpation, determined by noting how displaced the cardiac impulse is and how large is the area of the LV impulse.
   b) The greater and later the left parasternal movement, since this may represent the left atrium expanding during systole.
   c) The louder and longer the apical systolic murmur (with the exception of the descrescendo murmur caused by a very high left atrial pressure in acute MR).
   d) The more palpable the early rapid filling wave at the apex.
   e) The louder the S_3, since this is roughly porportional to the torrential diastolic flow.
   f) The longer and louder the diastolic flow murmur following the S_3.
   g) The wider the split of the S_2, unless the development of severe pulmonary hypertension narrows the split.

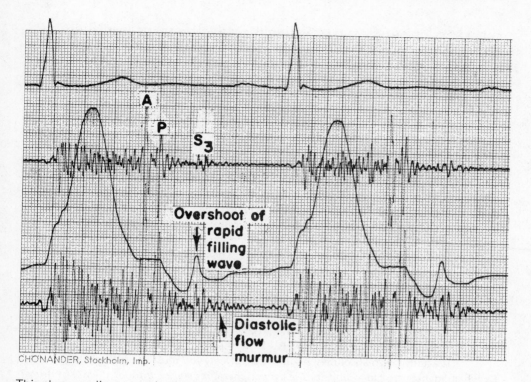

This phonocardiogram and apical pulse tracing is from the same 15-year-old girl with severe rheumatic MR as in the figure on p. 234. The pulse tracing was taken over the LV impulse in the supine position and is therefore an apex precordiogram instead of an apex cardiogram, which is taken in the left lateral decubitus position. The phonocardiograms are from the third left parasternal interspace. The upper one is taken at medium frequency; the lower one is a logarithmic tracing that brings out low and medium frequencies. Note the following signs of severe MR: (1) the widely split S_2 of 50 msec; (2) the diastolic flow murmur after the S_3, both of which are so loud that they can be recorded at the left sternal border (see figure on p. 234 for the same S_3 and diastolic flow murmur at the apex of this patient); (3) the exaggerated early rapid filling peak of the apical impulse (this would be palpable in the left lateral decubitus position).

*2.   How can you tell the degree of MR by a left parasternal precordiogram?

ANS.:   Since initial left parasternal movement is due mostly to the RV, and the late movement is due mostly to the left atrial expansion with the regurgitant volume, a ratio of late to early outward movement correlates with regurgitant volume [5]. If you draw a horizontal line at the onset of the initial outward movement, the amplitude of early and late movement above this line is made into a ratio of late outward movement over early outward movement. As the regurgitant volume increases, the ratio becomes larger, with an r value of 0.93 when correlated with angiographically determined regurgitation. The ratio is nullified by mixed mitral stenosis (MS) and MR or anything that causes RV movement, such as an atrial septal defect (ASD) or tricuspid regurgitation. (The time constant of the equipment may have to be at least 650 msec.) The regression equation for pure MR is:

$$\text{Regurgitant volume (in ml)} = \left(32 \times \frac{\text{late}}{\text{early}}\right) + 34$$

EFFECTS OF DRUGS AND MANEUVERS ON REGURGITANT MURMURS

Raising Peripheral Resistance

1. What happens to left-sided regurgitant murmurs if the peripheral resistance is increased? Why?

    ANS.:   They become louder, because with regurgitation there are two outlets for systole, and an increased resistance at the aortic outlet promotes more outflow through the other outlet.

2. How will a vasopressor agent such as methoxamine, phenylephrine, or angiotensin help to tell you whether a long systolic murmur at the apex is due to AS or MR?

    ANS.:   With increased peripheral resistance, the aortic murmur will be unchanged or become softer, but an MR murmur will become louder.

    Note: A vasopressor drug with a strong positive inotropic effect, such as norepinephrine, will only add a confusing variable. Phenylephrine and angiotensin have only weak inotropic effects. The dose of phenylephrine is 0.4—0.7 mg by slow intravenous infusion until a rise of about 20 mm Hg in systolic pressure is achieved [6].

    Angiotensin may be a preferable agent, not only because it is a natural humoral substance and thus has fewer side effects but also because its effects do not last as long as those of methoxamine [102]. The dose is 0.075 μg per kilogram, diluted to 20 ml and given intravenously. Nevertheless, if you wish to raise peripheral resistance with absolutely no inotropic effect, you must use methoxamine.

3. By which maneuvers can a subject raise his peripheral resistance without the use of drugs?

    ANS.:   a) By squatting, which not only increases venous return for a few beats but also causes a persistent increase in peripheral resistance.

    b) Handgrip, which will either decrease or have no affect on the murmur of AS [56].

    Note: a) Handgrip has little affect on the peripheral resistance of normal subjects. It will, however, increase the peripheral resistance in hypertensive patients who on ECG or x-ray have evidence of left ventricular hypertrophy [25]. Although at least 30% of maximum voluntary contraction is necessary to produce circulatory changes, 50% of maximum voluntary contraction will often produce a greater elevation of blood pressure. A voluntary contraction 75% of maximum will achieve a peak response in one minute [25].

    *b) Standing to increase peripheral resistance has different effects on the murmur of MR, depending on the cause of the MR. If the MR murmur is primarily dependent on dilatation, the smaller heart caused by the pooling effect of standing makes the murmur softer. But if dilatation is not a factor, the increased peripheral resistance caused by standing should make the murmur become louder. However, the decreased volume of regurgitation due to diminution of venous return on standing causes the murmur to stay about the same. (The MR murmur of the ballooned valve syndrome becomes louder on standing. See p. 313 for details.)

*4.   How can you bring out the type of MR murmur of papillary muscle dysfunction that is transient and is associated only with episodes of coronary insufficiency and angina?

ANS.:   Passive leg-raising to increase the LV volume can sometimes bring out this type of papillary dysfunction murmur [53].

Decreasing Peripheral Resistance with Nitrites

1.   How does amyl nitrite affect blood pressure and cardiac output? How do its effects differ from those of nitroglycerin?

ANS.:   Amyl nitrite causes an immediate and *marked* drop in blood pressure. After about 20 sec the cardiac output is *increased*. Nitroglycerin causes a *mild* drop in blood pressure and a *fall* in cardiac output.

2.   Why does amyl nitrite cause an increase in cardiac output while nitroglycerin causes a fall in cardiac output?

ANS.:   The rapid profound drop in blood pressure produced by amyl nitrite results in a strong reflex sympathetic outflow that constricts the veins [55]. The direct effect of amyl nitrite on the capillaries may open up shunts between the dilated arterioles and venules. The increased venous return, together with the reflex tachycardia, increases the cardiac output.

        Nitroglycerin, on the other hand, reduces venous return by causing venous pooling. This is because the mild drop in blood pressure produced by nitroglycerin is not strong enough to result in enough sympathetic outflow to cause venous constriction.

3.   How will amyl nitrite help to separate an aortic ejection murmur from an MR murmur at the apex?

ANS.:   By dropping the peripheral resistance, it makes the MR murmur softer. By causing an increased velocity of ejection through the aortic valve, it makes the aortic ejection murmur louder.

4.   How many inhalations of amyl nitrite are used?

ANS.:   A marked effect may be achieved with only three inhalations. If this does not lower the blood pressure adequately, inhalations may have to be continued for half a minute before a drop in pressure does occur.

        Note: The following precautions are helpful when using amyl nitrite:

a) Wear rubber gloves, or the odor may remain on your fingers for days. After use, flush the used capsule down the toilet, or it will impart its odor to your examining room for hours.

b) Never use it unless the patient is supine, or you may produce syncope.

c) Warn the patient that he will feel flushed and that his heart will pound for about 30 sec. Reassure the nervous patient by telling him that the drug was formerly used to take away "heart pain," but is no longer used because of the noise of cracking the capsule and its lingering odor.

d) An assistant should call out the systolic blood pressures throughout the entire procedure.

THE BALLOONED OR PROLAPSED MITRAL VALVE

Definitions and Terminology

1. What is meant by a ballooned or prolapsed mitral valve? What auscultatory findings does it cause?

    ANS.: It refers to the bulging of one or both mitral valve leaflets into the left atrium during systole, so that a crisp systolic sound or click and a later systolic MR murmur are commonly heard. The systolic murmur goes to the A_2.

    Note: Although the posterior leaflet is the one that most commonly balloons into the atrium, the anterior leaflet may also be involved.

2. What are all the names given to the ballooned or prolapsed mitral valve click and murmur complex?

    ANS.: a) Ballooned valve syndrome.

    b) Prolapsed mitral valve syndrome (the commonest term).

    c) Systolic click—murmur syndrome.

    d) Barlow's syndrome.

    e) Click, late-systolic murmur syndrome.

    f) Billowing mitral valve syndrome.

    Note: The word *syndrome* is applied because in this condition there are often symptoms of nonspecific chest pain, an ECG showing T wave abnormalities (negative T in aVF or the left precordium or abnormally notched T waves) and ventricular arrhythmias, which occasionally lead to sudden death.

3. Why may *ballooned valve* be preferable to the other terms?

    ANS.: a) *Prolapse* suggests to the novice a downward movement into the LV when actually it is a backward and upward movement into the left atrium.

    b) *Billowing* suggests that the normal valve does not billow, which is not true.

    c) *Barlow's syndrome* is not descriptive for the beginner.

    d) *Click—systolic murmur syndrome* ignores those patients with only the click or only the murmur and those in whom the systolic sound is not clicky.

    Note: The term *floppy valve syndrome* has been applied by some as a synonym for the ballooned valve syndrome. This is unfortunate, because it was originally meant to describe the most marked degree of myxomatous degeneration with elongated chordae, causing severe MR [69, 86]. In the usual ballooned valve syndrome, the MR is at most only moderate.

4. What can we call the click or sound that often precedes the delayed systolic murmur?

    ANS.: A nonejection click or sound. It cannot be called midsystolic because at times it may come as early as an ejection click and as late as a widely split S_2.

    Note: a) The click often comes slightly after the onset of the murmur.

    b) Multiple clicks are common.

    c) If the etiology is primarily myocardial infarction and papillary muscle dysfunction, it is not so likely to sound like a click.

Etiology, Pathology, and Physiology of the Ballooned Valve Syndrome

1. What is the usual mitral valve abnormality seen at surgery or necropsy when a ballooned mitral valve is examined?

    ANS.:   Myxomatous transformation. This may be recognized only on careful inspection, since the valve may appear grossly normal to casual examination by the pathologist.

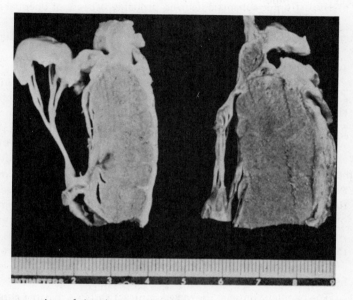

On the left is a cross section of the abnormal middle scallop of the posterior leaflet. On the right is the same area from a woman with left ventricular hypertrophy but no MR. (From J. K. Trent, A. G. Adelman, E. D. Wigle, and M. D. Silver. *Am. Heart J.* 79:539, 1970.)

Note: Although **Marfan's syndrome** is commonly associated with myxomatous valves, only rarely do patients with the ballooned valve syndrome have any of the other stigmata of Marfan's syndrome. However, 20-30% of patients with ballooned valves have joint laxity, high arched palates or other skeletal abnormalities such as scoliosis, **pectus excavatum**, and straight backs.

*2. Has the tricuspid valve been found to balloon with myxomatous transformation?

    ANS.:   Routine necropsy specimens, as well as RV angiocardiograms, have shown that the tricuspid valve can also balloon and show myxomatous changes. Whether or not this can occur in the absence of mitral ballooning is unknown.

3.   List the suspected etiologies of ballooning of the mitral valve.
       ANS.:   a) Congenital myxomatous transformation with elongated chordae.
                  Note: A significant percent have abnormal ventricular wall motion so that a
                  myocardial component may be important in many of these patients.
               b) Papillary muscle dysfunction due to myocardial infarction [91, 92].
              *c) Dysfunction of muscle adjacent to the posterior leaflet, as in myocardial infarc-
                  tion or congenital absence of the left circumflex coronary artery.
              *d) After mitral valve surgery, probably due to unequal length of the chordae [3].
              *e) Hypertrophic subaortic stenosis, probably because of unequal chordal length
                  due to asymmetric hypertrophy [18].

*4.   What congenital cardiac condition has been found to be commonly associated with the
       ballooned valve syndrome?
       ANS.:   Atrial septal defect.
                  Note: In the past, it was thought that MR was present only in the primum or
                  endocardial cushion type ASD, and that it was always due to cleft mitral valves.
                  Now it is conceded that MR can occur in secundum ASDs, not only due to a cleft
                  mitral valve (very rare) but also due to myxomatous degeneration of the valve,
                  with ballooning into the left atrium [57]. Occasionally, the MR is due to an
                  abnormally high insertion of the chordae near the top of the ventricular septum.

5.   What is the cause of the nonejection click preceding the delayed systolic murmur?
       ANS.:   Angiograms have shown a systolic bulge, ballooning, or prolapse of one leaflet
               (usually at the posterior cusp) or both leaflets into the left atrium at the moment
               of maximum ballooning. Therefore, a sudden stretch of the chordae as they give
               way with the peak pressure in midsystole seems to be an obvious explanation for
               the cause of the click [16]. It has therefore been called a "chordal snap." Plastic
               repair of mitral chordae tendineae rupture has produced a nonejection click. This
               has been used to defend the chordal snap theory.
                  The papillary muscles, however, contract early so that the chordae are under
               too much tension from the beginning of systole to "snap" during ventricular ejec-
               tion [74]. Therefore, this theory has been challenged by one that suggests that
               the click is a *valvular* sound, produced by the loss of support of one leaflet by its
               opposing leaflet, due to an abnormality of chordal length. Thus, a small piece of
               unsupported leaflet may suddenly flip upward to its full extent to produce a
               click [19].
                  Note: a) Most reports claim that the click always occurs at the point of *maximum*
                     ballooning, but this is controversial [24].
                        b) Although on auscultation the click usually seems to initiate the murmur,
                     on the phonocardiogram in many patients it may actually follow shortly
                     after the onset of the murmur.

*6.   What is the "contraction ring" theory for the cause of the nonejection click?
       ANS.:   Some investigators have found a posteroinferior area of excessive contraction in
               the LV during midsystole in most of their patients. This area is attached mainly
               to the posterior papillary muscle. Since this part of the LV contracts excessively,
               it pushes up the posterior papillary muscle and causes the chordae to become
               slack. Further systole then pulls the chordae taut, to produce the click [21].
               However, this type of contraction abnormality is not seen in all patients with the
               ballooned valve syndrome.

Note: To suggest further that ballooning of the mitral valve may sometimes be due to a primary myocardial abnormality, the following findings may be listed:

a) Angiograms have shown that at least 80% of patients with ballooned mitral valves have LV asynergy (abnormal areas of contraction or absence of contraction). At least six types of asynergy have been described [78]:

1) Reduction of extent or shortening of the inflow tract area around the mitral valve ring [51].

2) "Ballerina foot" pattern in right anterior oblique views (vigorous posteromedial contraction and anterior convexity).

3) "Hourglass," ringlike contraction of the middle of the ventricle.

4) Inadequate long axis shortening.

5) Posterior akinesis.

6) Cavity obliteration.

b) Late systolic clicks have been heard for the first time in patients during the course of their infarction [91, 92].

c) A late systolic murmur and click developed in one patient after radiopaque dye was inadvertently injected directly beneath the posterior leaflet.

d) Patients with coronary disease are sometimes found to have a click and late systolic murmur on squatting [14]. This is the opposite of what happens in the usual young patient with the ballooned valve syndrome.

7. How much MR is present if a delayed murmur to the S_2 is present?

ANS.: Since there is little or no regurgitation at the beginning of systole in these patients, only a mild to moderate amount of MR is likely to be present with this kind of murmur.

*8. What can cause the development of heart failure in a patient with mild MR secondary to the ballooned valve syndrome?

ANS.: a) Occasionally, chordae will rupture and produce severe MR [33, 54, 89].

b) Gradual progression from mild to severe MR can also occur, but this is rare [43].

c) Infective endocarditis on the mitral valve can occur.

Note: The first clue that a late systolic murmur was associated with MR was the infective endocarditis that occasionally developed in such patients.

*9. What is the commonest noncardiac cause of midsystolic clicks?

ANS.: A small left-sided pneumothorax. When loud, it may be heard at some distance from the patient. One theory claims that these clicks are produced by the heart flipping the lingula against the anterior thoracic wall [27]. (The fact that they often occur in diastole as well as systole helps to rule out a ballooned valve etiology.)

Note: For the first half of this century, midsystolic clicks were considered due to pleural-pericardial adhesions, probably because

a) Gallavardin described 4 cases in which autopsy evidence showed only pleural-pericardial adhesions as the apparent explanation [35].

b) When multiple clicks are heard with ballooned valves, they may mimic a pericardial friction rub [43].

Ballooned Valve Auscultatory Findings

Click and Murmur Shape and Loudness

1. What is the usual shape of delayed systolic murmurs in the ballooned valve syndrome?

   ANS.: To the ear, they often sound crescendo or plateau to the second sound.

   Note: Most of these murmurs actually are crescendo-descrescendo on a phonocardiogram [3]. They are rarely plateau, and although they seem to at first be crescendo to the S_2, they may often be seen to reach a peak near the S_2 if a phonocardiogram is run at fast paper speed.

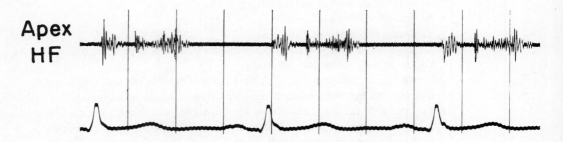

The midsystolic sound was a click heard loudest at the apex in this 45-year-old woman. The murmur following it is crescendo to the S_2. This is the classic ballooned valve click-murmur complex by auscultation.

2. What is the loudest grade of murmur in the ballooned valve syndrome?

   ANS.: If it is not a whoop or honk, which can be grade 6, it is almost never over grade 3/6.

   Note: a) Systolic musical honks or whoops are not an uncommon sign of a ballooned valve. They are usually transient and disappear with different positions and with different phases of respiration; and, when they have disappeared, a regurgitant murmur is almost always present, even if not due to a ballooned valve. The word *honk* refers to the honking of a goose.

   *b) Much more rarely, a loud, musical systolic murmur may be present in the left chest in the absence of a ballooned valve when an anomalous fibrous chord stretches across the ventricular cavity like the string of a musical instrument. When stretched by cardiac dilatation, it may become taut enough to produce a murmur [70].

3. Which components of the ballooned valve auscultatory findings may be missing?

   ANS.: Either the click or the murmur may be missing. However, certain maneuvers often bring them out.

Changing the Click and Murmur with Maneuvers or Drugs

1. What happens to the nonejection click and murmur when volume to the LV is decreased, as with standing, inspiration, or a Valsalva strain? Why?

   ANS.: They both come earlier and they often become louder. Indeed, they may only be heard on sitting or standing. The click may actually come so early on standing that it may fuse with the first sound and seem to disappear altogether [3].

Note: a) The click may also become louder in the left lateral decubitus position, perhaps because of the change of blood pressure that occurs in some patients in that position.

b) After the release of a Valsalva maneuver, the click may become louder because of the overshoot of blood pressure.

2. Why does the ballooned valve murmur become louder and begin earlier on standing or any maneuver that makes the heart smaller?

ANS.: Angiograms have shown an increase in ballooning in the upright position. This may occur because the redundant tissue acts like the dome of a parachute whose diameter is decreased if the edges are held down. That is, when the ventricle becomes smaller and the diameter is reduced, the center of the "parachute" is pushed up, due to the fixed length of chordae and papillary muscles in the smaller ventricle.

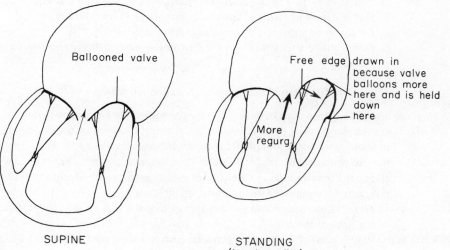

One of the diagnostic characteristics of the ballooned valve murmur is that it becomes louder and begins earlier when the heart is made smaller.

3. What maneuver can tell you that a crescendo systolic murmur to the S_2 is due to papillary muscle dysfunction rather than to the ballooned valve syndrome if the latter happens to have no click?

ANS.: Only the ballooned valve murmur will become louder and longer on sitting or standing.

*4. What happens to the (a) click and (b) murmur position and loudness with amyl nitrite?

ANS.: a) The click comes earlier and usually becomes softer or may even disappear. The smaller end-diastolic volume makes the click come earlier, and the low systolic pressure makes the click softer.

b) The murmur usually becomes softer immediately, and then after about 15 sec it may become louder, due to the overshoot of blood pressure. If the control murmur is only late systolic, amyl nitrite will usually cause it to become pan-systolic.

5. What is the effect of increasing blood pressure with phenylephrine or methoxamine on the position and loudness of (a) the click (b) the murmur?

ANS.: a) The click takes variable positions and usually becomes louder because of the greater force exerted on the mitral valve structure.

b) The murmur becomes louder, and you may even bring out a late systolic murmur if only a click is present.

*6. What is the effect on the click or murmur if the heart is made larger by slowing the rate with propranolol?

ANS.: Both the click and murmur may diminish or disappear.

*7. How do nonejection clicks following mitral valvotomy differ from other nonejection clicks?

ANS.: These clicks are

a) Lower in frequency and therefore less clicking in quality.

b) Louder.

c) Earlier in systole (more easily confused with an ejection sound).

d) Not constant in terms of the effect maneuvers have on them.

e) Likely to become single or multiple spontaneously.

f) Occasionally situated late in the murmur or even at the end of an early systolic murmur.

*The Apex Cardiogram with Ballooned Valves

*1. How can the apex cardiogram help to diagnose the ballooned valve syndrome?

ANS.: A midsystolic dip or retraction occurs at about the time of the nonejection click in about two-thirds of patients with the ballooned valve syndrome. The timing of the dip changes with maneuvers and thus keeps a constant relationship with the click. If the retraction is absent or slight, it can often be accentuated or brought out with standing or with amyl nitrite [90].

Note: Kinetocardiograms have shown that the late systolic movement can peak at the time of the click.

*2. What is the significance of midsystolic retraction on the apex cardiogram in ballooned valve syndromes?

ANS.: It implies that any MR that is present is mild. The actual cause of the retraction is unknown, but it may be due to a sudden rotation of the heart as the mitral leaflet bulges upward. Significant MR may be able to prevent this rotation effect by producing a recoil thrust toward the apex at the time of the click.

TRICUSPID REGURGITATION MURMURS

Site, Loudness, and Shape

1. Where is the murmur of tricuspid regurgitation (TR) usually heard best? In what other places may it occasionally be heard best?

ANS.: It is usually heard best at the left lower sternal border. It is occasionally heard best in the epigastrium, at the right sternal border and over the liver (in chronic obstructive pulmonary disease); or, if the RV is very large, it may be heard best over the mid-left thorax at the site of the usual LV apex area, which may be taken over by the RV.

Note: In chronic obstructive pulmonary disease, the TR murmur may be heard over the free edge of the liver, presumably because the diaphragm pushes the RV hard against the liver on inspiration.

2. What is the classic way of diagnosing TR by auscultation?

ANS.:   Listen for a pansystolic murmur at the left lower sternal border (or wherever a palpable RV lift is felt) that becomes louder with inspiration.

3. Why does the TR murmur usually increase in loudness on inspiration?

ANS.:   Because more blood is drawn into the RV and becomes available for regurgitation. Since the pulmonary artery pressure rises slightly on inspiration, there is increased resistance in that direction.

    Note: If the intrathoracic pressure drop on inspiration is not subtracted from the pulmonary artery pressure as taken with a manometer in the pulmonary artery, the pulmonary artery pressure will give the false impression of falling with inspiration.

*4. Does the murmur of TR remain louder on held inspiration (inspiratory apnea), or does it require moving respiration, as when one is looking for movement in the S_2 split?

ANS.:   It remains loud on inspiratory apnea, because as long as intrathoracic pressure is kept low by an expanded lung, more blood will be brought into the RV than on the expiration. An inadvertent Valsalva maneuver during held apnea will, however, counteract these effects by obstructing flow into the RV.

    Note: Occasionally, the TR murmur will not increase with inspiration. This may be because

    a) the regurgitation may be so severe that the slight increase in regurgitant volume on inspiration is unnoticeable.

    b) Inspiration may not bring much more blood into the RV because of a poor inspiratory effect secondary to a decreased vital capacity caused by such abnormalities as pulmonary congestion.

    c) In the absence of pulmonary hypertension, inspiration may so lower pulmonary vascular resistance that the extra blood drawn in on inspiration is ejected into the pulmonary artery rather than regurgitated.

    d) The RV may be so damaged that it is functioning near the plateau of the Starling curve, so that an increased volume and pressure in it cause little change in the strength of contraction.

5. How, besides by inspiration, can you increase the venous return in order to bring out a TR murmur?

ANS.:   a) By exercise.

    b) By having someone hold the patient's legs up or having the patient bend his knees up toward his chest.

    c) By amyl nitrite inhalation.

*6. When is a TR murmur decrescendo?

ANS.:   When the TR is very severe and the right atrium is not very enlarged, as in acute TR from rupture of tricuspid chordae. This is because the massive regurgitant volume produces so steep a rise in the V wave in the right atrium that it decreases the systolic gradient across a tricuspid valve as systole progresses and the V wave height becomes very high. (See figure on p. 302 for similar effect on left side.)

    Note: Occasionally, *no* murmur at all may be heard if free TR is present so that the atrium and ventricle are almost one chamber in systole.

*7.   What should you suspect if a tricuspid valve systolic whoop or honk is present?
        ANS.:   Tricuspid regurgitation, secondary to pulmonary hypertension.
                Note: This whoop or honk usually disappears if the pulmonary hypertension
                is relieved [46] .

Differential Diagnosis of Tricuspid and Mitral Regurgitation by Auscultation

1.   Why is it often difficult to tell TR from MR?
        ANS.:   a) The MR murmur transmitted to the left sternal border may sometimes increase
                on inspiration and so mimic TR. This is presumably due to some rotational
                phenomenon, which should be suspected if the heart sounds also increase with
                inspiration.
                b) The TR murmur may be loud at the usual apex area, which may be usurped by
                an enlarged RV. If it also does not increase on inspiration, it will mimic MR.

2.   What maneuver can help distinguish TR from MR on auscultation if the site of maximal
        loudness and the effect of respiration are questionable?
        ANS.:   A Valsalva maneuver can cause the TR murmur to return in the post-Valsalva
                state within about 1 sec [61] . An MR murmur should not return for at least about
                3 sec.

*3.   How can drugs help you distinguish between MR and TR?
        ANS.:   a) Methoxamine will only affect peripheral resistance and therefore will increase
                an MR murmur without affecting a TR murmur. (Norepinephrine cannot be
                used for this purpose, because it may raise pulmonary resistance in subjects
                with pulmonary hypertension [23] .)
                b) The administration of amyl nitrite is a useful method, because it does the oppo-
                site to the TR and MR murmur; i.e., it usually makes the TR murmur louder by
                increasing venous return, and the MR murmur softer by lowering peripheral
                resistance.
                Note: If the amyl nitrite causes a fall in pulmonary artery pressure because the
                pulmonary arteriolar constriction was vasoactive and not fixed, the RV will eject
                more blood into the pulmonary artery, so that the TR murmur will not increase,
                despite the increase in venous return.
                c) Serotonin (2 mg over 1 minute) will increase only pulmonary resistance and
                the TR murmur without affecting the MR murmur. It has not been used enough,
                however, to know whether or not it has dangerous side effects.

Causes of Tricuspid Regurgitation

1.   Does a hypertrophied RV alone, due to a high pressure in it (as in severe pulmonary stenosis
        or pulmonary hypertension) usually cause TR?
        ANS.:   No.

2.   Does a large RV volume alone (as in ASD) usually cause TR?
        ANS.:   No.

3.   What is necessary before secondary TR can be expected to occur, i.e., in the absence of
        primary tricuspid valve deformities?
        ANS.:   *Both* a high pressure and a large volume in the RV. The TR thus caused is *secondary TR.*
                Note: By *primary TR* is meant that occurring without pulmonary hypertension,
                as when the TR is due to trauma, to **Ebstein's anomaly**, or to infective endocarditis;
                the latter is seen primarily in heroin addicts.

4.   List the four common causes of both a high pressure and a large volume in the RV, so that TR is expected.

ANS.:   a) Mitral stenosis with secondary pulmonary hypertension.
        b) **Atrial septal defect** with pulmonary hypertension.
        c) Severe LV failure with secondary pulmonary hypertension, as well as an enlarged RV due to a high venous pressure and a small RV stroke volume.
        d) **Primary pulmonary hypertension** with true RV failure.
           Note: If the TR is secondary to chronic obstructive pulmonary disease with peripheral venous congestion, it is rarely severe enough to affect the form of the right atrial pressure curve; i.e., the TR is nearly always trivial [87].

*5.   Why may there be a large volume in the RV in MS in the absence of pulmonary regurgitation or primary TR?

ANS.:   Three theories may explain this:
        a) A sudden rise in pulmonary artery pressure occurs with exercise in patients with left atrial obstruction. One response of the RV to a sudden rise in resistance is to dilate. Perhaps, then, even at rest, it does not return to normal size, because in patients with left atrial obstruction there is always some slight increase in pulmonary artery pressure that may stimulate the RV to remain dilated.
        b) Pulmonary emboli may cause sudden episodes of dilatation. If the pressure remains high on exertion, the RV volume may never return to normal.
        c) The bronchial veins drain into the pulmonary veins to various degrees in different patients. If the left atrial and pulmonary venous pressures rise high enough, some pulmonary venous blood may flow from the pulmonary veins into the bronchial veins and thus via the azygos into the superior vena cava and RV. In patients with large connections between the bronchial and pulmonary veins, a significant left-to-right shunt may occur and may increase RV volume. This has not yet been proved or disproved.

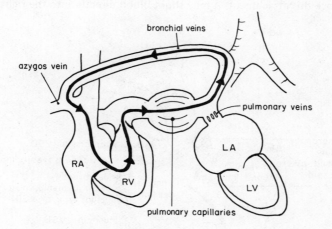

THE CARDIORESPIRATORY MURMUR

1.   What is meant by a cardiorespiratory (or cardiopulmonary) murmur?
     ANS.:   It is an extracardiac murmur, probably produced when the systolic motion of the
             heart compresses an expanded lung segment, perhaps via adhesions between the
             pericardium and pleura.
2.   What are the pitch and timing of this murmur?
     ANS.:   It is high-pitched, usually short, and may occur anywhere in systole and even in
             early diastole.
3.   How is the cardiorespiratory murmur recognized?
     ANS.:   It is heard only or best during deep inspiration. It tends to disappear near the end
             of expiration and during held inspiration.
4.   What are the most important differential diagnoses of the cardiorespiratory murmur?
     ANS.:   a) A late systolic MR murmur.
             b) A short aortic regurgitation (AR) murmur.
             c) A TR murmur.

VENTRICULAR SEPTAL DEFECT MURMURS

Shapes and Length

1.   Where is the usual VSD situated?
     ANS.:   In the membranous septum, i.e., in a small translucent area, extending about 1 or
             2 cm below the aortic valve. The attachment of the septal leaflet of the tricuspid
             valve bisects the membranous septum so that the usual VSD is below this attach-
             ment, i.e., in the intraventricular part of the membranous septum. If the VSD is
             above this attachment, it may shunt blood directly into the right atrium.

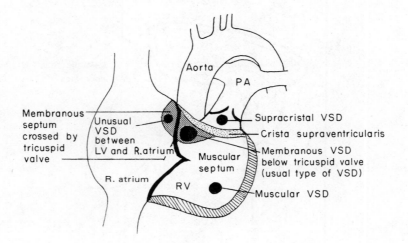

Defects in the membranous septum below the tricuspid valve are the most common.

2.   What are the various shapes of VSD murmurs?
     ANS.:

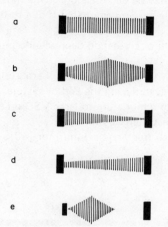

Unlike some MR murmurs, VSD murmurs probably always begin with the M_1.

3.   When is the VSD murmur mostly decrescendo?
     ANS.:   a) If it is of the muscular type, i.e., in the muscular part of the septum. Muscular
             contraction of the septum can close the VSD off toward the end of systole.
             Note: On a phonocardiogram, these murmurs may have a marked crescendo-
             decrescendo in the first third of systole, and careful scrutiny will usually show
             that they actually go to the S_2 [97].

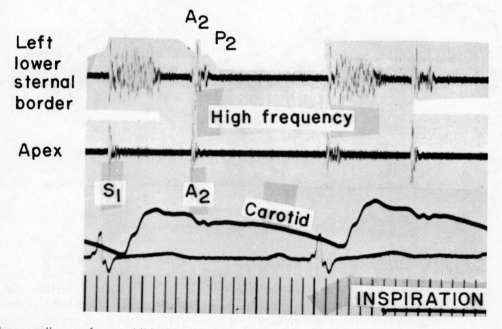

Phonocardiogram from a child with a muscular VSD. The murmur ends well before the S_2. Note
the normally moving split of S_2 on inspiration.

b) If moderate pulmonary hypertension is present with a large VSD, the murmur may end before the S₂ and may be decrescendo. (One must, however, avoid the area of the pulmonary ejection murmur that is due to the excess flow into the pulmonary artery.)

*4. How can you make the short decrescendo or crescendo-decrescendo murmur of a muscular VSD obviously pansystolic?

ANS.: By use of a vasopressor agent, which, by raising peripheral resistance to outflow, causes more left-to-right shunt even during the end of systole.

*5. What is the usual shape of the murmur of a moderate to large VSD on the phonocardiogram when the pulmonary artery pressure is less than 50 mm Hg?

ANS.: It is usually a pansystolic plateau (rectangular) murmur [40].

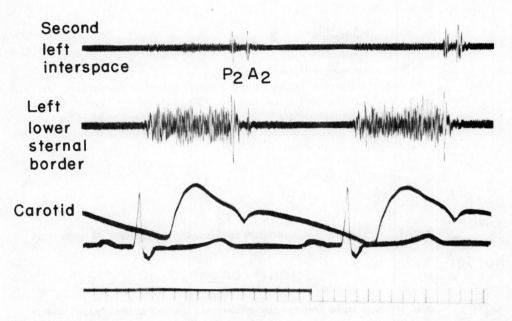

This murmur is plateau in the first cycle, suggesting a pulmonary artery pressure less than 50 mm Hg. The crescendo in the second cycle suggests that the VSD is not large, because small VSDs are the usual cause of murmurs that are crescendo to the S₂.

6. Why may a very large VSD produce a short ejection murmur or no murmur at all?

ANS.: It may create, in effect, a single ventricle, with the same systolic pressure in both RV and LV. When this pressure is transmitted to the pulmonary arterioles, the latter reflexly constrict in response. The raised resistance in the pulmonary circuit prevents much left-to-right flow through the VSD, and the shunt murmur may be soft or even disappear, so that the systolic murmur that you hear may only be an ejection murmur due to flow into a slightly dilated pulmonary artery.

Note: The syndrome of a VSD with pulmonary hypertension severe enough to cause a right-to-left shunt is called Eisenmenger's *complex,* because this is what Eisenmenger originally described. If the right-to-left shunt is at PDA or ASD levels, it is often called **Eisenmenger's syndrome**, an Eisenmenger reaction, or an Eisenmenger situation.

*7. When is the murmur of an uncomplicated VSD crescendo-decrescendo besides in muscular defects?

ANS.: a) In supracristal defects [94].

Note: a) The murmur of a very small VSD as recorded in the RV can be shown to be crescendo-decrescendo in the absence of any pulmonary stenosis (PS) [96]. These murmurs are, as expected, very high in pitch, since they are associated with a high gradient and low flow.

b) In many of these crescendo-decrescendo murmurs, especially if preceded by an early nonejection click, the VSD has been found on angiography to be at the apex of a membranous septum aneurysm that is protruding into the RV outflow tract but often producing no RV to pulmonary artery gradient [68]. However, most VSDs associated with an aneurysm of the ventricular septum produce a crescendo murmur to the S_2 [28].

b) If the VSD is very small. It is as if a small enough VSD acts like a valvular obstruction in that it produces the same shape as an ejection murmur.

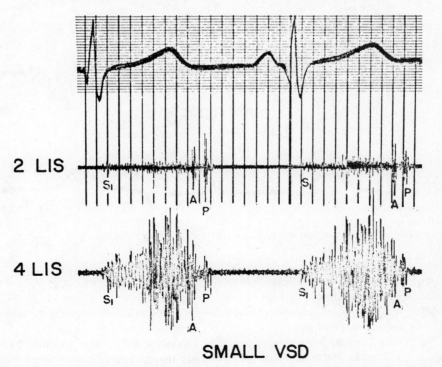

SMALL VSD

The crescendo-decrescendo effect of this small VSD is best recorded at the fourth left interspace (4 LIS) where the A_2 is obscured by the long murmur.

Loudness and Sites

1.   What is the relationship between the size of the VSD and the loudness of the murmur?
      ANS.:   If it is very small (pinhole VSD) or very large, the murmur may have any degree
               of loudness from grade 1–4/6. If it is moderately large, there is usually a very
               loud murmur. (Some of the loudest murmurs observed in cardiological practice
               are caused by moderately large VSDs.)

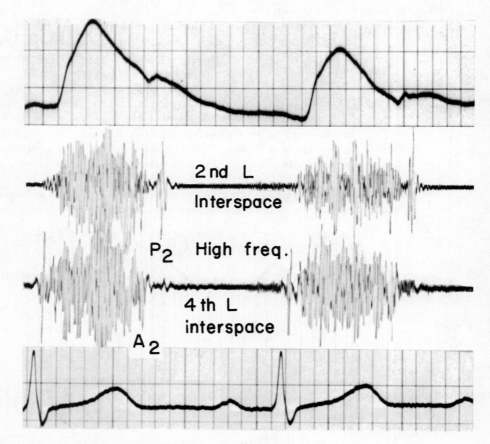

Loud pansystolic harsh murmur found in a patient with a large VSD.

2.   What auscultatory clues indicate that a soft VSD murmur is due to a large VSD with severe
      pulmonary hypertension?
      ANS.:   a) The murmur is often preceded by an ejection sound when pulmonary artery
                 pressure is high.
              b) The murmur will be followed by a loud single S_2 that in turn may be followed by
                 an early diastolic blow of pulmonary regurgitation (Graham Steell murmur).
              c) If a large flow is still present (the pulmonary hypertension is then said to be
                 hyperkinetic, vasoactive, or vasospastic), a mitral diastolic murmur due to excess
                 flow through the mitral valve may be heard.

Note: Beware of the long mitral diastolic murmur in patients with little flow but with coincidental rheumatic mitral stenosis [40].

3.   What is the usual site of maximal loudness of the VSD murmur?

ANS.:   The left lower sternal border.

4.   When may a VSD murmur be louder between the apex and the left lower sternal border than at the left sternal border?

ANS.:   Only very rarely,

a) When a large RV has displaced the LV to the left.

*b) When the VSD is in the muscular part of the septum near the apex. This is not an unusual site for a ruptured septum secondary to infarction [4].

*c) When the VSD shunts directly into the right atrium [40].

*5.   List the auscultation clues indicating that a VSD is ejecting blood directly into the right atrium.

ANS.:   a) The murmur may radiate loudly to the second right interspace.

b) If the shunt is large, the murmur may be loudest between the apex and the left sternal border. This may be because the enlarged right atrium rotates the heart slightly clockwise (as viewed from below).

c) If the shunt into the right atrium is large, there may be a tricuspid inflow murmur. If there is no ASD to cause this murmur, as judged by a normally moving S_2 split, a direct VSD shunt into the right atrium, or anomalous pulmonary venous drainage into the right atrium, should be suspected.

*6.   When can the murmur of a VSD be loudest at the second left interspace?

ANS.:   If it is supracristal, i.e., just under the pulmonary valve. The clue here is that the site where the murmur is heard next loudest is the first rather than the third left interspace.

Note: Since these patients have widely split second sounds, and their murmur may be slightly crescendo-decrescendo with a late peak, their murmurs can be confused with the murmur of PS [26, 94]. The crescendo shape to the major part of the murmur may be due to the fact that the defect tends to decrease in size during contraction, possibly due to late contraction of the infundibulum. This may increase the velocity of flow as systole progresses [26].

*7.   When should you suspect that PS is present with a VSD on auscultation?

ANS.:   a) When the split of the S_2 is very wide and the pulmonary component (P_2) very soft. The P_2 is usually of normal or increased loudness with a pure VSD.

b) When there is an area low on the chest near the epigastrium where the murmur becomes louder on inspiration with the patient either supine or standing. Like all left-sided murmurs, VSD murmurs usually become louder on expiration in all body positions.

c) When the murmur is loudest at the second left interspace. (However, the murmur of a supracristal VSD also is loudest here.)

d) When AR is also present; 50% in one series of VSD plus AR patients were found to have infundibular obstruction [45].

*8.   Why is it important to try to diagnose the type of VSD as being subpulmonic, i.e., supracristal?

ANS.:   Very commonly, AR develops in these patients because of prolapse of the right coronary cusp of the aortic valve through the defect. These defects, although anatomically large, are often functionally small because the aortic leaflet prolapse partially closes them off.

Note: When AR is present, the combination of a second left interspace crescendo murmur to the A_2 followed by a decrescendo murmur may imitate a PDA continuous murmur.

*9. What should you suspect if a large VSD is suggested by such x-ray signs as pulmonary plethora (shunt vascularity) and some cardiomegaly, and yet the murmur is less than grade 4/6, i.e., has no thrill despite a normal chest configuration?

ANS.: a) Severe pulmonary hypertension.

b) Another source of shunt flow through a PDA or an ASD.

c) Multiple VSDs.

Note: The patient with multiple VSDs (Swiss cheese defect) usually has a softer murmur than expected, i.e., grade 3/6 or less, even though such patients usually have a large shunt [29]. This may be because

a) They are muscular defects and thus tend to close off during the end of systole. Each one may close off at a different time in systole.

b) Each individual hole may produce a soft or moderately loud murmur. Two moderately loud murmurs may not necessarily summate to make a louder murmur, because each one may transmit its sound to an independent place on the chest wall or be maximally loud at a different frequency.

10. What is meant by "maladie de Roger"?

ANS.: In 1861, the French pediatrician Henri Roger presented the first comprehensive description of an *asymptomatic* VSD and described the murmur through the defect as loud and long, with its maximum intensity over the upper third of the medial precordial area [101]. The expression is now used to refer to a small VSD with a loud murmur at the left lower sternal border. Roger, however, neither specified the size of the VSD nor placed the murmur at the lower sternal border.

The Ventricular Septal Defect Murmur Versus the Mitral Regurgitation Murmur

*1. When does the effect of amyl nitrite on the VSD murmur differ from that on the MR murmur?

ANS.: It differs only in the presence of hyperkinetic or vasospastic pulmonary hypertension. Amyl nitrite usually does not affect pulmonary artery pressure unless there is vasospastic constriction. Amyl nitrite will ordinarily lower systemic resistance much more than pulmonary resistance, thus decreasing the left-to-right shunt and making the VSD murmur softer.

In the presence of pulmonary artery constriction, however, amyl nitrite may dilate the pulmonary arterioles and diminish pulmonary resistance *even more than systemic resistance.* The murmur will therefore then become louder or stay the same. This may be used as a test for fixed pulmonary resistance with VSDs, because severe pulmonary hypertension fixed by hypertrophy or obliteration will not be affected by amyl nitrite and the murmur will become softer due to the fall in systemic resistance [98].

2. How can the shape of the murmur differentiate a VSD murmur from that due to MR?

ANS.: a) In MR, the murmur may have a delayed onset with a crescendo to the S_2. This delayed onset is not seen with VSDs. A small VSD that has a crescendo to the S_2 will begin at the S_1.

b) An early crescendo-decrescendo murmur, on the other hand, is not characteristic of MR, but is expected in very small congenital muscular VSDs.

*3.   How can you distinguish an MR from a VSD murmur by phonocardiogram plus a simul-
taneous carotid tracing?

ANS.:   The isovolumic contraction time (from the mitral component of the S_1 to the
onset of carotid upstroke) is usually shorter in VSD than in MR. In uncomplicated VSD, it is 10–40 msec. (The normal range is 30–40 msec.)

Note: The combination of a VSD and MR is so rare that when it is found,
you should strongly suspect the presence of a corrected transposition in which
the left AV valve (tricuspid valve) is incompetent [60].

CONTINUOUS MURMURS

Definitions and Causes

1.   What are the two definitions of a continuous murmur?

ANS.:   There are two definitions:

a) It never stops; i.e., it is truly continuous throughout systole and diastole.

b) A murmur that waxes to the S_2, wanes after it, and stops before the next S_1;
i.e., it is not truly continuous, but does envelop the second sound and go more
than slightly beyond it.

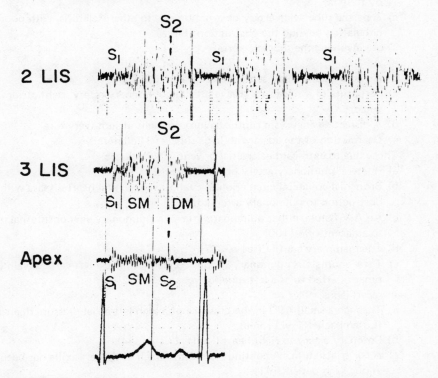

Phonocardiograms from a patient with a PDA. The S_2 at the apex marks the beginning of diastole
for the tracings of the continuous murmur, which envelops and obliterates the second sound at
the left sternal border. This murmur did not sound truly continuous at the third left interspace
(3 LIS) since it seemed to end in mid-diastole. The pulmonary artery systolic pressure was 35 mm
Hg. The pulmonary flow was slightly more than twice the systemic flow.

2. What is a systolic and diastolic murmur heard in the same area called if it is not continuous?

    ANS.:   A to-and-fro murmur. This implies that the systolic component is due to blood going in one direction and the diastolic murmur is due to flow in the opposite direction, e.g., an AS ejection murmur and an AR murmur. (See figure on p. 363.) A continuous murmur, on the other hand, implies a murmur due to continuous flow in the same direction in both systole and diastole.

    Note: The systolic murmurs of a VSD or MR plus an AR diastolic murmur have also been called to-and-fro murmurs even though they are not back and forth through the same orifice.

*3. Are all continuous murmurs regurgitant?

    ANS.:   No. Continuous murmurs may be caused by a

    a) Partial obstruction to a vessel, as in bilateral peripheral pulmonary artery stenosis.

    b) Excessively rapid flow through a vessel, as in collateral circulation secondary to a coarctation of the aorta.

4. List the causes of continuous murmurs primarily in or transmitted to the chest.

    ANS.:   Those due to transmission from above the clavicle:

    a) The venous hum in children (see p. 331).

    b) An arteriovenous (A-V) fistula in the neck, either congenital or acquired (usually by trauma).

    *c) A partial subclavian artery obstruction due to atherosclerosis, with poor collateral circulation beyond the obstruction [84].

    Those involving the thoracic aorta:

    a) A PDA.

    b) An aortic-pulmonary septal defect (see p. 330).

    c) A rupture of a **sinus of Valsalva** into the pulmonary artery, right atrium, or ventricle.

    *d) A dissecting aneurysm rupturing into the right atrium (very rare).

    e) Coarctation of the aorta with large subcostal collaterals.

    Those due to extracardiac arterial or venous turbulence:

    *a) Bilateral pulmonary artery branch stenosis.

    b) Bronchial collateral circulation in cyanotic congenital heart disease with severe obstruction to pulmonary arterial flow.

    c) An A-V fistula, either pulmonary artery to pulmonary vein or internal mammary to adjacent vein [100].

    d) The mammary souffle (see p. 337).

    *e) Total anomalous pulmonary venous connection into a left vertical vein (sometimes referred to as a left superior vena cava) [42].

    Intracardiac:

    *a) Through a small ASD in the presence of a high left atrial pressure due to MS (Lutembacher's syndrome).

    *b) Coronary artery to right heart fistulas (see p. 334).

    *c) A **cor triatriatum**. A continuous murmur high in the left axilla has been noted in one such patient [41].

5. Why should you search for a continuous murmur in the arms, legs, or abdomen in any patient in congestive failure of obscure etiology?

    ANS.:   A search must be made for an A-V fistula, congenital or traumatic. If large (1 cm or more in diameter), failure signs and symptoms may occur over a period of years.

Note: This is a high output type of failure without actual myocardial insufficiency. The A-V shunt causes a low peripheral resistance for which the body tries
to compensate by increasing blood volume and **filling pressure** [65]. The sympathetic outflow that causes the high venous pressure may increase peripheral resistance. This in turn creates more shunt flow, causing a vicious cycle of more
increase in blood volume and venous pressure until peripheral edema occurs. A
high left atrial pressure also results and can cause pulmonary congestion and
dyspnea despite a normal cardiac output.

6.   What is the commonest cause of a continuous murmur?
      ANS.:   Patent ductus arteriosus.

THE PATENT DUCTUS ARTERIOSUS

Shape and Duration

1.   What are some of the other names for the continuous murmur of PDA when it is truly
      continuous?
      ANS.:   a) Machinery murmur.
               b) Gibson murmur [30].
2.   Why is a PDA murmur continuous?
      ANS.:   Because there is a continuous aortic-pulmonary pressure gradient throughout
               both systole and diastole (if the pulmonary artery pressure is not far from normal).
3.   When is the continuous murmur of PDA not "machinery" in quality or duration?
      ANS.:   When it is not truly continuous, i.e., when it begins slightly after the S_1 and cre-
               scendos to the S_2, to end after a short decrescendo in early or mid-diastole.
               Note: About half of PDA murmurs in children are not truly continuous, and
               many are merely pansystolic, exactly mimicking a VSD murmur.
*4.   Why may there be no diastolic component to the PDA murmur in some children?
      ANS.:   Because with the pulmonary vasoconstriction secondary to the shunt, there is often
               moderate pulmonary hypertension, which decreases the aortic-pulmonary artery
               gradient more in diastole than in systole. The low aortic pressures of infants and
               children, plus the reflex low diastolic pressure caused by the ejection of a large
               volume of blood into the aorta, tends to decrease the gradient further. When only
               a long systolic murmur is present, differentiation from a VSD is difficult [32].
               Note: a) Raising aortic pressure with methoxamine or ephedrine is an excellent
                          way of bringing out the continuous nature of the murmurs. However,
                          if norepinephrine is used, the murmurs may disappear altogether, because
                          the pulmonary artery pressure may increase more than systemic pressure,
                          presumably because reactive pulmonary hypertensive arterioles are
                          extremely sensitive to norepinephrine.
                       b) In any child with a VSD type of pansystolic murmur, a bounding pulse
                          with a pulse pressure of over 50 should make you strongly suspect
                          either only a PDA or a PDA in addition to a VSD [77].
                       c) The combination of clenched fists, overlapping fingers, rocker-bottom
                          feet, and excessively wrinkled skin of infants with trisomy 16–18 sug-
                          gests that both a PDA and VSD are present.

*5.   Until what age is the aortic-pulmonary gradient usually small enough to prevent the con-
        tinuous murmur with PDA, so that only a VSD-like pansystolic murmur is heard?
        ANS.:   Up to age 1 year, the thick fetal pulmonary arterioles may not have involuted
                enough to keep the pulmonary artery pressure normal as it tries to accommodate
                the increased shunt flow. Despite this, about a third of newborns with PDA are
                said to have a continuous murmur for at least a few hours while the fetal ductus
                is still patent, and many typical PDA murmurs begin at age 6 weeks [9]. After
                the first few hours, a systolic murmur due to a small left-to-right shunt may be
                present during the first half-day. In cities at high altitudes, the hypoxia causes
                the pulmonary hypertension to be too great for even a systolic murmur to occur.
                Note: a) The ductus arteriosus is normally patent in the newborn for about a
                            week.
                        b) A bidirectional or right-to-left shunt occurs in about 12% of newborns
                            for a few hours, especially when crying [65].
                        c) The continuous murmur heard in the first 24 hours has only a short
                            diastolic component, due to the high pulmonary artery pressure in the
                            newborn.

*6.   Where in systole does the typical PDA murmur reach its maximum intensity by phono-
        cardiograms?
        ANS.:   It is crescendo to a peak at or slightly before the S_2, and then is decrescendo to
                beyond the S_2.
                Note: The aortic-pulmonary gradient does not accurately reflect the shape of
                the murmur, since the gradient is maximum in midsystole, but the murmur is
                maximum in late systole. The reason for the late murmur peak is unknown, but
                in the absence of stenosis, a murmur shape is more related to acceleration of flow
                than it is to velocity of flow or gradient. There is some suggestion that the earlier
                the systolic peak, the greater the caliber of the ductus.

*7.   If the PDA is in the low pressure area distal to the site of coarctation of the aorta, may a
        continuous murmur still be present? Why?
        ANS.:   Yes. The mean pressure beyond the coarctation is almost the same as normal
                aortic mean pressure. The only difference from normal is in the pulse pressure.
                However, if a coarctation is present together with a PDA, a continuous murmur
                may be absent. This probably occurs when the ductus is very small and opens
                very near the coarcted segment [15].

Loudness and Site

1.   Where is the PDA murmur heard (a) loudest and (b) next loudest?
        ANS.:   a) Loudest in the second left interspace.
                b) Next loudest in the first left interspace.
                    Note: With a right-sided aortic arch, the PDA murmur may be best heard in
                    the first or second *right* interspace.

*2.   What can make a PDA murmur transiently disappear without any change in pulmonary
        artery pressure?
        ANS.:   Some ducti are thought to have an unusual attachment that allows them to kink
                and so close off. One such ductus murmur paradoxically diminished with methox-
                amine [73]. Another one intermittently disappeared with no constant maneuver.
                A slightly angulated course was found at surgery [85]. Another one had a valve-
                like structure inside the ductus [47].

Note: a) Permanent closure of PDAs can occur with endarteritis due to infective endocarditis and with atheromatous thrombosis.

  b) A PDA murmur may not be heard if the ductus is small and the patient is obese. It may also be masked by an unimportant aortic stenosis and regurgitation to-and-fro murmur [1].

*3. What is the most difficult differential diagnosis between a to-and-fro murmur and a continuous PDA murmur?

ANS.: A small VSD with a crescendo murmur to the A_2, together with AR with its decrescendo murmur after the A_2. Both murmurs may occasionally be maximally loud at the second left interspace. The clue here is that the harsh quality of the VSD murmur may suddenly give way to the breathy blow of the AR murmur. The quality of the PDA murmur does not suddenly change in diastole.

*4. How much pulmonary hypertension is necessary to completely eliminate a PDA murmur?

ANS.: Moderate pulmonary hypertension can completely eliminate the shunt murmur, despite at least a moderate left-to-right shunt. This is probably because a shunt with moderate flow and little gradient produces mostly low frequencies, which are easily dissipated at the upper chest area, where there is much air between the stethoscope and the heart.

OTHER AUSCULTATORY SIGNS OF PATENT DUCTUS ARTERIOSUS

*1. Explain the effect on the typical PDA murmur of (a) a vasopressor agent such as methoxamine and (b) a vasodilator such as amyl nitrite.

ANS.: a) A vasopressor increases the murmur because it increases the gradient.

  b) Amyl nitrite decreases the murmur because it decreases the aortic-pulmonary gradient.

  Note: In the presence of hyperkinetic pulmonary hypertension, amyl nitrite can increase the PDA murmur because it may relax hyperactive pulmonary arterioles more than it diminishes peripheral systemic resistance.

*2. List the auscultatory signs of a large PDA shunt flow besides the continuous murmur.

ANS.: a) A paradoxically split S_2.

  b) A diastolic mitral murmur or even an opening snap due to an excess flow through the mitral valve.

  c) Multiple systolic clicks or crackles (sometimes called "eddy sounds"), especially in the second half of systole and in early diastole.

  Note: When the shunt is large, a phonocardiogram will often show that the peak of the murmur comes well before the A_2.

PATENT DUCTUS ARTERIOSUS WITH
HIGH PULMONARY ARTERY PRESSURE

1. How by inspection can you tell a reversed shunt through a PDA from reversed shunts at the atrial or ventricular level, i.e., how can you differentiate between the Eisenmenger syndromes?

ANS.: The feet may be more cyanotic and clubbed than the hands. This is known as "differential **cyanosis** and **clubbing**."

Note: The differential cyanosis can be brought out by raising pulmonary artery pressure still more with exercise.

2.   What causes differential cyanosis in a PDA Eisenmenger situation, and why may the left hand be more cyanotic and clubbed than the right hand?

ANS.:   The ductus often joins the pulmonary artery to the aorta just beyond the left subclavian artery. Unsaturated pulmonary artery blood will then pass beyond the left subclavian artery, and both hands will be less clubbed and cyanotic than the feet. (Remember that with pulmonary hypertension, unsaturated blood flows through a ductus from the pulmonary artery to the aorta.) If, however, the ductus is at the junction of aorta and left subclavian artery, this artery may also receive unsaturated blood, and the left hand will be as cyanotic and clubbed as the feet.

3.   Which component of the murmur is the first to disappear as pulmonary artery pressure rises, due to pulmonary hypertension?

ANS.:   The diastolic component first disappears because the diastolic gradient first disappears.

4.   Why may there still be a diastolic decrescendo murmur at the left sternal border even if a PDA has a reversed shunt and no aortic-pulmonary gradient during diastole?

ANS.:   This may be the murmur of pulmonary regurgitation due to the high pressure beyond a dilated pulmonary artery (Graham Steell murmur). *(See p. 368 for explanation of the occasional loud diastolic murmur without decrescendo in PDA with reversed shunt.)

*5.   Why may there be either a systolic regurgitant or short ejection-type murmur at the left sternal border in a reversed shunt PDA?

ANS.:   The regurgitant murmur may be due to TR, and the ejection murmur may be due to turbulence produced as blood flows into a dilated pulmonary artery.

6.   When will a right-to-left shunt (reversed ductus flow due to pulmonary hypertension) produce a murmur?

ANS.:   It is a general rule that right-to-left shunts do not produce murmurs.

Patent Ductus Arteriosus Versus Aortic-Pulmonary Septal Defect Murmurs

1.   What is meant by an aortic-pulmonary septal defect (sometimes called "aortic-pulmonary window")?

ANS.:   It is an opening between the ascending aorta and pulmonary artery about 1 cm above the pulmonary valves.

2.   What auscultatory clues are there to differentiate a PDA from an aortic-pulmonary septal defect murmur?

ANS.:   Even though the site of maximum loudness may be at the second left interspace in both, the next loudest site in PDA is usually one interspace higher, while the aortic-pulmonary septal defect murmur is more likely to be second loudest one interspace lower.

*3.   In which is there more likely to be a continuous murmur, in an aortic-pulmonary septal defect or in a PDA? Why?

ANS.:   In a PDA. Only about 15% of aortic-pulmonary septal defects are small enough to have pulmonary artery pressures sufficiently low to allow a continuous murmur [64].

THE VENOUS HUM

1. Where is a venous hum best heard?

    ANS.:   Low in the neck, just medial to the sternomastoid and just above the clavicle.

2. What does a venous hum sound like?

    ANS.:   Sometimes it is like a continuous roar; at other times it is like "the sound of the sea" heard by putting a seashell to the ear. Sometimes it is a whining sound. The diastolic component is often higher pitched and louder than the systolic. Probably the only quality that is never present is that of an actual hum.

3. What causes the venous hum?

    ANS.:   Two theories have been proposed:

    a) Turbulence caused by a confluence of flow through internal jugular and sub-clavian veins as they pour into the superior vena cava.

    b) Anterior angulation of the internal jugular vein by the transverse process of the atlas [17]. (This angulation and also the murmur can be shown to increase by turning the head away from the side of the hum.)

4. How can you elicit a venous hum if one is not heard by merely placing the stethoscope on the neck?

    ANS.:   a) Sit the patient up with his feet on the bed to bring maximum blood volume to the heart from the legs as well as from the head.

    b) Apply the smallest stethoscope bell lightly to the right side of the neck, as closely as possible to the clavicle and anterior border of the sternomastoid muscle. A small bell may be necessary in order to maintain a good air seal without excess pressure. Too much pressure will eliminate the hum.

    c) Ask the patient to turn his head away gradually. When maximum rotation is reached, ask him to raise his head as high as possible.

    d) When a continuous roar or whine is heard, test for the presence of a hum by applying moderate pressure with the fingers a few inches above the stethoscope. A venous hum will disappear with moderate pressure on the internal jugular vein.

A small bell is invaluable in enabling you to apply airtight light pressure anterior to the sternomastoid muscle.

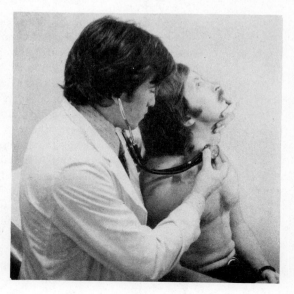

5. What is the significance of a venous hum that can be elicited without much head-turning?

ANS.: It suggests that the circulation time is at least normal and may even be faster than normal.

Note: An unelicited venous hum is found commonly in young children, but in only about 10% of normal subjects over age 50. However, in about half of subjects over 50, it can be elicited by rotating and raising the head. The unelicited venous hum is of most help in confirming hyperthyroidism in the young and in suggesting the diagnosis of apathetic hyperthyroidism in the elderly, i.e., hyperthyroidism with no apparent symptoms or signs of thyrotoxicosis and often with gross failure, TR, and atrial fibrillation [20]. The nonelicited venous hum is also common in severe uremia with a low hematocrit.

6. How is the venous hum eliminated besides by applying pressure above the stethoscope?

ANS.: a) Decrease venous return from the jugular veins by placing the patient in a supine position.

b) Turn the patient's head toward the side of the hum.

7. What is suggested by a venous hum that is difficult to obliterate?

ANS.: It suggests more strongly than even a nonelicited venous hum that there is a very rapid **circulation time**, as in thyrotoxicosis or in chronic renal failure with a low hematocrit.

Note: Chronic renal disease with severe uremia can produce both true and false AR murmurs. The false ones are elicited in the approximately 10% of subjects with severe uremia and anemia who have a venous hum with a diastolic component that is transmitted to the second right interspace and mimics AR.

8. Why is a venous hum usually more likely to be heard on the right than on the left?

ANS.: The right jugular vein is larger than the left, possibly because about two-thirds of intracranial venous drainage is via the right internal jugular vein.

9. What besides the venous hum might cause a supraclavicular continuous murmur?

ANS.: a) A traumatic or congenital A-V fistula.

b) Partial obstruction of any of the arteries arising from the aorta (aortic arch syndromes).

Note: A continuous murmur due to aortic branch stenosis means that there is poor collateral circulation distal to the obstruction. Good collateral circulation would raise the pressure distal to the obstruction enough to prevent a continuous gradient across the obstruction.

10. When will a venous hum mimic a PDA?

ANS.: In some children, the venous hum is transmitted downward to the upper chest, and since it sounds like a continuous murmur, it has been mistaken for the murmur of a PDA.

Note: When the diastolic component is high-pitched, it can be transmitted to the upper chest to mimic AR. This hum is especially likely to be mistaken for AR because the systolic component of the hum may not be transmitted downward.

*11. When can a venous hum be heard lower on the chest wall than the second left interspace?

ANS.: In patients with total anomalous pulmonary venous connection with a left vertical vein (which in turn drains into the innominate vein), the torrential flow may produce a continuous murmur like a venous hum that may be loudest slightly lower than the second left interspace [13]. This may sometimes be due to partial obstruction of the vertical vein between the pulmonary artery and the left main bronchus [

*CONTINUOUS MURMURS OF PULMONARY ARTERY AND PULMONARY ARTERY BRANCH STENOSIS

*1.   What is necessary before a pulmonary artery stenosis can produce a continuous murmur? (This does not refer to pulmonary *valve* stenosis.)

   ANS.:   The pulmonary artery stenosis must be multiple, so that there is pulmonary hypertension proximal to the obstruction. Experimentally, a continuous murmur can only be produced by stenosis in a pulmonary artery if the opposite one is clamped [22].

   Note: a) You should suspect multiple pulmonary artery branch stenosis if you diagnose severe pulmonary hypertension with or without cyanosis and hear a continuous murmur over the posterior chest as well as anteriorly, especially if there is a normal pulmonary artery on the roentgenogram [84]. Cyanosis may be present if there is a right-to-left shunt through an ASD, VSD, or PDA.

   b) If there is severe multiple pulmonary artery stenosis, the continuous murmur may be due to enlarged, tortuous bronchial arteries supplying the lungs [50].

*2.   Where is a continuous murmur sometimes heard if a large pulmonary embolus causes partial obstruction of a left pulmonary artery?

   ANS.:   Under the left scapula.

   Note: It may increase with inspiration.

*3.   How can a thoracic aortic aneurysm cause a continuous murmur?

   ANS.:   An aneurysm can compress a pulmonary artery so that there is a gradient across the narrowed area in both systole and diastole.

PULMONARY ARTERIOVENOUS FISTULAS

1.   What is meant by a pulmonary A-V fistula?

   ANS.:   A right-to-left shunt from the pulmonary artery to the pulmonary vein. This is usually congenital.

*2.   What is the effect of respiration and body position on the continuous murmur of a pulmonary A-V fistula?

   ANS.:   The effect of respiration is variable. However, it usually makes the murmur louder, because inspiration increases the pulmonary artery—pulmonary vein pressure gradient. Compression of the fistula by lying on the side of the malformation, or elevation of the diaphragm by lying supine, may attenuate or eliminate the murmur [36].

   Note: A continuous murmur is heard in only about two-thirds of patients with this fistula.

3.   By inspection alone, what clues indicate that the continuous murmur is due to a pulmonary A-V fistula?

   ANS.:   a) Cyanosis and clubbing.

   b) Telangiectasis on the skin or mucous membranes.

*CONTINUOUS MURMURS OF BRONCHIOPULMONARY ANASTOMOSES

*1. What should you suspect as a cause of a continuous murmur heard bilaterally in a patient
with cyanosis and a roentgenogram suggestive of no pulmonary artery at all?
ANS.: Large bronchial arteries supplying the lungs in a patient with
a) A persistent truncus arteriosus with small pulmonary arteries, or
b) A solitary arterial trunk or an aorta with pulmonary atresia.
Note: Pulmonary plethora (shunt vascularity) on chest x-ray examination in a
cyanotic patient does not deny that a continuous murmur is due to bronchial
artery collateral circulation, because bronchial collaterals can produce excessive
flow to the lungs.
*2. What is suggested as the cause of a *unilateral* continuous murmur in a cyanotic patient with
a PS murmur?
ANS.: A tetralogy of Fallot with
a) An absent pulmonary artery on one side. The continuous murmur may then
be due to bronchial collateral circulation on that one side.
b) One pulmonary artery arising from the aorta.
c) A PDA. However, a continuous murmur with uncomplicated tetralogy of Fallot
is more likely to be due to the bronchial collateral circulation associated with
pulmonary atresia because a PDA with an uncomplicated tetralogy of Fallot is
very rare [11, 66].
Note: A continuous murmur in a cyanotic newborn may be due to mitral atresia
with a forced left-to-right flow through a small ASD or stretched foramen ovale.

CONTINUOUS MURMURS OF CORONARY ARTERY OR
AORTA-TO-RIGHT-HEART FISTULAS

1. What besides an aortic-pulmonary septal defect are the great-vessel or intracardiac causes of
a continuous murmur with maximum intensity lower than the second left interspace?
ANS.: a) A left or right coronary artery (usually dilated) communicating with the coronary
vein, right atrium, RV, or pulmonary artery.
b) Rupture of a sinus of Valsalva into the right atrium or RV.
Note: Both these lesions will tend to produce diastolic accentuation of the murmur, especially in early diastole. But the rupture of the sinus of Valsalva murmur
tends to be much louder than the coronary artery murmur and often has a cooing or
musical quality. Look for a dicrotic pulse (see p. 44), which is very common in
subjects with rupture of a sinus of Valsalva [63].
2. Why will the anomalous coronary artery to right heart fistula usually produce diastolic accentuation of the continuous murmur?
ANS.: There is more coronary flow in diastole than systole.
*3. Which coronary artery abnormal drainage areas are suggested by a continuous murmur
loudest at the (a) second or third right interspace, (b) second left interspace, (c) left lower
sternal border, (d) upper sternum, (e) apex, (f) third or fourth right interspace, or (g) lower
sternum? (This is for reference purposes and not for memorization.)

ANS.:   a) Right coronary artery to right atrium [37, 49, 50].

b) Left coronary artery to pulmonary artery [49].

c) Left coronary or circumflex artery to coronary sinus [49]. Left coronary artery or circumflex artery to RV [62], or via right coronary artery to pulmonary artery [62, 99].

d) Right coronary artery to RV [49].

e) Circumflex artery to coronary sinus [48]. Left coronary artery to pulmonary artery or to apex of RV [49].

f) Right coronary artery to coronary sinus or to right atrium [48, 60].

g) Left coronary artery to RV [60].

Note: Even if the murmur is loudest at the left lower sternal border, if it transmits well to the *right* lower sternal border, or if only the diastolic component is louder to the right of the sternum, it should still suggest a shunt from the right coronary artery to the right atrium or ventricle [12, 37].

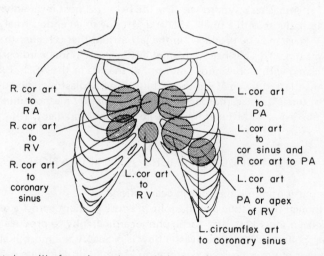

Coronary artery fistulas will often give a clue to their site of drainage by the site of the loudest murmur.

4.   Why may a rupture of a sinus of Valsalva into the RV produce diastolic accentuation of the continuous murmur?

ANS.:   The muscular walls encircling the orifice of the communication may relax in diastole to allow more regurgitation [10]. (The murmur is usually loudest in early diastole, when the aortic pressure is still high.)

*5.   Where is the continuous murmur loudest if a sinus of Valsalva ruptures into (a) the right ventricle or (b) the right atrium?

ANS.:   a) If into the RV, the murmur is loudest at the third left or right interspace or at the left sternal border.

b) If into the right atrium, the murmur is loudest in the lower left or right sternal border or in the epigastrium.

Note: If on turning the patient into the right lateral decubitus position, the murmur is directed into the right chest, a communication with the right atrium is likely.

*CONTINUOUS MURMURS OF TOTAL ANOMALOUS
PULMONARY VENOUS CONNECTION AND ATRIAL SEPTAL DEFECT

*1.   Why will total anomalous pulmonary venous drainage into the right atrium occasionally produce a continuous murmur? Where is this murmur heard?

ANS.:   a) Torrential flow from the persistent left superior vena cava into the dilated right superior vena cava may produce a continuous murmur under the right clavicle.

b) The venous return from a persistent left superior vena cava may be compressed between the pulmonary artery and the left main bronchus [13, 42]. This murmur is heard around the second left interspace.

*2.   Under what conditions besides the presence of total anomalous pulmonary venous drainage will there be a continuous murmur in a patient with an ASD?

ANS.:   a) When MS is also present, bringing about an elevation in left atrial pressure that causes a persistent gradient across a small ASD. An ASD plus MS is known as Lutembacher's syndrome. The MS here is almost invariably rheumatic.

b) In patients with a small ASD and MR due to an endocardial cushion defect, a V wave may be produced in the left atrium that is higher than that in the right atrium. This has been shown by intracardiac phonocardiography to be associated with a continuous murmur at the site of the ASD. Externally, this is manifested by an MR murmur plus an early diastolic, mixed-frequency murmur at the left sternal border. It is made louder by methoxamine, which increases the degree of MR and the intra-atrial V wave gradient.

CONTINUOUS MURMURS OF COARCTATION

1.   What causes the continuous murmur in coarctation?

ANS.:   Although the systolic and diastolic pressure gradient across a severe coarctation has been shown by intra-aortic phonocardiography to produce a continuous murmur, collateral intercostal vessel flow is probably the most likely cause of a continuous murmur heard in coarctation. In mild or moderate coarctation, there is only a systolic murmur over the area of actual coarctation.

*2.   What is the clue for differentiating a PDA murmur from a coarctation murmur by auscultation of the posterior chest?

ANS.:   If the murmur is heard just as easily or even more easily over the posterior chest, it is much more likely to be due to coarctation, i.e., either to the collateral circulation on the chest wall or to the coarctation itself.

Note: If a continuous murmur is heard only over the lower two or three ribs posteriorly, you should suspect an abdominal coarctation [83].

THE MAMMARY SOUFFLE

1. What is the cause of the mammary souffle?

    ANS.: It is an arterial murmur due to a large flow of blood into the breast during pregnancy and lactation in a minority of pregnant women.

    Note: That the murmur arises in the superficial arteries of the breast is shown by the observation that firm pressure with the stethoscope or pressure lateral to the stethoscope can abolish the murmur. Palpable arterial pulsations in the relevant intercostal spaces are present in most cases. Its high pitch, the systolic accentuation, and the absence of any effect of a Valsalva maneuver suggest further that it is an arterial rather than a venous murmur [81].

2. What is characteristic of the timing of the mammary souffle?

    ANS.: There is a delay between the S_1 and the murmur, which often spills over the S_2 into early diastole [95]. Therefore, it must be distinguished from other causes of continuous murmurs.

    *Note: If there is little difference between the loudest and softest parts of the murmur, suspect an internal mammary A-V fistula and expect the murmur to be present permanently.

3. In which trimester of pregnancy does the mammary souffle begin?

    ANS.: In the second or third trimester. However, it may not begin until the first postpartum week.

4. What is the usual site and loudness of the mammary souffle?

    ANS.: It is usually heard along the left sternal border, and it is rarely more than grade 4/6.

    Note: It may disappear when the patient sits up.

5. How long does the postpartum souffle last if the patient continues to lactate?

    ANS.: From several weeks to 2½ months.

REFERENCES

1. Abbott, J. A., and Shively, H. H. Auscultatorily silent patent ductus arteriosus. *Chest* 63:371, 1973.
2. Aravanis, C. Silent mitral insufficiency. *Am. Heart J.* 70:620, 1965.
3. Barlow, J. B., Bosman, C. K., Pocock, W. A., and Marchand, P. Late systolic murmurs and nonejection ("mid-late") systolic clicks. *Br. Heart J.* 30:203, 1968.
4. Barnard, P. M., and Kennedy, J. H. Postinfarction ventricular septal defect. *Circulation* 32:76, 1965.
5. Basta, L. L., Wolfson, P., Eckberg, D. L., and Abboud, F. M. The value of left parasternal impulse recordings in the assessment of mitral regurgitation. *Circulation* 48:1055, 1973.
6. Beck, W., Schrire, V., Vogelpoel, L., Nellen, M., and Swanepoel, A. Hemodynamic effects of amyl nitrite and phenylephrine on the normal human circulation and their relation to changes in cardiac murmurs. *Am. J. Cardiol.* 8:341, 1961.
7. Bergland, J. M., Rucker, W. R., Reeves, J. T., and Surawicz, B. Pre-excitation as a cause of appearance and increased intensity of systolic murmurs. *Circulation* 33:131, 1966.
8. Burch, G. E., DePasquale, N. P., and Phillips, J. H. Clinical manifestations of papillary muscle dysfunction. *Arch. Intern. Med.* 112:158, 1963. Classic article.

9. Burnard, E. D. A murmur from the ductus arteriosus in the newborn baby. *Br. Med. J.* 1:806, 1958.

10. Buzzi, A. Evaluation of a precordial continuous murmur. *Am. J. Cardiol.* 4:551, 1959.

11. Campbell, M., and Deuchar, D. C. Continuous murmurs in cyanotic congenital heart disease. *Br. Heart J.* 12:173, 1961.

12. Carmichael, D. B., and Davison, D. G. Congenital coronary arteriovenous fistula. *Am. J. Cardiol.* 8:846, 1961.

13. Carter, R. E. B., Capriles, M., and Noe, Y. Total anomalous pulmonary venous drainage. *Br. Heart J.* 31:45, 1969.

14. Cheng, T. O. Late systolic murmur in coronary artery disease. *Chest* 61:346, 1972.

15. Crevasse, L. E., and Logue, R. B. Atypical patent ductus arteriosus. *Circulation* 19:332, 1959.

16. Criley, J. M., Lewis, K. B., Humphries, J. O., and Ross, R. S. Prolapse of mitral valve. *Br. Heart J.* 28:488, 1966.

17. Cutforth, R., Wiseman, J., and Sutherland, R. D. The genesis of the cervical venous hum. *Am. Heart J.* 80:488, 1970.

18. Desser, K. B., and Benchimol, A. The apexcardiogram in patients with the syndrome of midsystolic click and late systolic murmur. *Chest* 62:739, 1972.

19. Dock, W. Production mode of systolic clicks due to mitral cusp prolapse. *Arch. Intern. Med.* 132:118, 1973.

20. Dougherty, M. J., and Craige, E. Apathetic hyperthyroidism presenting as tricuspid regurgitation. *Chest* 63:767, 1973.

21. Ehlers, K. H., Engle, M. A., Levin, A. R., Grossman, H., and Fleming, R. J. Left ventricular abnormality with late mitral insufficiency and abnormal electrocardiogram. *Am. J. Cardiol.* 26:333, 1970.

22. Eldridge, F., Selzer, A., and Hultgren, H. Stenosis of a branch of the pulmonary artery. *Circulation* 15:865, 1957.

23. Endrys, J., and Bartova, A. Pharmacological methods in the phonocardiographic diagnosis of regurgitant murmurs. *Br. Heart J.* 24:207, 1962.

24. Engle, M. A. The syndrome of apical systolic click, late systolic murmur, and abnormal T waves. *Circulation* 39:1, 1969.

25. Ewing, D. J., Irving, J. B., Kerr, F., and Kirby, B. J. Static exercise in untreated systemic hypertension. *Br. Heart J.* 35:413, 1973.

26. Farru, O., Duffau, G., and Rodriguez, R. Auscultatory and phonocardiographic characteristics of supracristal ventricular septal defect. *Br. Heart J.* 33:238, 1971.

27. Fox, M. B. Clicking pneumothorax. *Lancet* 1:210, 1948.

28. Freedom, R. M., White, R. D., Pieroni, D. R., Varghese, P. J., Krovetz, L. J., and Rowe, R. D. The natural history of the so-called aneurysm of the membranous ventricular septum in childhood. *Circulation* 49:375, 1974.

29. Friedman, W. F., Mehrizi, A., and Pusch, A. L. Multiple muscular ventricular septal defects. *Circulation* 32:35, 1965.

30. Gibson, G. A. Clinical lectures on circulatory affections. *Edinb. Med. J.* 8:1, 1900.

31. Giuliani, E. R. Mitral valve incompetence due to flail anterior leaflet. *Am. J. Cardiol.* 20:784, 1967.

32. Gonzalez-Cerna, J. L., and Lillehei, C. W. Patent ductus arteriosus with pulmonary hypertension simulating ventricular septal defect. *Circulation* 18:871, 1958.

33. Goodman, D., Kimbiris, D., and Linhart, J. W. Chordae tendineae rupture complicating the systolic click-late systolic murmur syndrome. *Am. J. Cardiol.* 33:681, 1974.

34. Goodman, D. J., and Hancock, E. W. Secundum atrial septal defect associated with a cleft mitral valve. *Br. Heart J.* 35:1315, 1973.

35. Hancock, E. W., and Cohn, K. The syndrome associated with midsystolic click and late systolic murmur. *Am. J. Med.* 41:183, 1966.

36. Hazlett, D. R., and Medina, J. Postural effects on the bruit and right-to-left shunt of pulmonary arteriovenous fistula. *Chest* 60:89, 1971.

37. Heidenreich, R. P., Leon, D. F., and Shaver, J. A. A case of anomalous right coronary artery to right atrial fistula presenting as atypical aortic insufficiency. *Am. J. Cardiol.* 23:453, 1969.

38. Heikkila, J. Mitral incompetence complicating acute myocardial infarction. *Br. Heart J.* 29:162, 1967.

39. Hider, C. F., Taylor, D. E. M., and Wade, J. D. The effect of papillary muscle damage on atrio-ventricular valve function in the left heart. *Q. J. Exp. Physiol.* 50:15, 1965.

40. Hollman, A., Morgan, J. J., Goodwin, J. F., and Fields, H. Auscultatory and phonocardiographic findings in ventricular septal defect. *Circulation* 28:94, 1963.

40a. January, L. E., Fisher, J. M., and Ehrenhaft, J. L. Mitral insufficiency resulting from rupture of normal chordae tendineae. *Circulation* 26:1329, 1962.

41. Jegier, W., Gibbons, J. E., and Wiglesworth, F. W. Cor triatriatum: Clinical hemodynamic and pathological studies: Surgical correction in early life. *Pediatrics* 31:255, 1963.

42. Jensen, J. B. Total anomalous pulmonary venous return. *Am. Heart J.* 82:387, 1971.

43. Jeresaty, R. M. Mitral valve prolapse-click syndrome. *Prog. Cardiovasc. Dis.* 15:623, 1973.

44. Karliner, J. S., O'Rourke, R. A., Kearney, D. J., and Shabetai, R. Haemodynamic explanation of why the murmur of mitral regurgitation is independent of cycle length. *Br. Heart J.* 35:397, 1973.

45. Keck, E. W. O., Ongley, P. A., Kincaid, O. W., and Swan, H. J. C. Ventricular septal defect with aortic insufficiency. *Circulation* 27:203, 1963.

46. Keenan, T. J., and Schwartz, M. J. Tricuspid whoop. *Am. J. Cardiol.* 31:642, 1973.

47. Keith, T. R., and Sagarminaga, J. Spontaneously disappearing murmur of patent ductus arteriosus. *Circulation* 24:1235, 1961.

48. Kimbiris, D., Kasparian, H., Knibbe, P., and Brest, A. N. Coronary artery-coronary sinus fistula. *Am. J. Cardiol.* 26:532, 1970.

49. Koops, B., Kerber, R. E., Wexler, L., and Greene, R. A. Congenital coronary artery anomalies. *J. A. M. A.* 226:1425, 1973.

50. Lees, M. H., and Dotter, C. T. Bronchial circulation in severe multiple peripheral pulmonary artery stenosis. *Circulation* 31:759, 1965.

51. Liedtke, A. J., and Gault, J. H. Systolic click syndrome. *Circulation* 58:453, 1973.

52. Lindgren, K. M., and Epstein, S. E. Idiopathic hypertrophic subaortic stenosis with and without mitral regurgitation. *Br. Heart J.* 34:191, 1972.

53. Lipp, H., Gambetta, M., Schwartz, J., de la Fuente, D., and Resnekov, L. Intermittent pansystolic murmur and presumed mitral regurgitation after acute myocardial infarction. *Am. J. Cardiol.* 30:690, 1972.

54. Marchand, P., Barlow, J. B., DuPlessis, L. A., and Webster, I. Mitral regurgitation with rupture of normal chordae tendineae. *Br. Heart J.* 28:746, 1966.

54a. Markiewicz, W., Amikam, S., Roguin, N., and Riss, E. Changing hemodynamics in patients with papillary muscle dysfunction. *Br. Heart J.* 37:445, 1975.

55. Mason, D. T., and Braunwald, E. The effects of nitroglycerin and amyl nitrite on arteriolar and venous tone in the human forearm. *Circulation* 32:755, 1965.

56. McCraw, D. B., Siegel, W., Stonecipher, H. K., Nutter, D. O., Schlant, R. C., and Hurst, J. W. Response of heart murmur intensity to isometric (handgrip) exercise. *Br. Heart J.* 34:605, 1972.

57. McDonald, A., Harris, A., Jefferson, K., Marshall, J., and McDonald, L. Association of prolapse of posterior cusp of mitral valve and atrial septal defect. *Br. Heart J.* 33:383, 1971.

58. Merendino, K. A., and Hessel, E. A. The "murmur on top of the head" in acquired mitral insufficiency. *J. A. M. A.* 199:142, 1967.

59. Mittal, A. K., Langston, M., Jr., Cohn, K. E., Selzer, A., and Kerth, W. J. Combined papillary muscle and left ventricular wall dysfunction as a cause of mitral regurgitation. *Circulation* 44:174, 1971.

60. Morgan, J., Pitman, R., Goodwin, J. F., Steiner, R. E., and Hollman, A. Anomalies of the aorta and pulmonary arteries complicating ventricular septal defect. *Br. Heart J.* 24:279, 1962.

61. Morgan, J. R., and Forker, A. D. Isolated tricuspid insufficiency. *Circulation* 43:559, 1971.

62. Morgan, J. R., Forker, A. D., O'Sullivan, M. J., Jr., and Fosburg, R. G. Coronary arterial fistulas. *Am. J. Cardiol.* 30:433, 1972.

63. Morgan, J. R., Rogers, A. K., and Fosburg, R. G. Ruptured aneurysms of the sinus of Valsalva. *Chest* 61:640, 1972.

64. Morrow, A. G., Greenfield, L. J., and Braunwald, E. Congenital aortopulmonary septal defect. *Circulation* 25:463, 1962.

65. Moss, A. J., Emmanouilides, G., and Duffie, E. R., Jr. Closure of the ductus arteriosus in the newborn infant. *Pediatrics* 32:25, 1963.

66. Ongley, P. A., Rahimtoola, S. H., Kincaid, O. W., and Kirklin, J. W. Continuous murmurs in tetralogy of Fallot and pulmonary atresia with ventricular septal defect. *Am. J. Cardiol.* 18:821, 1966.

67. Phornphutkul, C., et al. Cardiac manifestations of Marfan syndrome in infancy and childhood. *Circulation* 45:596, 1973.

68. Pombo, E., Pilapil, V. R., and Lehan, P. H. Aneurysm of the membranous ventricular septum. *Am. Heart J.* 79:188, 1970.

68a. Ranganathan, N., Lam, J. H. C., Wigle, E. D., and Silver, M. D. Morphology of the human mitral valve. *Circulation* 41:459, 1970.

69. Read, R. C., Thal, A. P., and Wendt, V. E. Symptomatic valvular myxomatous transformation (the floppy valve syndrome). *Circulation* 32:897, 1965.

70. Roberts, W. C. Anomalous left ventricular band. *Am. J. Cardiol.* 23:735, 1969.

71. Roberts, W. C., and Perloff, J. K. Mitral valvular disease. *Ann. Intern. Med.* 77:939, 1972.

72. Rotem, C. E., and Hultgren, H. N. Corrected transposition of the great vessels without associated defects. *Am. Heart J.* 70:305, 1965.

73. Sakamoto, T., Takabatake, Y., Uozumi, A., and Kawai, N. Atypical response of intermittent continuous murmur of patent ductus arteriosus to vasoactive agents, with particular reference to the external and intracardiac phonocardiography. *Jap. Heart J.* 8:318, 1967.

74. Salisbury, P. F., Cross, C. E., and Rieben, P. A. Chorda tendinea tension. *Am. J. Physiol.* 205:385, 1963.

75. Salomon, J., Augen, M., and Levy, M. J. Secundum type atrial septal defect with cleft mitral valve. *Chest* 58:540, 1970.

76. Sanders, C. A., Scannell, J. G., Harthorne, J. W., and Austen, G. Severe mitral regurgitation secondary to ruptured chordae tendineae. *Circulation* 31:506, 1965.

77. Sasahara, A. A., Nadas, A. S., Rudolph, A. M., Wittenborg, M. H., and Gross, R. E. Ventricular septal defect with patent ductus arteriosus. *Circulation* 22:254, 1960.

78. Scampardonis, G., Yang, S. S., Maranhao, V., Goldberg, H., and Gooch, A. S. Left ventricular abnormalities in prolapsed mitral leaflet syndrome. *Circulation* 48:287, 1973.

79. Schlesinger, Z., Kraus, Y., Deutsch, V., Yahini, J. H., and Neufeld, H. N. An unusual form of mitral valve insufficiency simulating aortic stenosis. *Chest* 58:385, 1970.

80. Schrire, V., Vogelpoel, L., Nellen, M., Swanepoel, A., and Beck, W. Silent mitral incompetence. *Am. Heart J.* 61:723, 1961.

81. Scott, J. T., and Murphy, E. A. Mammary souffle of pregnancy. *Circulation* 18:1038, 1958.

82. Shapiro, H. A., and Weiss, D. R. Mitral insufficiency due to ruptured chordae tendineae simulating aortic stenosis. *N. Engl. J. Med.* 261:272, 1959.

83. Shapiro, M. J. Coarctation of the abdominal aorta. *Am. J. Cardiol.* 4:547, 1959.

84. Shapiro, W. Unusual experiences with precordial continuous murmurs. *Am. J. Cardiol.* 7:511, 1961.

85. Shapiro, W., Said, S. I., and Nova, P. L. Intermittent disappearance of the murmur of patent ductus arteriosus. *Circulation* 22:226, 1960.

86. Sherman, E. B., Char, F., Dungan, W. T., and Campbell, G. S. Myxomatous transformation of the mitral valve producing mitral insufficiency. *Am. J. Dis. Child.* 119:171, 1970.

87. Sherman, W. T., Ferrer, I., and Harvey, R. M. Competence of the tricuspid valve in pulmonary heart disease (Cor pulmonale). *Circulation* 31:517, 1965.

88. Sleeper, J. C., Orgain, E. S., and McIntosh, H. D. Mitral insufficiency simulating aortic stenosis. *Circulation* 26:428, 1962.

89. Sloman, G., Stannard, M., Hare, W. S. C., Goble, A. J., and Hunt, D. Prolapse of the posterior leaflet of the mitral valve. *Isr. J. Med. Sci.* 5:727, 1969.

90. Spencer, W. H., III, Behar, V. S., and Orgain, E. S. Apex cardiogram in patients with prolapsing mitral valve. *Am. J. Cardiol.* 32:276, 1973.

91. Steelman, R. B. Midsystolic clicks in arteriosclerotic heart disease. *Circulation* 45:1145, 1972.

92. Steelman, R. B., White, R. S., Hill, J. C., Nagle, J. P., and Cheitlin, M. D. Midsystolic clicks in arteriosclerotic heart disease. *Circulation* 44:503, 1971.

93. Steinfeld, L., Dimich, I., and Park, S. C. The late systolic murmur of rheumatic mitral regurgitation (MR). *Circulation* 44:106, 1971.

94. Steinfeld, L., Dimich, I., Park, S. C., and Baron, M. G. Clinical diagnosis of isolated subpulmonic (supracristal) ventricular septal defect. *Am. J. Cardiol.* 30:19, 1972.

95. Tabatznik, B., Randall, T. W., and Hersch, C. The mammary souffle of pregnancy and lactation. *Circulation* 22:1069, 1960.

96. Van der Hauwaert, L., and Nadas, A. S. Auscultatory findings in patients with a small ventricular septal defect. *Circulation* 23:886, 1961.

97. Vogelpoel, L., Schrire, V., Beck, W., Nellen, M., and Swanepoel, A. The atypical systolic murmur of minute ventricular septal defect and its recognition by amyl nitrite and phenylephrine. *Am. Heart J.* 62:101, 1961.

98. Vogelpoel, L., Schrire, V., Beck, W., Nellen, M., and Swanepoel, A. Variations in the response of the systolic murmur to vasoactive drugs in ventricular septal defect, with special reference to the paradoxical response in large defects with pulmonary hypertension. *Am. Heart J.* 64:169, 1962.

99. Wald, S., Stonecipher, K., Baldwin, B. J., and Nutter, D. O. Anomalous origin of the right coronary artery from the pulmonary artery. *Am. J. Cardiol.* 27:677, 1971.

100. Wells, B. G., and Hurt, R. L. Congenital arteriovenous fistula of the internal mammary vessels. *Br. Heart J.* 19:135, 1957.

101. Willius, F. A., and Keys, T. E. *Cardiac Classics.* St. Louis: Mosby, 1941. Pp. 623–638.

102. Yamamoto, H., Arakawa, K., Yamashita, T., Murakami, H., Sakai, T., Torii, S., and Nakamura, M. A new pharmacologic phonocardiography by the use of angiotensin. *Am. Heart J.* 81:29, 1971.

15

Diastolic Murmurs

DIASTOLIC ATRIOVENTRICULAR VALVE MURMURS

Mitral Stenosis Murmurs

Timing and Shape

1. When in the cycle does the diastolic murmur of mitral stenosis (MS) begin? How does it relate to the S_2?

    ANS.: It begins just after the opening snap (OS). This means that there must be a pause between the A_2 and the diastolic murmur, a pause due to isovolumic relaxation time of the left ventricle (LV).

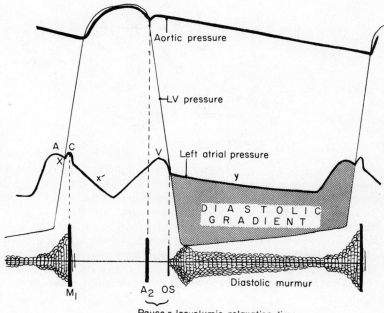

Pause = Isovolumic relaxation time

There should be no mitral murmurs between the A_2 and the OS because this is isovolumic relaxation time. Note the slow Y descent of the left atrium due to the difficulty in emptying the left atrium through the stenotic valve. This accounts for the pressure gradient and murmur, both of which are decrescendo except for the very beginning and end.

---

*indicates material that is for electives or fellows in cardiology, or concerns rare phenomena, of interest primarily to cardiologists.

Boldface type indicates that the term is explained in the Glossary.

Note: There is often a slight pause between the OS and the diastolic murmur of MS when listening with the stethoscope. This is probably because although flow begins as soon as the mitral valve opens, the gradient increases for a short period, since the LV is still rapidly expanding after the OS. This increase in gradient is reflected in the phonocardiogram which often shows that the MS murmur has a short, early crescendo. We hear the OS, and then the peak of the crescendo, as though there were a pause between the OS and the beginning of the murmur.

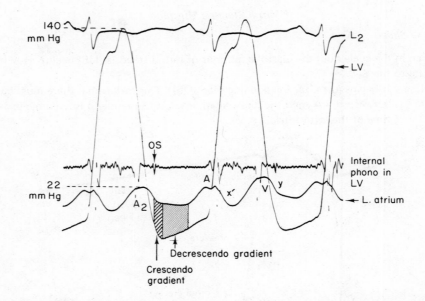

Phonocardiogram, left atrial and LV pressure tracings from a slightly hypertensive 50-year-old man with a mitral valve that was not calcified, but which barely admitted the surgeon's finger. These tracings were taken with equisensitive micromanometers at the tips of the catheters to eliminate any time delays due to tubing. The diastolic murmur (not shown here) follows the gradient and therefore should have a short early crescendo before the decrescendo. This gives a rhythm of "one — — — two-du huuu" to the heart sounds, opening snap and murmur. The distance between the "two" and the "du" is the time for isovolumic relaxation. The distance between the "du" and the "huuu" is the time to the peak of the early crescendo. The long 2—OS interval of about 90 msec (0.09 sec) in this patient is probably due to his hypertension. (See p. 213 for explanation.)

2.   Does the most rapid filling occur in early diastole in the presence of significant MS as it does in normal hearts?

ANS.:   Yes, although there is more rapid filling in early than in later diastole even in MS, the rate of filling is slower than normal.

Note: An apex cardiogram can show that the rate of LV filling during the early filling phase is usually slower than normal in MS because the early filling phase either has a slower slope than normal or is shorter than normal.

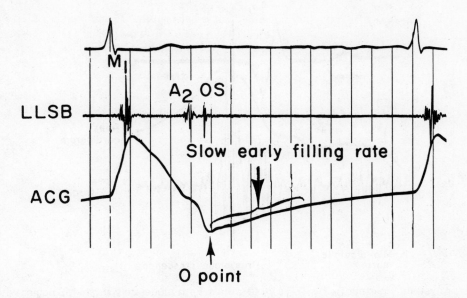

On an apex cardiogram (ACG), the mitral valve opens at the 0 point and is followed by an early, steep rapid filling wave. In MS, the rapid early filling wave is usually replaced by a slowly rising wave. Occasionally, a steep, early rapid filling rise is present, but it is shorter than normal.

Note that the 0 point here follows the OS. The relation between the OS and the 0 point depends on the time constant of the pulse unit; the shorter the time constant, the earlier the 0 point.

That this is from a patient with severe MS is shown by the lateness of the M_1 on the upstroke of the apex cardiogram, and because with the A_2—OS interval about 70 msec and the Q—M_1 interval 110 msec, the Q—1 minus 2—OS = 40 msec, which signifies severe MS (see p. 220).

3.   What is the typical shape of the diastolic murmur of MS on auscultation? Why?
   ANS.:   After a short crescendo, it is decrescendo, followed by a late crescendo to the M_1.
           The decrescendo reflects the decrescendo **gradient** between the left atrium and the
           LV. The late crescendo has a more complicated explanation which follows.

The Crescendo Murmur to the M_1 in Mitral Stenosis (the "Presystolic" Murmur)

1.   What should a murmur look like if it is produced by atrial contraction forcing blood through
   a stenotic mitral valve?
   ANS.:   It should follow the curve of atrial pressure rise and fall; i.e., it should be crescendo-
           decrescendo.
2.   What is the actual shape of the diastolic murmur produced by atrial contraction at the end
   of diastole in MS?
   ANS.:   It produces a crescendo murmur to the first sound. This murmur is often called
           "late diastolic" or "presystolic accentuation."
3.   Does the "presystolic" crescendo murmur of MS reach to the M_1?
   ANS.:   Yes.

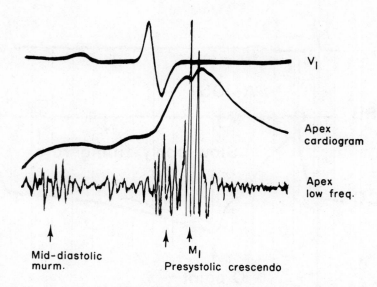

V_I

Apex
cardiogram

Apex
low freq.

Mid-diastolic
murm.

M_I

Presystolic crescendo

The "presystolic" murmur in this 45-year-old woman with moderately severe MS begins with the onset of ventricular contraction, as shown by the simultaneous apex cardiogram tracing taken at very fast speed. However, blood is still flowing from the left atrium to the LV until mitral valve closure (M_1). Therefore, cardiologists prefer to consider this period as part of diastole.

4.   Does the ventricle contract before the M_1?
      ANS.:   Yes. (The time between ventricular contraction and closure of the mitral valve is the preisovolumic contraction period. This period is prolonged in MS because of both the high left atrial pressure and the stiffness of the mitral valve that has to be overcome before the mitral valve can be closed.)

5.   If the "presystolic" crescendo murmur occurs during the preisovolumic LV contraction period, i.e., during LV contraction, is its murmur really presystolic?
      ANS.:   Not all of it. Although it may begin at the time of peak atrial contraction before the ventricle contracts, most of it is actually an early systolic murmur, provided *systolic* is defined as beginning with ventricular contraction.
      Note: a) The following tells us that the crescendo murmur to the M_1 is mostly a systolic murmur by the definition of the beginning of systole just given.
               1) Most of it occurs after the QRS.
               2) In simultaneous LV pressure and phonocardiographic studies, most of it occurs with the LV pressure rise.
               3) Most of it occurs with LV movement on the apex cardiogram when taken with simultaneous phonocardiograms.
               4) Since it ends with the M_1, which is mitral closure, it must have occurred during the time the LV pressure was rising to close the mitral valve; i.e., it must occur during the preisovolumic contraction period of LV systole.

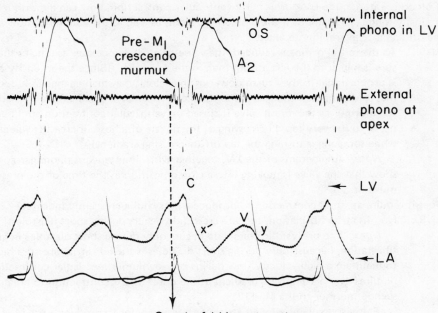

Pre-M₁
crescendo
murmur

Onset of LV contraction

These simultaneous phonocardiograms and left atrial and LV pressure tracings were taken with catheter-tip micromanometer pressure transducers to eliminate any time delays due to tubing. Note that the "presystolic" crescendo of the MS murmur occurs during ventricular systole. This is from a 43-year-old man, mildly symptomatic, with severe MS, but only a small amount of calcium in his mitral valve. His left atrial A wave was 32 mm Hg, but his cardiac index was 2.7, which is low-normal. He had a grade 3/6 diastolic rumble at the apex, of which only the presystolic component is seen well in these phonocardiograms.

b) When the LV begins to contract, the left atrial pressure is slightly higher than that in the LV, and as long as it remains higher, blood will flow from the left atrium to the LV even though the LV is contracting. Since blood is still flowing into the LV while it is beginning to contract, cardiologists prefer to call the period of LV contraction before the mitral valve closes "diastole" or "presystole." Thus, the cardiologist's systole is defined as beginning with mitral valve closure, even though the physiologist's systole has begun slightly earlier. This is consistent with the auscultation definition of the beginning of diastole, which, although physiologically beginning with the end of actual ventricular contraction, is accepted as beginning with the second sound. The second sound is, in fact, not the end of ventricular systole, but is at the end of a period of reduced ejection or the "prodiastole" of Wiggers. Thus, there is the physiologist's ventricular systole, which begins and ends with active ventricular contraction, and the auscultator's systole, which begins with the first sound and ends with the second. By a "presystolic" murmur, then, the auscultator means "just before the first sound."

6. If blood is entering the LV during early ventricular contraction, how can a murmur become gradually louder (crescendo) if the pressure gradient, as well as the volume of flow across the orifice, is being rapidly reduced?

    ANS.:   As the mitral orifice is reduced, the velocity of flow increases as long as the pressure is higher in the left atrium than in the LV [12]. (Since the intensity of sound is proportional to the fourth power of the velocity, a small change in blood velocity may cause marked changes in intensity of a murmur.) The increase in loudness of the murmur as the mitral valve is closed by ventricular contraction could be compared to the very rapid narrowing of the nozzle of a hose (increasing velocity) while someone is turning the tap off (decreasing gradient).

    Note: Angiograms of the LV, together with simultaneous phonocardiograms, show that the valve is moving into a closed position at the time of the presystolic murmur.

*7.   Does it require an atrial contraction to produce a presystolic crescendo murmur?

    ANS.:   No. In atrial fibrillation, the late crescendo occurs during short diastoles [12].

    Note: The presystolic crescendo occurs only during short diastoles in atrial fibrillation, because only during short diastoles is the left atrial pressure high enough to maintain a high-velocity flow during preisovolumic ventricular contraction. It requires over a 10-mm Hg gradient at the onset of LV contraction to create a crescendo murmur to the M_1 [12].

    This also explains why an atrial contraction helps to produce a pre-M_1 crescendo. An atrial contraction can elevate left atrial pressure sufficiently to create the necessary increased velocity of forward flow as the mitral valve orifice is reduced by ventricular contraction.

*8.   What does the presence of a crescendo murmur to the M_1 tell you about the mitral valve in MS?

    ANS.:   The valve must be sufficiently flexible to change the size of the orifice, i.e., must not be rigidly calcified (although it may be too fibrosed or calcified for a valvotomy) [30].

    Note: a) Important mitral regurgitation (MR) can eliminate this pre-M_1 accentuation despite sinus rhythm [66]. The cause is unknown, but it may be partly due to the marked dilatation of the left atrium associated with severe MR. This dilatation may almost paralyze the atrium. Perhaps it contracts poorly because of the greater rheumatic damage to a left atrium seen in this combined lesion.

    b) Before an excellent result can be expected from a valvotomy, the presystolic crescendo should have been eliminated by the surgery, provided that it was not eliminated by the inadvertent production of severe MR.

Pitch and Quality

1. Is the mitral diastolic murmur of MS high or low in pitch? Why?

    ANS.:   Low. This is because a murmur that is produced more by flow than by gradient produces low frequencies. The gradient across the mitral valve in diastole is relatively low as gradients go, no matter how severe the stenosis is; i.e., in the usual severe MS, the maximum diastolic gradient would be about 30 mm Hg at the beginning of diastole and about 10 mm Hg at the end. Peak systolic gradients with significant obstructions during systoles, as in aortic stenosis (AS), are at least 50 mm Hg.

2.   What are some of the descriptions given to the mitral diastolic murmur that help to symbolize the low frequencies?

ANS.:   a) Rumbling.

b) Like distant thunder.

c) Like a ball rolling down a bowling alley.

d) Blubbering (Austin Flint used this word in 1884).

3.   Under what circumstances are there high frequencies in a mitral diastolic murmur?

ANS.:   If the force across the orifice is strong, due to either a good **circulation time**, a strong LV expansion, a strong atrial contraction, or some mitral regurgitation (MR) in the previous systole that increases the volume crossing the valve in the following diastole. The presystolic crescendo to the M_1 part of the murmur is usually rich in high frequencies.

Note: A wide, rough S_1 is often confused with a MS presystolic crescendo. This can usually be separated out if you know that the pre-M_1 crescendo murmur almost always contains many high frequencies [33]. Therefore, firm pressure with the diaphragm will not make this murmur disappear, but will instead bring out the high-pitched crescendo whiff to the M_1. A rough S_1, on the other hand, will with firm diaphragm pressure separate into split sound components.

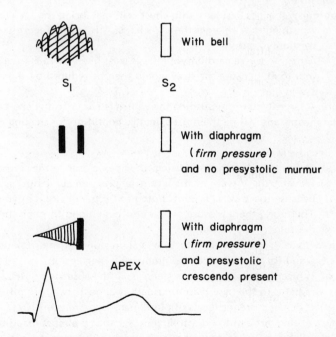

A wide, rough first sound due to many low-frequency components can be differentiated from a presystolic murmur of MS plus M_1 by eliminating the low frequencies as much as possible with firm pressure.

Factors That Increase Loudness of Mitral Stenosis Murmurs

1. What tends to make a MS murmur loud?
   ANS.:   a) Anything that causes a good flow across the obstructed mitral valve.
   b) Anything that brings the LV closer to the stethoscope.

2. Does the MS murmur become louder on inspiration or expiration? Why?
   ANS.:   On expiration, because
   a) The stethoscope is closer to the heart during expiration.
   b) Blood from the lungs is forced into the left side of the heart during expiration.
   (It is useful to think of the lungs as a sponge that expels its blood into the left atrium during the squeezing effect of expiration.)

3. What besides mild MS can cause good flow across the obstructed valve at rest?
   ANS.:   a) A high left atrial pressure, as in severe MS, together with powerful forces pulling the blood into the LV.
   b) Concomitant MR during the previous systole.

4. What powerful forces can pull the left atrial blood into the LV despite severe MS?
   ANS.:   A very healthy LV, especially with the addition of digitalis. (There is still controversy about the ability of a ventricle to actively "pull" or "suck" blood during diastole.)

5. What anatomical changes besides a thin chest wall may bring the LV close to the stethoscope?
   ANS.:   a) Anything that enlarges the LV such as MR, aortic regurgitation (AR), or a **cardiomyopathy**.
   Note: A severe cardiomyopathy is least likely to make the mitral diastolic murmur loud, because the flow would then be reduced by the poorly functioning LV in diastole.
   b) A large left atrium pushing the ventricle closer to the chest wall by displacement.

*6. Why will concomitant MR be the most effective condition for making the MS murmur louder?
   ANS.:   Because MR
   a) Makes the LV larger and brings the apex closer to the stethoscope.
   b) Elevates the V wave of the left atrial pressure curve during systole. This is because the V wave is contributed to by the regurgitant volume during systole. Therefore, there is more pressure forcing blood through the mitral valve in diastole.

*7. What does a grade 4/6 (i.e., with a thrill) mitral diastolic murmur tell us about the severity of (a) the MS and (b) the presence of pulmonary hypertension?
   ANS.:   a) It means at least moderate stenosis, in the absence of MR. If, however, it radiates to the base (very unusual), it almost always signifies severe MS [4].
   b) It denies systemic levels of pulmonary hypertension [67].

8. How can you bring out a mitral diastolic murmur that is almost inaudible?
   ANS.:   a) Bring the LV closer to the stethoscope by turning the patient into the **left lateral decubitus position** and listen during end-expiration over the site where your finger felt the apex beat.
   b) Use very light pressure with the largest bell available that will allow a good air seal. (If the murmur is soft, firm pressure can completely obliterate the low frequencies of a MS rumble.)
   c) Increase the flow across the mitral valve.

9.   How can you increase the flow across the mitral valve?
     ANS.:   a) Have the patient cough a few times, or listen after a Valsalva straining maneuver.
                 In the post-Valsalva state, the obstructed vena caval venous flow is released to
                 flood the lungs and pour into the LV.
             b) Have someone raise the patient's legs as high as possible as you listen, or have
                 the patient bend his knees up toward his chest.
             c) If the heart rate is too fast, or if the patient is in failure, listen after digitalis
                 has slowed the rate and increased the force of ventricular expansion.
             d) Listen with the patient squatting or during handgrip. Cardiac output is increased
                 for a few beats after squatting. During handgrip, the diastolic gradient has been
                 shown to increase as a result both of the increase in cardiac output and increase
                 in heart rate [18].
             e) Have the patient exercise. When you turn the patient into the left lateral decubi-
                 tus position, you should listen immediately, before the effect of the exercise of
                 turning is lost.
                 Note: The maximally effective time for supine straight leg-raising exercise,
                 beyond which there is probably not much increase in cardiac output, is 3
                 minutes or, at the most, 4 minutes; i.e., some physiologists consider 3 or 4
                 minutes of moderate exercise sufficient to reach a steady state. The more
                 vigorous the exercise, the longer it takes to reach a steady state.
             f) Administer amyl nitrite.
10. Why does amyl nitrite make the MS murmur louder?
     ANS.:   Amyl nitrite has two actions: it not only decreases peripheral resistance but it
             also increases cardiac output. It does the latter by producing a powerful sympa-
             thetic outflow in response to the drop in blood pressure. The sympathetic outflow
             increases venous tone, and thus venous return is increased. There is also a possi-
             bility that it opens up shunts between the arterial and venous circulation, thus
             further increasing venous return. The sympathetic tone also causes a reflex tachy-
             cardia. The increased venous return plus the tachycardia causes an increase in
             cardiac output. The tachycardia also shortens diastole, allowing less emptying
             time for the left atrium. This raises the left atrial pressure and increases the
             gradient across the valve.

Factors That Make the Mitral Stenosis Murmur Softer

1.   What besides a thick or emphysematous chest wall can make a diastolic murmur soft in the
     presence of tight MS?
     ANS.:   a) Low flow.
             b) A large right ventricle (RV) pushing the LV posteriorly. Remember that the
                 RV is an anterior chamber, and, if it enlarges, it pushes the LV away from the
                 anterior chest wall.
            *c) A coincidental atrial septal defect (ASD) [21].
2.   What besides the mitral obstruction itself can cause a low flow in MS?
     ANS.:   a) Severe pulmonary hypertension. This causes an additional obstruction to flow
                 for which right ventricular hypertrophy may not compensate completely.
             b) Other valves causing obstruction, i.e., tricuspid or aortic stenosis.
             c) A cardiomyopathy, usually on either a rheumatic or coronary basis.

d) Atrial fibrillation. Atrial fibrillation often causes too fast a rate for good diastolic flow through an obstruction, but even when the heart rates are normal, the loss of atrial contraction reduces flow. It has been shown that a well-placed atrial contraction can increase cardiac output by about 25% in the presence of significant MS [26].

Note: In atrial fibrillation, the murmur of MS may disappear at the end of a long diastole for two opposite reasons:

   a) There may be such *mild* MS that the gradient disappears by the end of diastole.

   b) There is such *severe* MS that although the gradient is still high at the end of a long diastole, the flow is too low to permit a murmur to be heard. If the diastolic murmur is heard at the end of a long diastole, both a high gradient and a fair flow are likely to be present.

3. What is peculiar about the site of some soft MS murmurs that may make them difficult to hear?

   ANS.: They may occasionally be so localized that the murmur may disappear a few millimeters away from the exact area. You can best locate the exact area for listening by palpating the apex beat with the patient in the left lateral decubitus position and placing the stethoscope bell only at the area of the apex beat or just medial to it.

*4. What anatomical factors have been thought to correlate with completely silent MS, i.e., no apical diastolic rumble at any time even when the patient is not in failure?

   ANS.: Any one or combination of the following:

   a) Almost completely immobile mitral valves [61].

   b) Adhesions, thickening, and shortening of the chordae causing a second area of stenosis below the valve [61].

   c) A posteromedially deviated mitral valve orifice [61].

   d) A large left atrial thrombus, deviating the stream away from the apex [61].

   e) A large ASD (Lutembacher's syndrome) [21].

   Note: If a large ASD flow occurs, left atrial blood will choose the ASD rather than the obstructed mitral valve, and so the MS murmur will diminish. (If, however, pulmonary hypertension develops and decreases the left-to-right shunt through the ASD, the MS murmur may become louder again.)

Etiology and Differential Diagnosis

1. What is the usual etiology of MS?

   ANS.: Rheumatic fever, which causes a chronic process of valvular fibrosis and fusion as well as calcification, together with shortened, thickened chordae tendineae.

*2. What are some unusual causes for MS?

   ANS.: a) Congential MS. This is very rare in the adult because about 90% of such patients die by age 2 if not treated surgically. Even the exceptional patients who live until adolescence have been in failure since infancy [56]. One case has been reported in which the patient had no heart failure symptoms except for fatigue until age 18, probably because of anomalous pulmonary venous drainage that offered some protection against an excessively high left atrial pressure [1].

Note: The valves in one form of congenital MS, known as a "parachute" mitral valves (one papillary muscle sending chordae to fused, thickened, and fibrosed leaflets), may function normally or even be purely regurgitant [22].

b) Calcified bacterial vegetations, as large as 2 cm in diameter, have obstructed a mitral valve in a patient who had only MR prior to the infective endocarditis [5].
Note: Verrucous endocarditis (Libman-Sacks valvulitis of disseminated lupus) does not usually cause enough mitral obstruction even to produce a diastolic murmur [28].

c) Mitral ring constriction due to localized constrictive pericarditis of the atrio-ventricular (AV) ring (very rare).

d) A left atrial myxoma.
Note: A left atrial myxoma can have a grade 4/6 diastolic murmur, i.e., with a thrill. A piece of myxoma may embolize and the murmur disappear [52].

3.   What can imitate the MS diastolic murmur despite no significant diastolic gradient across the mitral valve? What auscultatory clues can indicate that it is not the murmur of MS?

ANS.:   a) A diastolic flow murmur due to excessive flow across the mitral valve, as in severe MR or **ventricular septal defect** (VSD).

*b) Hypertrophic subaortic stenosis. The reason is unknown [51].

c) The Austin Flint murmur.

The auscultatory clues to the absence of true MS are as follows:

1) a) An S_3 usually precedes the murmurs listed, and a true S_3 thud never precedes a MS murmur [50]. This can be a problem, however, when the MS murmur begins loudly.

b) The murmurs listed tend to be short.

The Austin Flint Versus the Mitral Stenosis Murmur

1.   What is the Austin Flint murmur?

ANS.:   An apical diastolic rumble imitating the murmur of MS but due to an AR stream affecting the mitral valve.

Note: A right-sided Austin Flint murmur due to pulmonary regurgitation has been reported [23].

2.   What are some theories concerning the mechanical cause of the Austin Flint murmur?

ANS.:   There are several theories:

a) The aortic regurgitant flow may create a negative pressure on the ventricular surface of the septal leaflet of the mitral valve. This would tend to pull that leaflet downward. The forward flow through the mitral valve, however, creates eddy currents on the underside of the septal leaflet that produce a negative pressure on the ventricular side of the valve and tend to close it. These opposing forces may make the septal leaflet and its chordae attachments vibrate.

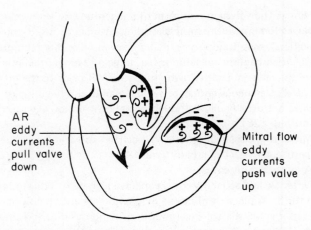

AR
eddy
currents
pull valve
down

Mitral flow
eddy
currents
push valve
up

Even though this mechanism could cause fluttering of the mitral anterior leaflet, it is doubtful whether such a fluttering could by itself produce a murmur.

Note: Angiocardiograms and echocardiograms often show vibrations of the septal leaflet in patients with Austin Flint murmurs. This theory of murmur production is weakened by the fact that some patients with the vibrating leaflets have no Austin Flint murmur, and some with the Austin Flint murmur have no leaflet vibrations.

b) A more plausible theory makes use of the idea that the aortic regurgitant flow may impinge on the undersurface of the septal leaflet of the mitral valve and push it up, to create a relative MS. (A yellow plaque has been seen on the anterior leaflet of the mitral valve of some patients with the Austin Flint murmur. This may be a jet lesion [38, 60] .)

*3.   What suggests that the apical diastolic murmur in severe AR is at least sometimes due merely to a transmission of the low-frequency components of the AR murmur?

ANS.:   a) It sometimes appears to start with the S_2, i.e., before the mitral valve has had a chance to open.

b) If AR is severe, its murmur is rich in low frequencies, which can be transmitted downstream to the apex.

*4.   What was Austin Flint's explanation for the apical diastolic rumble in AR?

ANS.:   The ventricular volume is so great due to double filling (from both the normal mitral flow and AR flow) that it floats the mitral valves upward into a nearly closed position, thus producing a relative MS [19] .

Note: Austin Flint's theory is difficult to defend because all mitral valves tend to float rapidly into a semiclosed position during rapid filling, but no diastolic murmur is normally produced unless there is excess flow through the mitral valve, as in subjects with severe MR. His theory also requires the development of a high LV pressure early in diastole. This does not occur.

5.   How did Austin Flint describe the quality and position of this murmur in diastole? Why?
ANS.:   He described it as a blubbering presystolic murmur. It sounded to him exactly the
same in timing and quality as the murmur of MS. Since he thought that the atrium
contracted just after the early filling phase, he considered almost all of diastole as
presystolic except for this very early filling phase. He recommended that all MS
diastolic murmurs also be called presystolic.

Note: Only a small portion of the Austin Flint murmur is actually presystolic
in the modern sense. In one study, a definite presystolic accentuation was not
demonstrable in any patient in an entire series of 17 patients [38]. In another
study, a presystolic component was completely absent in 2 of 15 patients with an
Austin Flint murmur [60]. The pre-M_1 accentuation of the Austin Flint murmur,
even when present, is often a very subtle finding. The diastolic murmur, far from
being presystolic, usually begins at or before the time of an S_3. It sometimes
begins even earlier than the diastolic murmur of MS.

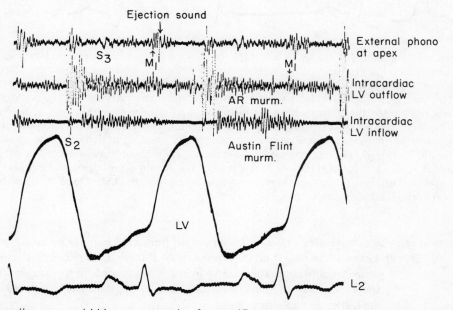

Phonocardiograms and LV pressure tracing from a 45-year-old man with marked orthopnea who
had an Austin Flint murmur due to severe AR due to a previous infective endocarditis. Note that
the diastolic rumble at the apex begins even before the S_3 was recorded externally. Note also the
absence of a presystolic crescendo and the soft M_1.

In severe AR, there is often a reversal of pressure gradient across the mitral valve
in late diastole. Since angiograms in such patients have shown some late diastolic MR,
the presystolic component of the Austin Flint murmur in severe AR has been said to
be due to this late diastolic regurgitation [31]. Intracardiac phonocardiograms, however, have shown that although a reversed gradient can produce a recordable presystolic murmur in the left atrium, this murmur cannot be recorded either on the surface
or LV inflow tract phonocardiogram. In severe AR the presystolic component of the
Austin Flint murmur is usually absent [20].

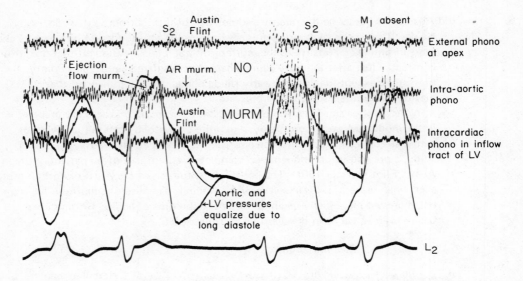

Phonocardiograms, aortic and LV pressure tracings from a 51-year-old man who had severe AR with dyspnea on exertion and paroxysmal nocturnal dyspnea following infective endocarditis two months prior to this tracing. He had a grade 3/6 aortic ejection murmur due to excessive forward flow, a grade 3/6 aortic diastolic blowing murmur at the left sternal border, and a grade 3/6 diastolic rumble (Austin Flint murmur) at the apex.

Note the sudden pause (due to sinus suppression secondary to a premature ventricular contraction with retrograde conduction) that allowed the LV pressure to rise as high as aortic pressure. The Austin Flint murmur stopped, even though the LV pressure must have exceeded left atrial pressure; i.e., late MR is not the cause of any part of the Austin Flint murmur. Note also how the amount of AR is limited by the rapid rate of rise of pressure in the LV. This is why, with sudden, severe AR, the diastolic murmur may be short.

6.   How can you differentiate an Austin Flint murmur from a MS murmur by auscultation?
   ANS.: a) Listen for an OS. If no OS is present, see if there is heavy calcification on image-amplification fluoroscopic examination to account for its absence. If there is no calcium in the mitral valve and no OS, the chances that MS is present are markedly diminished.
   b) If an S_3 is heard, it is most likely to be an Austin Flint murmur, provided you are certain that the S_3 is not a RV S_3 or a loud beginning to the MS murmur.
   c) Amyl nitrite will produce a louder MS murmur, while an Austin Flint murmur becomes softer or even disappears.
   Note: a) Amyl nitrite makes the Austin Flint murmur disappear because in AR there are two outlets for the blood in the aorta during diastole. One outlet is backward into the LV; the other is forward into the peripheral arteries. If you lower the resistance in one outlet, blood will tend to flow preferentially toward that outlet. Amyl nitrite lowers peripheral resistance, thus increasing the peripheral runoff and therefore decreasing the amount of AR. (In the presence of severe congestive failure, amyl nitrite may have no effect [50].)

   b) An echocardiogram of the mitral valve is a definitive way of differen-
      tiating the MS from the Austin Flint murmur.

7. When can the detection of an Austin Flint murmur be clinically useful?
   ANS.:   When it is heard despite the presence of only a grade 1/6 murmur. It may then
           be the only auscultatory clue to the marked degree of AR.

8. How much AR is present when an Austin Flint murmur is heard?
   ANS.:   Although a regurgitant volume of at least 50 ml is usually found, the Austin Flint
           murmur has been present in not more than moderate AR [41, 44].
               Note: The Austin Flint murmur usually means a high left atrial mean pres-
           sure and a high LV end-diastolic pressure [38, 41].

Mitral Diastolic Flow Murmurs (Inflow Murmurs)

1. What is meant by a mitral diastolic flow murmur?
   ANS.:   One that is produced by a relative MS, i.e., by an excessive flow through a normal
           mitral valve.

2. List some common causes of excessive flow through a mitral valve that can produce a
   diastolic flow murmur.
   ANS.:   a) Mitral regurgitation (moderate to severe).
           b) A hyperkinetic state, e.g., severe thyrotoxicosis.
           c) A very slow rate with a healthy heart, e.g., congenital complete **atrioventricular
              (AV) block** [3, 42].
           d) A left-to-right shunt flow, e.g., VSD or **patent ductus arteriosus** (PDA) with at
              least a 2:1 shunt, i.e., at least twice as much blood going through the pulmonary
              artery per minute as through the aorta.
               Note: The advantage of hearing a flow murmur in the presence of a VSD with
           signs of pulmonary hypertension is that it tells you that the condition is operable,
           i.e., the pulmonary hypertension is not fixed (no pulmonary vascular disease), but
           is caused instead by an excessive flow into the pulmonary arterioles (hyperkinetic
           pulmonary hypertension).

3. In what way is a diastolic flow murmur similar to a MS murmur?
   ANS.:   a) They are both low-pitched rumbles.
           b) They both occur after a delay following the S_2.
           c) They both are best heard over the apex beat in the left lateral decubitus position.

4. In what way does a mitral diastolic flow murmur differ from a MS murmur?
   ANS.:   A flow murmur usually starts with an S_3, is shorter, and has no late diastolic or
           presystolic component. (See figures on pp. 305 and 234.)

5. Why does the diastolic flow murmur not start with the opening of the mitral valve?
   ANS.:   Probably because the mitral valve in its immediate opening makes too large an
           orifice for a murmur to be produced. At the time of the S_3, however, the mitral
           cusps are moving up and are rapidly becoming more opposed to one another; a
           murmur then occurs while rapid flow is still continuing for a short time. The
           murmur is thus probably due to increasing velocity of flow as a result of a dynami-
           cally narrowing mitral orifice, much like the effect of narrowing the nozzle of a hose.
               Note: Echocardiograms have shown that immediately after an opening move-
           ment of the mitral valve, a closing movement occurs that flips the valve rapidly into a
           semiclosed position, probably as a result of eddy currents. After the S_3, the closing
           movement accelerates.

6.   How can heart sounds imitate a mid-diastolic murmur?
       ANS.:   An S_3 plus an S_4 close together can occasionally mimic a mid-diastolic murmur [59].

*7.   What is meant by a Carey Coombs murmur?
       ANS.:   It is the diastolic inflow murmur usually ushered in by an S_3, heard in subjects with
                cardiomegaly *and MR* due to acute rheumatic fever [10, 11].

                Note: Many modern writers tend to ignore the MR and imply that the inflow
                murmur is a special type of mitral murmur caused by the valvulitis itself rather
                than being an expected flow murmur heard in any patient with much MR and
                torrential flow through a mitral valve that is in a semiclosed position. Even Carey
                Coombs thought that it was due to dilatation of the LV.

                Since even a physiological S_3 can sometimes be followed by a short flow mur-
                mur, the term *Carey Coombs murmur* should probably not be used in the absence
                of at least moderate MR.

TRICUSPID DIASTOLIC FLOW MURMURS

1.   What is the site of the tricuspid inflow murmur?
       ANS.:   Anywhere over the RV area. This includes all the mid-lower chest area, which
                means the right and left parasternal area, as well as the epigastrium. When the RV
                is very large, the entire left lower chest area can become the RV area.

2.   List the common causes of increased flow through the tricuspid valve.
       ANS.:   a) Shunt flows, e.g., in **atrial septal defects** (ASDs) and **anomalous pulmonary
                   venous connection** into the right atrium.
                b) Tricuspid regurgitation (TR).

3.   How can a tricuspid inflow murmur be exaggerated besides by exercise?
       ANS.:   a) By holding the legs up, or bending the knees up toward the chest.
                b) By deep inspirations or by panting, rapid respirations for a few beats.
                c) By amyl nitrite inhalation.

*4.   With what is a tricuspid inflow murmur confused?
       ANS.:   The murmur of tricuspid stenosis (TS).

                Note: In the presence of normal sinus rhythm, the TS murmur is almost always
                only presystolic or has a presystolic component and has many high frequencies in
                it. The tricuspid inflow murmur usually has only low frequencies and occurs at
                about the time that an S_3 would occur.

*5.   How does an ASD tricuspid diastolic flow murmur differ in timing from the VSD mitral
       diastolic flow murmur?
       ANS.:   In an ASD, it starts earlier, at about the time of the opening of the tricuspid valve,
                and is not preceded by an S_3 [36]. It may occasionally be presystolic as well [17].
                (In a VSD, it not only starts later but is almost always initiated by an S_3.)

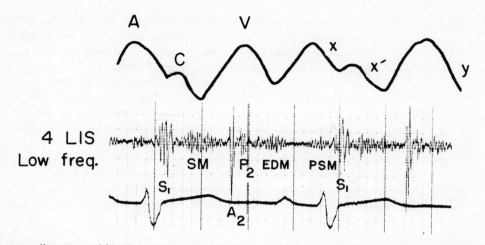

Phonocardiogram and jugular pulse tracing from a teenaged girl with an ostium primum ASD. The presystolic murmur (PSM) is unusual in ASDs, but, when present, is crescendo-decrescendo and not crescendo to the first sound, as in MS.

Note that the Y descent in the jugular tracing is almost equal to the combination of X + X′ descents. This is due to the high V wave, which results from the addition to the right atrium of blood from some additional source, i.e., not only from the venae cavae but here also from the left atrium and even from the LV because of MR, which is expected with primum defects.

> *Note:* If with an ASD there is anomalous pulmonary venous connection with the right atrium, a tricuspid flow murmur may persist despite pulmonary hypertension high enough to decrease the shunt through the ASD considerably. This is probably because the pulmonary venous pressure remains higher than right atrial pressure, and an increased flow into the right atrium is maintained [43].

TRICUSPID STENOSIS DIASTOLIC MURMURS

1. What is the site of the tricuspid stenosis (TS) murmur?
   ANS.:   The same as that of the tricuspid inflow murmur, i.e., the RV area.
2. How does the TS murmur differ from the MS murmur in normal sinus rhythm?
   ANS.:   a) There is no presystolic crescendo with the TS murmur, i.e., the presystolic murmur is nearly always a crescendo-decrescendo murmur. In MS, a presystolic crescendo-decrescendo occurs only if there is a long P—R interval.

   b) There is only occasionally an early or mid-diastolic component, unless atrial fibrillation is present [16].

   c) It always increases with inspiration, often markedly, while the MS murmur characteristically increases with expiration [44].

   *d) The presystolic TS murmur begins at about 60 msec from the onset of the P wave. Because the left atrium contracts later than the right atrium, the MS crescendo murmur to the M_1 begins later, at about 120—200 msec after the P.

e) The MS murmur is louder in the left lateral decubitus position. The TS murmur is characteristically accentuated in the right lateral decubitus position [29].

f) The MS murmur is usually predominantly low-pitched (with soft high frequencies added); the TS presystolic murmur is often scratchy.

Note: Rheumatic TS is probably never present without MS, even though on rare occasions the TS may be the dominant significant lesion [35]. Therefore, if no MS can be diagnosed, a presystolic murmur at the left sternal border should make you suspect either a right atrial myxoma, an ASD, or carcinoid stiffening of the tricuspid valve [2].

3. When one says that the TS murmur increases with inspiration, does this mean moving inspiration, as when checking for splits of S_2, or does it mean held inspiration?

ANS.:   It means both during moving inspiration and during inspiratory apnea. Be careful that a Valsalva maneuver is not performed during the inspiratory apnea, or the TS murmur will become softer.

4. Why does the TS murmur become louder on inspiration?

ANS.:   Inspiration lowers all intrathoracic pressures, including right atrial and RV pressures. This increases inflow into the right heart. Since RV inflow is restricted by the TS, the volume in the RV is not increased as much as in the right atrium, where venous inflow is unrestricted [68]. The mean right atrial pressure tends to remain unchanged with inspiration, while RV pressure drops [16]. The relatively higher pressure in the right atrium increases the gradient across the tricuspid valve.

*5. What should you think of besides TS if an inspiration-accentuated mid-diastolic tricuspid inflow murmur or a presystolic murmur is heard?

ANS.:   a) Ebstein's anomaly.

b) An ASD with large flow.

c) A right atrial myxoma [58, 64].

Note: Some patients with a right atrial myxoma and a mid-diastolic inflow murmur also have a murmur between the M_1 and the second component of a widely split S_1 [5, 27]. The second component is probably a T_1, i.e., the tricuspid component of the first sound. This murmur may be due to TR with upward movement of the tumor through the tricuspid valve before the valve closes.

DIASTOLIC SEMILUNAR VALVE MURMURS

Aortic Regurgitation Murmurs

Etiologies of Aortic Regurgitation

1. What are the commonest causes of severe AR (a) in the child and (b) in the adult?

ANS.:   a) In the young child, a VSD with aortic valve prolapse may be the commonest cause of severe AR.

b) In the adult, rheumatic heart disease is the commonest cause of severe AR, and syphilis (lues) is the next commonest cause.

Note: Since lues does not cause AS, the diagnosis of concomitant AS tends to rule out lues.

2.   What is the commonest cause of *mild* AR in the adult? Why?

ANS.:   Severe hypertension. In one series of severe hypertensive patients, 60% had AR [32]. Three causes have been suggested.

a) Dilatation of the aortic ring.

b) High pressure above a bicuspid or a fenestrated aortic valve. Fenestrations are common in both aortic and pulmonary valves. An aortic valve with the normal three cusps but no fenestrations may explain the absence of AR murmurs in many patients with very severe hypertension.

Note: a) Bicuspid aortic valves occur in about 2% of males and 1% of females.

b) If the AR murmur is due to hypertension and the diastolic pressure is brought below 115 mm Hg, the AR may disappear.

*3.   List some rare causes of AR (a) with arthritis and (b) without arthritis.

ANS.:   a) With arthritis:

1) Ankylosing spondylitis. (The cusps are shortened and thickened by fibrous tissue and may occasionally produce AR a few years before the spondylitis. However, the incidence rises with the duration of the arthritis [6].)

2) Reiter's syndrome. The AR may occur from 1 to 20 years later in about 5% of patients with this syndrome.

3) Rheumatoid arthritis.

4) Psoriatic arthritis.

5) Disseminated lupus erythematosus.

6) Arthritis associated with ulcerative colitis.

b) Without arthritis:

1) A bicuspid aortic valve.

2) Osteogenesis imperfecta. The AR here is due to dilatation of the aortic root [13].

3) Marfan's syndrome. The AR here is due to dilatation of the aortic root and myxomatous degeneration of the valves [46].

Note: Although both males and females have MR with Marfan's syndrome, AR develops only in males (usually under age 40). Myxomatous transformation and spontaneous rupture of an aortic cusp can occur without Marfan's syndrome [39]. When some features of Marfan's syndrome are found, cystic medial necrosis of the aorta with or without dissecting aneurysm is usually an associated lesion [45].

4) Dissecting aneurysm of the ascending aorta.

5) Supravalvular AS. The AR here is due either to fusion of a cusp with the supravalvular membrane or to the valve leaflets adhering to the aortic wall [57].

6) Uremia.

7) Aortitis syndrome, or Takayasu's disease. The AR here is due to dilatation of the aortic ring [62].

8) Rupture of a sinus of Valsalva.

9) Infective endocarditis on a bicuspid valve. (It is probable that the bicuspid valve that caused the infective endocarditis to occur was slightly regurgitant in the first place.)

4.   What should make you suspect that a bicuspid aortic valve is the cause of the AR?
      ANS.:   If the AR is mild in the presence of an ejection click followed by an early ejection
               murmur that is loudest in the second right interspace.
                    *Note: The following theory may explain the incompetence of a bicuspid
               valve. If the valve edges were straight between their attachments, the valves would
               be obstructive as they opened. The only way to avoid obstruction is for at least
               one of the leaflets to have a voluminous or redundant free-edge distance that is
               greater than the straight-line distance between its attachments. This redundant
               valve tissue may allow free forward flow in systole, but may prolapse downward
               during diastole, to produce at least a mild regurgitation, especially if only one
               leaflet has the extra length [15].

*5.   Why may uremia cause AR?
      ANS.:   Occasionally what appears to be AR is due to a loud venous hum commonly heard
               with the severe anemia in some uremic patients. The accentuated diastolic com-
               ponent of the hum may be transmitted down to the base of the heart. However,
               it is not always due to this, as shown by its often being a Cole-Cecil type of AR
               murmur (see p. 365) [34]. That it is not always due to a bicuspid or rheumatic
               valve that happens to produce an audible murmur because of hypertension or
               volume overload is shown by the fact that it can occur when the blood pressure
               has been made normal by dialysis and when the valves are found to be normal at
               autopsy. It is also not related to the level of uremia. It is correlated only with
               the presence of at least two of the three conditions commonly seen in uremia:
               severe anemia, volume overload, or diastolic pressure of 120 mm Hg or more [34].
                    Note: Severe anemia can bring out the murmur of trivial aortic (and mitral)
               regurgitation by increasing the blood volume and by causing cardiomegaly.

Timing and Shape

1.   When in the cycle does the AR murmur begin, and what is its shape?
      ANS.:   It begins with the aortic component of the second sound (A_2). Although in gen-
               eral it is decrescendo, there is often an early short crescendo-decrescendo.
                    Note: This crescendo-decrescendo is due to the shape of the aortic-ventricular
               gradient, which increases as ventricular pressure drops below aortic pressure to
               nearly zero in early diastole. A good dicrotic wave may also be partly responsible
               for this crescendo-decrescendo, but the presence of a good dicrotic wave in AR
               suggests mild or, at the most, moderate AR. Therefore, a marked crescendo-
               decrescendo effect in the early part of the murmur probably suggests that the AR
               is not severe.

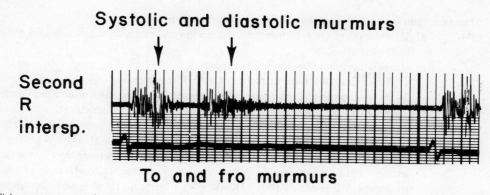

Systolic and diastolic murmurs

Second R intersp.

To and fro murmurs

This murmur was due to mild syphilitic AR. It was loudest at the second and third right inter-spaces. Note the slight early crescendo-decrescendo. A systolic murmur due to blood going in one direction, together with a diastolic murmur due to blood going in the opposite direction, is called a to-and-fro murmur.

*2.   What is the auscultatory effect of the early crescendo-decrescendo?

ANS.:   If soft, sometimes only the delayed decrescendo part is heard, and it appears to start only after a short silent period following the A_2. The peak of the crescendo occurs at about 50—200 msec after the A_2. The background rhythm is:

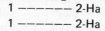

1 —————— 2-Ha
1 —————— 2-Ha

3.   What is the significance of a pandiastolic murmur in comparison with the short one that finishes before the end of diastole?

ANS.:   A pandiastolic murmur suggests that the AR is at least moderate in degree, pro-vided that the heart rate is not so fast that any diastolic murmur would be pandiastolic.

Quality and Loudness

1.   What is the dominant frequency or pitch of the usual AR murmur? Why?

ANS.:   This depends on whether the AR is mild, moderate, or severe. If mild, then the murmur is due more to a large gradient than to flow. Therefore, the murmur is purely high-pitched. If moderate, the murmur is due to a mixture of flow and high gradient, and it will have mixed frequencies. If severe, the murmur may be very rough, due to an excess of low and medium frequencies.

2.   How can you best imitate with the voice the sound of a typical mild AR murmur, i.e., purely high-pitched?

ANS.:   In Mexico, this has been called the classic "aspirative" AR murmur in imitation of noisily breathing *in* through the mouth. If you breathe *out* quickly with the mouth open or whisper "ah," you can just as easily imitate the classic AR mur-mur.

Note: Since it sounds so much like a breath sound, you may find it helpful to have the patient hold his breath in expiratory apnea in order for you to perceive this murmur better.

3.   How can you increase the loudness of the very soft AR murmur?

ANS.:   a) Sit the patient up, lean him forward, and press hard with the diaphragm during held expiration.

b) Increase peripheral resistance as follows:

*1) By intravenous administration of a vasopressor drug.

2) By having the patient squat. The increase in venous return for a few beats will help increase the murmur loudness on immediate auscultation.

   Note: Squatting is effective in bringing out a grade 1/6 murmur, but has little effect on the murmur of moderate to marked AR [63]. The slight increase in peripheral resistance caused by removing the blood-pressure-lowering effect of the force of gravity on the leg circulation is inadequate to affect an already moderate degree of AR [40]. (Kinking of arteries is probably unimportant in the squatting effect on blood pressure, since drawing the knees up to the chest in the lying position has little effect on blood pressure.)

c) Increase the blood pressure by isometric exercise, i.e., handgrip.

*4.   When can moderate AR be associated with a soft murmur, i.e., grade 1–2/6, despite a normal chest diameter and wall thickness?

ANS.:   In the presence of low flow due to MS.

   Note: In the presence of significant MS, the AR is probably trivial if the diastolic pressure is over 70 mm Hg and the pulse pressure is less than 40 mm Hg [8].

*5.   What is the timing and shape of musical AR murmurs, and what is their significance?

ANS.:   a) Pandiastolic decrescendo after the usual initial crescendo.

b) The musical parts may occur only in early diastole and then be followed by the usual high-frequency decrescendo murmur for the rest of diastole.

c) Either of the above, plus mid- or late-diastolic crescendo-decrescendo components.

   Musical aortic diastolic murmurs are often seen in patients with perforated valves, torn everted valves (often luetic), or ruptures of the aortic sinuses. The ruptures are usually secondary to myxomatous transformation or infective endocarditis.

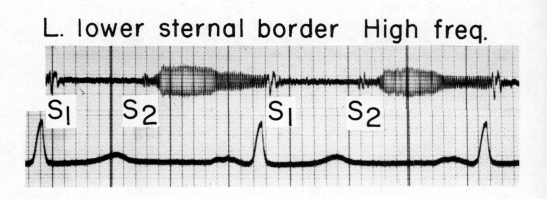

Luetic AR was suspected as the cause of this aortic diastolic murmur. Note the regular vibrations seen in all phonocardiograms of musical murmurs.

Site

1. Where, as a rule, is the AR murmur best heard?

    ANS.:   Over the midsternum or just to the left of the sternum at the level of the third or fourth intercostal space.

2. When is the AR murmur best heard to the right of the sternum?

    ANS.:   It is occasionally heard best in the second or third right interspace in the presence of marked poststenotic dilatation of the aorta, or when marked atherosclerotic tortuosity pushes the ascending aorta anteriorly and to the right. However, it is only under very unusual circumstances that it is best heard in the fourth right interspace. It is heard there only if it is due to nonrheumatic conditions that cause peculiar directions of the regurgitant stream; e.g., when it is secondary to an aortic aneurysm, lues, prolapsed aortic valve, or ruptured **sinus of Valsalva.**

3. What other unusual radiation to the left is occasionally found in AR?

    ANS.:   The murmur may be loud at the left sternal border, diminish as one approaches the apex, and then become louder again as one listens more toward the axilla. Thus, it may even be as loud or louder in the midaxillary line as at the sternal edge. Occasionally, it may even be heard *only* in the axillary area or at the apex. This has been called the Cole-Cecil murmur [9] . The cause for this unusual radiation is unknown. This may have been one of the causes of the "silent" AR reported in 16 patients with significant AR on cineangiography; i.e., the murmur may only have been present in the mid-left thorax, axilla, or apex, and when in the latter, may have been obscured by the murmur of MS [49] .

Sudden, Severe Aortic Regurgitation

1. What are the most likely causes of sudden, severe AR?

    ANS.:   a) Infective endocarditis.

    b) Rupture of an **aneurysm** of the sinus of Valsalva.

2. What are the auscultatory signs of sudden, severe AR at the apex?

    ANS.:   A soft or absent S_1 at the apex and a loud S_3 [65] .

    Note: a) The soft or absent S_1 in sudden, severe AR is due to a rise in LV pressure in diastole so rapid that it rises above left atrial pressure in mid-diastole and closes the mitral valve prematurely.

    b) The loud S_3, which occurs at the moment LV pressure becomes higher than left atrial pressure, may be the result of tensing of the chordae tendineae and papillary muscles by mitral valve closure [65] .

3. Why will sudden, severe AR often cause diastole to equal, or even be shorter than, systole, so that it is difficult to tell systole from diastole by auscultation?

    ANS.:   While ejection is prolonged by the severe volume overload in the LV, the diastolic period is shortened by tachycardia.

*4. Why should an exaggerated atrial hump occur on the apex cardiogram of some patients with severe AR? Why should the atrial hump disappear in sudden severe AR?

    ANS.:   In severe AR the atrial hump enlarges probably because of a relative myocardial ischemia. Dogs with severe AR have been found to have high levels of myocardial oxygen extraction, leading to relative ischemia. Relative ischemia is thought to be the cause of the loss of compliance of the LV in patients with angina, in whom large atrial humps also develop during angina attacks.

The A wave of the apex precordiogram may disappear in sudden, severe AR when the LV diastolic pressure is very high at the end of diastole. This is because when LV pressure becomes higher than left atrial pressure, the mitral valve closes and stays closed despite left atrial contraction. (On echocardiogram, the A wave, or atrial mitral valve opening movement, disappears in very severe AR.)

*5.   Why will an AR murmur not be pandiastolic in sudden, severe AR even despite diastoles that are shorter than normal?

   ANS.:   In sudden, severe AR the LV does not expand as well as in chronic AR, i.e., it is less distensible. Therefore, the LV pressure in diastole may rise so high so fast that it may reach the aortic diastolic pressure level (which also falls to very low levels) in mid-diastole. This equalization of aortic and ventricular pressures will eliminate the diastolic pressure gradient and murmur at the end of diastole. (This will also limit the actual amount of AR that can occur. See figure on p. 356.)

   Note: You may make the presystolic component of the AR murmur disappear with very severe AR by the handgrip maneuver or a vasopressor agent. These may result in enough increase in the AR so that slightly more regurgitation will cause LV end-diastolic pressure to exceed left atrial pressure.

Differential Diagnosis

1.   What can imitate an AR murmur?

   ANS.:   a) A pulmonary regurgitation (PR) murmur caused by a high pressure in the pulmonary artery (Graham Steell murmur).

   b) High-frequency components of MS murmurs transmitted to the left sternal border.

   *c) The soft, AR-like diastolic murmur heard at the second or third left interspace in some patients with severe but incomplete obstruction of the anterior descending coronary artery [7].

   *d) A loud venous hum. In about 10% of patients with severe uremia and anemia on dialysis, the louder diastolic component of the venous hum may be transmitted downward to the second right interspace, where the systolic component is not heard.

*THE MURMUR OF ANTERIOR DESCENDING CORONARY ARTERY STENOSIS

*1.   Why is the coronary artery obstruction murmur best heard in diastole?

   ANS.:   Maximum flow in the coronary arteries is in diastole.

*2.   What are the characteristics of the diastolic murmur of coronary artery stenosis?

   ANS.:   It is

   a) High-pitched [47].

   b) Crescendo-decrescendo, corresponding to the pattern of diastolic coronary flow, which is maximum in the first quarter of diastole [24, 47].

   c) Most easily heard with the patient sitting upright.

   Note: It has been observed to disappear after infarction and after aortocoronary bypass surgery.

*3.   What does the presence of the diastolic murmur of coronary artery stenosis suggest about the degree of obstruction?

  ANS.:   It suggests a good enough flow to produce enough turbulence to cause a diastolic murmur. Therefore, it is not surprising that not over a 50% obstruction has been found in those cases that have been reported.

PULMONARY REGURGITATION MURMURS

Murmurs with High Pressure in the Pulmonary Artery (Graham Steell Murmur)

1.   Does the pulmonary artery pressure have to be very high to produce a PR murmur?

  ANS.:   Usually very high, i.e., at nearly systemic levels. Pulmonary regurgitation murmurs are rarely present with pulmonary artery pressures below 80 mm Hg.

    Note: If a patient with a VSD has pulmonary hypertension and a Graham Steell murmur, this tells you nothing about the pulmonary vascular resistance. A PR murmur may occur even with normal pulmonary vascular resistance if the pulmonary pressure reaches about 100 mm Hg.

2.   How does the Graham Steell murmur differ from the AR murmur?

  ANS.:   It may not differ; i.e., both may be from grade 1 to 6, both may have an early crescendo-decrescendo, and both may become louder on expiration [48]. The Graham Steell murmur, however, often increases with inspiration when it is loud.

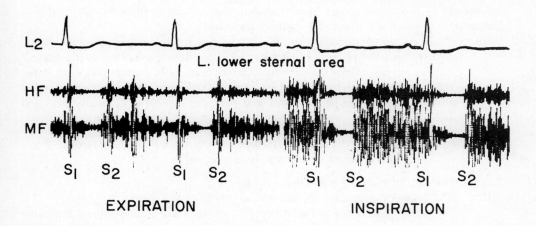

These phonocardiograms are from a patient with a PDA whose pulmonary artery pressure was 145 mm Hg, with an aortic pressure about the same. This loud diastolic murmur (Graham Steell murmur) increased markedly on inspiration. A soft Graham Steell murmur may not increase with inspiration.

3. Why does the Graham Steell murmur often decrease with inspiration despite the increase in pulmonary artery flow in inspiration?

   ANS.: The PR murmur is best heard in the second left interspace, where the effect of inspiration in pushing the stethoscope away from the heart is most marked and will overcome all other effects on the murmur.

   There is also a probability that inspiration may not increase flow to the lungs in patients with severe pulmonary hypertension because of the concomitant TR commonly present.

4. How can a Valsalva strain help in determining whether a PR or an AR murmur is present?

   ANS.: Immediately on release, the PR murmur will resume its pre-Valsalva loudness. The AR murmur will take four or five beats to return to normal intensity. However, this post-Valsalva effect depends on the murmur's becoming softer during the straining, which, unfortunately, is not always the case.

   Note: All high-frequency decrescendo murmurs starting with the P_2 at the left sternal border are not necessarily due either to AR or to PR if they are short. In patients with a dilated pulmonary artery, there can be an early, short diastolic decrescendo scratch without AR or PR. Such murmurs may sometimes result from an extracardiac effect of adhesions between the pulmonary artery and the surrounding lung.

5. Is the Graham Steell murmur rare or common in patients with MS?

   ANS.: It is rare. However, it used to be thought common because the murmur of AR was misinterpreted as being due to PR.

*6. When can a PDA with pulmonary hypertension produce a loud diastolic murmur that is produced at the ductus and not at the pulmonary valve?

   ANS.: There are reports of grade 4 or more diastolic murmurs due to such a rapid drop in pulmonary artery pressure because of PR that flow through the ductus occurs only in diastole. Since the pulmonary artery pressure in diastole may drop faster than aortic pressure, the murmur may even be crescendo to the first sound [69]. In every one of these patients who died, necropsy showed an unusually short and wide ductus [46].

Pulmonary Regurgitation Murmurs with Normal Pressure in the Pulmonary Artery
(Primary Pulmonary Regurgitation)

1. List five causes of primary PR murmurs.

   ANS.: a) Congenital absence of the pulmonary valves.

   Note: A tetralogy of Fallot with PR not surgically induced almost invariably has no pulmonary valves, and the pulmonary obstruction is due to a constricted valve ring.

   b) Infective endocarditis involving a pulmonary valve.

   c) The postoperative effect of surgery for pulmonary stenosis.

   d) Idiopathic dilatation of the pulmonary artery. (In some series, about a third of patients with idiopathic dilatation have PR.)

   e) Disproportionately dilated pulmonary arteries associated with increased flow, as in ASD or VSD. This might really be another instance of coincidental idiopathic dilatation of the pulmonary artery. In one series of 21 patients with uncomplicated ASD, 4 had an early basal diastolic murmur recorded externally and only in the outflow tract of the RV (see **inflow and outflow tract** of the RV) by internal phonocardiography [17].

Note: An "immediate" diastolic murmur at the left lower sternal border that begins with the P_2 in some ASD patients with normal pulmonary artery pressures has been shown sometimes to originate at the ASD. It may be the diastolic component of a continuous murmur at the ASD caused by a high left atrial pressure due to MR, plus a small to moderate-sized ASD [53].

2. How does the shape, length, and pitch of a primary PR murmur differ from that of the Graham Steell murmur?

ANS.: With high pressures in the pulmonary artery, the shape, length, and pitch of the murmur is the same as that of AR, i.e., a high-pitched decrescendo murmur with a tendency to a very early crescendo-decrescendo. In the murmur of PR with *normal* pressures in the pulmonary artery, there is often a slight delay after the P_2 before any murmur is heard at all. However, even if it starts with the P_2, the murmur tends to be short and rough, due to dominant medium and low frequencies.

Note: Intracardiac phonocardiograms have shown no pause between the P_2 and the murmur.

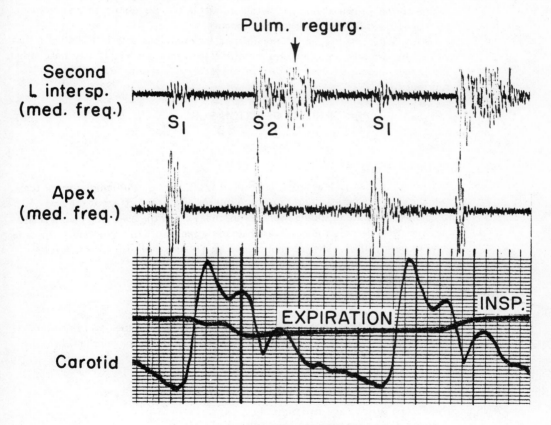

PRIMARY PR

This murmur of primary PR in a teenaged boy was early diastolic and had many low and medium frequencies in it. It did not increase with inspiration at the second left interspace because too much air was interposed between heart and stethoscope in that area. The murmur was softer at the left lower sternal border, where, however, it did become louder with inspiration.

3. How does respiration affect the murmur of primary PR?

 ANS.: It increases with inspiration, unlike most Graham Steell murmurs (unless the latter is loud).

4. What does the PR murmur with low pulmonary artery pressure resemble most? Why?

 ANS.: The murmur of TS, because

 a) Both are usually of low and medium pitch.

 b) Both may begin after a slight pause following the P_2.

 c) Both may be loudest along the left lower sternal border.

 d) Both increase with inspiration.

 e) Both are short.

 Note: An early diastolic murmur alone in TS usually is heard only in the presence of atrial fibrillation. In normal sinus rhythm, there is almost always a presystolic component.

*5. Why is the primary PR murmur short?

 ANS.: The diastolic pressure in the pulmonary artery falls rapidly because it started off with a normal pressure and has diastolic runoff in two directions, so that pulmonary artery and RV pressures rapidly equalize.

 Note: When the PR is mild, the murmur may have characteristics between that of the Graham Steell murmur and the primary PR murmur; i.e., it may start earlier, last longer, and have higher frequencies than the moderate to severe primary PR murmur [37].

PERICARDIAL FRICTION RUBS

Etiology

1. What causes friction rubs?

 ANS.: Pericarditis, either generalized or diffuse. It is assumed that inflammation of the two layers of the pericardium causes the rub sounds by the effect of the two roughened membranes sliding over one another. When the overlying pleura is also involved, then perhaps the noises are caused by the pleura rubbing against the outer layer of pericardium. The rub then would be a pleuro-pericardial friction rub.

2. What are three of the commonest causes of a generalized pericarditis?

 ANS.: Viral pericarditis, disseminated lupus erythematosis, and uremia.

3. What is the commonest cause of a localized pericarditis?

 ANS.: Acute myocardial infarction.

 Note: If there has been neither infarction nor trauma to the heart (including radiation to the chest), then consider a metastatic tumor involving the heart.

How to Recognize a Pericardial Friction Rub

1. How many murmurs are heard in most friction rubs?

 ANS.: Three: one systolic and two diastolic.

 Note: Even though the heart sounds may also be replaced by rubs, you may still hear in the background a rhythm of one systolic and two diastolic accentuations.

2.   What adjectives and analogies have been used to describe the quality of friction rubs?

ANS.:   They usually sound crunching, scraping, creaking, grating, crackling, or scratching. They often sound like squeaky shoes or like two pieces of sandpaper rubbed against one another. Occasionally, however, they sound no different from any mixed-frequency murmur. They often sound surprisingly superficial, so that increased stethoscope pressure seems to make them unexpectedly louder.

   Note: A rub that increases with inspiration, but did not on a previous examination, may signify the collection of pericardial fluid. A softening rub may also indicate fluid accumulation.

3.   At what times in diastole do the two diastolic rubs occur?

ANS.:   a) In early diastole, near the end of early rapid expansion of the ventricle, at the time when an S_3 would occur.

   b) At the end of diastole, when atrial contraction produces sudden ventricular expansion. This is the moment when an S_4 would occur.

4.   Where in systole may the systolic rub occur?

ANS.:   Anywhere. It may replace a heart sound or only occur in midsystole. There is therefore the possibility of three rubs in systole.

5.   With one major rub replacing the first sound in systole and two in diastole, what is the rhythm or cadence of a friction rub that is heard as a background, even if they are not distinctly separate?

ANS.:   The same as a quadruple rhythm due to a double gallop, i.e., "sh-dup-sh-sh——sh-dup-sh-sh." This rhythm must be practiced at a rapid rate because most patients with friction rubs have a tachycardia. Since the systolic rub often replaces both the S_1 and S_2, it is common to hear the rhythm as: "shsh-sh-sh——shsh-sh-sh." When one of the diastolic rubs is absent, it is usually the S_3; i.e., an S_4 rub is the last to disappear.

6.   Is the friction rub usually louder during inspiration or expiration? Why?

ANS.:   In about a third of patients, it increases during inspiration [14, 54]. This may be due to:

   a) The downward pull of the diaphragm on the pericardium, drawing it more tautly over the heart. This is the most likely cause, because the diaphragm is attached to the pericardium, and it is conceivable that a small amount of fluid between the two layers of the pericardium could be squeezed out by the tightening of the two layers with inspiration. This might partly account for the fact that the pericardial rub is not always absent when pericardial effusion is present.

   b) The expanded lung pressing on the pericardium.

   c) The greater expansion of the RV during inspiration than the expansion of the LV during expiration. This would stretch the pericardium more during inspiration.

7.   Of the three major rub components, which one is almost always present? Which is the next commonest component?

ANS.:   The systolic component is almost always present. The atrial systolic component is next in frequency of occurrence, but almost always occurs together with the systolic component. Only rarely does an atrial systolic rub occur alone as the only rub sound.

   Note: A systolic rub alone is more likely to occur in atrial fibrillation than in sinus rhythm [25].

8.   Where are most friction rubs best heard?
        ANS.:   At the left sternal border, at about the third or fourth left interspace.
9.   When is the friction rub transient?
        ANS.:   During the course of acute myocardial infarction when it may last only a few hours.
                    Note: In the **postmyocardial infarction syndrome** (Dressler's syndrome) it may
                last for weeks.
*10.   What can imitate a friction rub?
        ANS.:   A noisy pneumothorax. A shallow pneumothorax at the left lung apex (occasionally
                only seen on a film taken on full expiration) can apparently cause some air pockets
                on the medial aspect of the left lung. The contraction of the LV against these bubble
                of air may produce varying sounds at the apex synchronous with ventricular systole
                and diastole [50]. They have been described as grinding, clicking, and crunching
                and may be heard at a distance from the patient. They do not occur with a right-
                sided pneumothorax and for some reason seem to occur almost entirely in young,
                healthy males.
                    Note: A mixture of fluid and air in the pericardium, as when a few milliliters
                of air are introduced into the pericardium to replace fluid withdrawn, produces a
                metallic tinkle synchronous with systole. A large amount of injected air can pro-
                duce a churning, splashing sound (mill wheel murmur) [55].

REFERENCES

1. Aldridge, H. E., and Wigle, E. D. Partial anomalous pulmonary venous drainage with intact
    interatrial septum associated with congenital mitral stenosis. *Circulation* 31:579, 1965.
2. Ashman, H., Zaroff, L. I., and Baronofsky, I. Right atrial myxoma. *Am. J. Med.* 28:487,
    1960.
3. Ayers, C. R., Boineau, J. P., and Spach, M. S. Congenital complete heart block in children.
    Am. Heart J. 72:381, 1966.
4. Bardet, J., and Bardet, A. Phonocardiographie du rétrécissement mitral. *Arch. Mal. Coeur*
    59:917, 1966.
5. Barlow, J., Fuller, D., and Denny, M. A case of right atrial myxoma. *Br. Heart J.* 24:120,
    1962.
6. Benisch, B. M. Mitral stenosis and insufficiency: A complication of healed bacterial endo-
    carditis. *Am. Heart J.* 82:39, 1971.
7. Burg, J. R., Weaver, K. A., Russell, T., II, and Kassebaum, D. G. Disappearance of coronary
    artery stenosis murmur after aortocoronary bypass. *Chest* 63:440, 1973.
8. Cohn, L. H., Mason, D. T., Ross, J., Jr., Morrow, A. G., and Braunwald, E. Preoperative
    assessment of aortic regurgitation in patients with mitral valve disease. *Circulation* 34
    (Suppl. 31):76, 1966.
9. Cole, R., and Cecil, A. B. The axillary diastolic murmur in aortic insufficiency. *Bull. Johns
    Hopkins Hosp.* 19:353, 1908.
10. Coombs, C. F. *Rheumatic Heart Disease.* Bristol, England: Wright, 1924. P. 203.
11. Coombs, C. F. Rheumatic myocarditis. *Quarterly J. Med.* 2:26, 1908.
12. Criley, J. M., and Hermer, A. J. The crescendo presystolic murmur of mitral stenosis with
    atrial fibrillation. *N. Engl. J. Med.* 285:1284, 1971.

13. Criscitiello, M. G., Ronan, J. A., Jr., Besterman, E. M. M., and Schoenwetter, W. Cardiovascular abnormalities in osteogenesis imperfecta. *Circulation* 31:255, 1965.

14. Dressler, W. Effect of respiration on the pericardial friction rub. *Am. J. Cardiol.* 7:130, 1961.

15. Edwards, J. E. The congenital bicuspid aortic valve. *Circulation* 23:485, 1961.

16. El-Sherif, N. Rheumatic tricuspid stenosis; a haemodynamic correlation. *Br. Heart J.* 33:16, 1971.

17. Feruglio, G. A., and Sreenivasan, A. Intracardiac phonocardiogram in thirty cases of atrial septal defect. *Circulation* 20:1087, 1959.

18. Fisher, M. L., Nutter, D. O., Jacobs, W., and Schlant, R. C. Haemodynamic responses to isometric exercise (handgrip) in patients with heart disease. *Br. Heart J.* 35:422, 1973.

19. Flint, A. On cardiac murmurs. *Am. J. Med. Sci.* 44:29, 1962.

20. Fortuin, N. J., and Craige, E. On the mechanism of the Austin Flint murmur. *Circulation* 45:558, 1972.

21. Garbagni, R., Angelino, R., and Tartara, D. Lutembacher's syndrome: Clinical and hemodynamic studies before and after operation. *Arch. Mal. Coeur* 54:511, 1961.

22. Glancy, D. L., Chang, M. Y., Dorney, E. R., and Roberts, W. D. Parachute mitral valve. *Am. J. Cardiol.* 27:309, 1971.

23. Green, E. W., Agruss, N. S., and Adolph, R. J. Right-sided Austin Flint murmur. *Am. J. Cardiol.* 32:370, 1973.

24. Gregg, D. E. *Coronary Circulation in Health and Disease.* London: Kimpton, 1950.

25. Harvey, W. P. Auscultatory findings in diseases of the pericardium. *Am. J. Cardiol.* 7:15, 1961.

26. Heidenreich, F. P., Thompson, M. E., Shaver, J. A., and Leonard, J. J. Left atrial transport in mitral stenosis. *Circulation* 40:545, 1969.

27. Kaufmann, G., Rutishauser, W., and Hegglin, R. Heart sounds in atrial tumors. *Am. J. Cardiol.* 8:350, 1961.

28. Kong, T. Q., Kellum, R. E., and Haserick, J. R. Clinical diagnosis of cardiac involvement in systemic lupus erythematosus. *Circulation* 26:7, 1962.

29. Laake, H. Rheumatic tricuspid stenosis. *Acta Med. Scand.* 161:109, 1958.

30. Lakier, J. B., Pocock, W. A., Gale, G. E., and Barlow, J. B. Haemodynamic and sound events preceding first heart sound in mitral stenosis. *Br. Heart J.* 34:1152, 1972.

31. Lochaya, S., Igarashi, M., and Shaffer, A. B. Late diastolic mitral regurgitation secondary to aortic regurgitation: Its relationship to the Austin Flint murmur. *Am. Heart J.* 74:161, 1967.

32. Luisada, A. A., and Argano, B. The phonocardiogram in systemic hypertension. *Chest* 58:598, 1970.

33. Luisada, A. A., and diBartole, G. High frequency phonocardiography. *Am. J. Cardiol.* 8:51, 1961.

34. Matalon, R., Moussalli, A. R. J., Nidus, B. N., Katz, L. A., and Eisinger, R. P. Functional aortic insufficiency — a feature of renal failure. *N. Engl. J. Med.* 285:1522, 1972.

35. Morgan, J. R., Forker, A. D., Coates, J. R., and Myers, W. S. Isolated tricuspid stenosis. *Circulation* 44:729, 1971.

36. Nadas, A. S., and Ellison, R. C. Phonocardiographic analysis of diastolic flow murmurs in secundum atrial septal defect and ventricular septal defect. *Br. Heart J.* 29:684, 1967.

37. Nemickas, R., Roberts, J., Gunnar, R. M., and Tobin, J. R., Jr. Isolated congenital pulmonic insufficiency. *Am. J. Cardiol.* 14:456, 1964.

38. O'Brien, K. P., and Cohen, L. S. Hemodynamic and phonocardiographic correlates of the Austin Flint murmur. *Am. Heart J.* 77:603, 1969.

39. O'Brien, K. P., Hitchcock, G. C., Barratt-Boyes, B. G., and Lowe, J. B. Spontaneous aortic cusp rupture associated with valvular myxomatous transformation. *Circulation* 37:273, 1968.

40. O'Donnell, T. V., and McIlroy, M. B. The circulatory effects of squatting. *Am. Heart J.* 64:347, 1962.

41. Parker, E., Craig, E., and Hood, W. P., Jr. The Austin Flint murmur and the a wave of the apexcardiogram in aortic regurgitation. *Circulation* 43:349, 1971.

42. Paul, M. H., Rudolph, A. M., and Nadas, A. S. Congenital complete atrioventricular block: Problems of clinical assessment. *Circulation* 18:183, 1958.

43. Perloff, J. K. Auscultatory and phonocardiographic manifestations of pulmonary hypertension. *Prog. Cardiovasc. Dis.* 9:303, 1967.

44. Pridie, R. B., Benham, R., and Oakley, C. M. Echocardiography of the mitral valve in aortic valve disease. *Br. Heart J.* 33:296, 1971.

45. Read, R. C., Thal, A. P., and Wendt, V. E. Symptomatic valvular myxomatous transformation (the floppy valve syndrome). *Circulation* 32:897, 1965.

46. Rosenthal, T., and Kariv, I. A pathognomonic murmur of "atypical" patent ductus arteriosus. *Chest* 56:350, 1969.

47. Sangster, J. F., and Oakley, C. M. Diastolic murmur of coronary artery stenosis. *Br. Heart J.* 35:840, 1973.

48. Schwab, R. H., and Killough, J. H. The phonocardiographic differentiation of pulmonic and aortic insufficiency. *Circulation* 32:352, 1965.

49. Segal, B. L., Likoff, W., and Kaspar, A. J. "Silent" rheumatic aortic regurgitation. *Am. J. Cardiol.* 14:628, 1964.

50. Semple, T., and Lancaster, W. M. Noisy pneumothorax. *Br. Med. J.* 1:1342, 1961.

51. Shabetai, R., and Davidson, S. Asymmetrical hypertrophic cardiomyopathy simulating mitral stenosis. *Circulation* 45:37, 1972.

52. Silverman, J., Olwin, J. S., and Graettinger, J. S. Cardiac myxomas with systemic embolization. *Circulation* 26:99, 1962.

53. Somerville, J., and Resnekov, L. The origin of an immediate diastolic murmur in atrioventricular defects. *Circulation* 32:797, 1965.

54. Spodick, D. H. Pericardial friction. *N. Engl. J. Med.* 278:1204, 1968.

55. Spodick, D. H. Acoustic phenomena in pericardial disease. *Am. Heart J.* 81:114, 1971.

56. Starkey, G. W. B. Surgical experiences in the treatment of congenital mitral stenosis and mitral insufficiency. *J. Thorac. Cardiovasc. Surg.* 38:336, 1959.

57. Starr, A., Dotter, C., and Griswold, H. Supravalvular aortic stenosis: Diagnosis and treatment. *J. Thorac. Cardiovasc. Surg.* 41:134, 1961.

58. Tai, A., Gross, H., and Siegelman, S. S. Right atrial myxoma and pulmonary hypertension. *N.Y. State J. Med.* 70:2996, 1970.

59. Taquini, A. C., Massell, B. F., and Walsh, B. J. Phonocardiographic studies of early rheumatic mitral disease. *Am. Heart J.* 20:295, 1940.

60. Ueda, H., Sakamoto, T., Kawai, N., Watanabe, H., Uozumi, A., Okada, R., Kobayashi, T., Yamada, T., Inoue, K., and Kaito, G. The Austin Flint murmur. *Jap. Heart J.* 6:294, 1965.

61. Ueda, H., Sakamoto, T., Kawai, N., Watanabe, H., Uozumi, A., Okada, R., Kobayashi, T., and Kaito, G. "Silent" mitral stenosis. *Jap. Heart J.* 6:206, 1965.

62. Ueda, H., Sugiura, M., Ito, I., Saito, Y., and Morooka, S. Aortic insufficiency associated with aortitis syndrome. *Jap. Heart J.* 8:107, 1967.

63. Vogelpoel, L., Nellen, M., Beck, W., and Schrire, V. The value of squatting in the diagnosis of mild aortic regurgitation. *Am. Heart J.* 27:709, 1969.

64. Waxler, E. B., Kawai, N., and Kasparian, H. Right atrial myxoma: Echocardiographic, phonocardiographic, and hemodynamic signs. *Am. Heart J.* 83:251, 1972.

65. Wigle, E. D., and Labrosse, C. J. Sudden, severe aortic insufficiency. *Circulation* 32:708, 1965.

66. Wood, P. An appreciation of mitral stenosis. I. Clinical features. *Br. Med. J.* 1:1051, 1954. Classic article.

67. Wood, P. An appreciation of mitral stenosis. II. Investigation and results. *Br. Med. J.* 1:1113, 1954. Classic article.

68. Wooley, C. F., Levin, H. S., Leighton, R. F., Goodwin, R. S., and Ryan, J. M. Intracardiac sound and pressure events in man. *Am. J. Med.* 42:248, 1967.

69. Wunsch, C. M., and Tavel, M. E. Patent ductus arteriosus and pulmonary valve insufficiency: Unusual clinical manifestations. *Chest* 57:572, 1970.

16

Abdominal Murmurs

1. List the known causes of abdominal murmurs.
   ANS.: a) Normal arterial and venous flow murmurs, usually only in young people.
   b) Renal artery stenosis.
   c) Hepatic, due to
   1) Anastomoses between portal and systemic veins in cirrhosis with portal hypertension.
   2) Hepatic malignancies.
   3) Alcoholic hepatitis [4].
   d) Splenic artery aneurysms.
   e) Aortic obstruction due to atheromas [5].
   f) Splenic, superior mesenteric, or common or external iliac artery stenosis from within or by pressure from an extrinsic mass [4].
   g) Mesenteric, due to increased flow to the inflamed bowel of acute infectious intestinal disease.

NORMAL ABDOMINAL MURMURS

1. How common are abdominal murmurs in normal subjects?
   ANS.: Almost half of subjects under 25, but only about 5% over 50, have abdominal flow murmurs. Thus, an abdominal murmur in an adult, for all practical purposes, should be considered as probably an abnormal finding [2, 5].
2. Where are (a) normal and (b) abnormal abdominal murmurs heard?
   ANS.: a) Normal murmurs are heard
   1) In the epigastrium.
   2) Over the inferior vena cava, 2–3 cm to the right and above the umbilicus. This is the equivalent of the venous hum and is heard in about 5% of normal subjects [2].
   b) Abnormal abdominal murmurs are heard anywhere except over the inferior vena cava.
3. What is the value of being aware of epigastric murmurs in normal subjects?
   ANS.: In very thin patients, the murmur may radiate to the left lower sternal border of the chest and be confused with a cardiac murmur. Since an epigastric murmur may be continuous, it may imitate a regurgitant type of murmur.

---

*indicates material that is for electives or fellows in cardiology, or concerns rare phenomena, of interest primarily to cardiologists.

4.   Are epigastric murmurs early systolic, pansystolic, or continuous?
    ANS.:   They may be of any length.
5.   How can amyl nitrite inhalation tell you the degree of stenosis producing the arterial murmur?
    ANS.:   With mild or moderate stenosis, the arterial murmur is intensified in about 25 sec by causing an increased cardiac output and flow through the stenotic area. With severe stenosis, on the other hand, the murmur may soften, because amyl nitrite can dilate ample collateral vessels to the area beyond the obstruction, so that flow will preferentially pass through collaterals. It is also possible that distal to a severely obstructed artery, the arterioles are already maximally dilated, so that after amyl nitrite, the blood will escape through other arteries dilated by the drug [3].

RENAL ARTERY STENOSIS MURMURS

1.   What is the pitch and timing of the stenosing renal vascular lesion murmur?
    ANS.:   High-pitched. It is sometimes a to-and-fro murmur, i.e., systolic and diastolic (with systolic accentuation), sometimes only short systolic, and sometimes continuous. The short systolic murmur is especially common in severe stenosis.
        *Note: Even though the most likely cause of a renal artery murmur is atherosclerotic obstruction, the kind of renal artery lesion most likely to have an arterial murmur is fibromuscular dysplasia.
2.   Where are the best sites for hearing renal vascular murmurs?
    ANS.:   a) Beneath the costal margin anteriorly, lateral to the aorta and lumbar spine.
        b) Just above the umbilicus, usually to the left of the midline. If it is heard at the sides or back, it is usually transmitted from the anterior abdomen.
3.   How can you suspect renal hypertension by auscultation besides listening over the abdomen?
    ANS.:   In the presence of severe hypertension, a murmur over one or both femoral arteries due to atherosclerosis of the femoral arteries also suggests renal artery stenosis.

MISCELLANEOUS ABDOMINAL MURMURS

1.   What does a venous hum over the abdominal wall suggest?
    ANS.:   If it is not the normal venous hum in a young person, it suggests cirrhosis with portal hypertension and an anastomosis between the portal and systemic veins. However, a continuous murmur rather than a hum is more likely to mean either an arteriovenous fistula of the portal system or renal artery stenosis.
2.   What should a systolic murmur in the left hypochondrium suggest?
    ANS.:   a) Splenic abnormalities:
            1) Aneurysm of the splenic artery or a tortuous and calcified splenic artery.
            2) A huge spleen.
            3) A traumatized spleen.
        b) Carcinoma of the body of the pancreas, compressing the splenic artery.
        c) Renal artery stenosis.
3.   What does a friction rub over the splenic area suggest?
    ANS.:   Splenic infarction due to embolism, as in infective endocarditis.

4.   What is probably the commonest cause of an epigastric murmur in patients referred for abdominal aortography for any reason?

   ANS.:   Celiac artery stenosis. Even in younger hypertensive patients with abdominal murmurs, one study found that asymptomatic celiac compression was a more likely cause of the murmur than renal artery stenosis [1].

   Note: An abdominal murmur commonly accompanies a complete occlusion of the celiac artery, and is likely caused by flow through collateral channels [1].

REFERENCES

1. McLoughlin, M. J., Cotapinto, R. F., and Hobbs, B. B. Abdominal bruits. *J. A. M. A.* 232:1238, 1975.
2. Rivin, A. U. Abdominal vascular sounds. *J. A. M. A.* 221:688, 1972.
3. Ueda, H., Sakamoto, T., Yamada, T., Uozumi, Z., Kobayashi, T., Kawai, N., Inoue, K., and Kaito, G. Quantitative assessment of obstruction of the aorta and its branches in "aortitis syndrome": The value of functional phonoarteriography using vasoactive drugs. *Jap. Heart J.* 7:3, 1966.
4. Zoneraich, S., and Zoneraich, O. Diagnostic significance of abdominal arterial murmurs in liver and pancreatic disease. *Angiology* 22:197, 1971.
5. Zoneraich, S., and Zoneraich, O. Value of auscultation and phonoarteriography in detecting atherosclerotic involvement of the abdominal aorta and its branches. *Am. Heart J.* 83:620, 1972.

17
Prosthetic Valve Sounds

NORMAL BALL VALVE SOUNDS AND RHYTHMS

1. Does a Starr-Edwards ball valve produce a sound both on opening and closing?
    ANS.:   Yes. When it opens, it strikes the cage struts to produce an opening click (OC). When it closes, it strikes the cage ring to produce a closing click (CC).

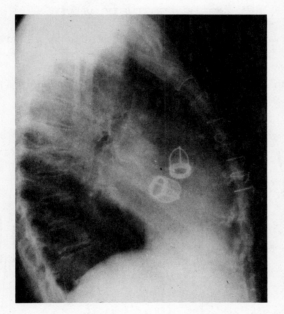

The lower larger cage is mitral. The balls, or poppets, are not radiopaque enough to tell their position.

2. Which *normal* heart sounds are heard in the presence of (a) an aortic ball valve and (b) a mitral ball valve?
    ANS.:   a) With an aortic prosthesis, the M_1 will be the only normal heart sound not replaced by an aortic OC and CC.

_____
*indicates material that is for electives or fellows in cardiology, or concerns rare phenomena, of interest primarily to cardiologists.

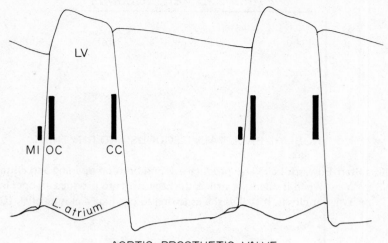

AORTIC PROSTHETIC VALVE

The aortic prosthetic valve will sound like a normal heart that has a loud ejection click and loud S_2.

b) With a mitral prosthesis, the S_2 will be the only normal heart sound heard.

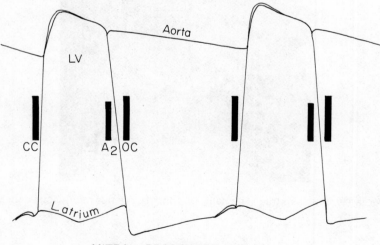

MITRAL PROSTHETIC VALVE

The only normal sound expected with a mitral prosthetic valve is the S_2. Any aortic component of the S_1 would be masked by the loud CC. The rhythm with the OC is exactly like that heard in mitral stenosis with an opening snap.

3. What is the rhythm or cadence produced by an OC or CC of an aortic prosthetic ball valve together, with the normal M_1 included?

ANS.: The order of sounds is M_1—OC ————— CC. Therefore, the rhythm is duclick ———— click . . . . duclick ———— click.

Note: In the presence of an aortic prosthetic valve, the M_1 is rarely heard well away from the apex area because

a) Most patients with a prosthetic aortic valve have some myocardial damage, thus producing a softer M_1.

b) The loud click following a soft sound may mask the soft sound (backward masking). Therefore, an aortic prosthetic valve rhythm often consists only of an opening and closing click, resulting in a rhythm of

click ———— click . . . . click ———— click.

4. What is the rhythm or cadence of a mitral ball valve together with its normal S_2?

ANS.: The order of sounds is CC ———— S_2—OC. Therefore, the rhythm is click ———— duclick . . . . click ———— duclick.

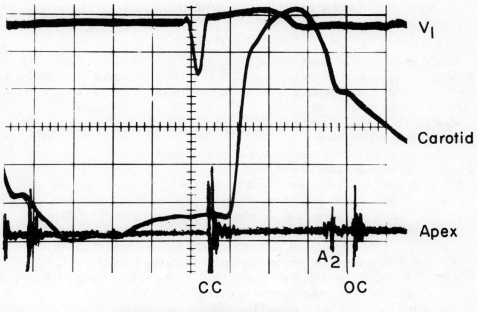

CC   A2   OC

MITRAL PROSTHESIS

With a mitral prosthetic valve, the first sound is replaced by the CC, but the second sound is the patient's own (at the apex it is only an A_2). The opening of the prosthetic valve (OC) will be heard at the same time as would an opening snap.

Note: a) This is a very important rhythm to recognize, because it is the same as the rhythm of a patient with mitral stenosis and an opening snap, i.e., S_1 ———— S_2–OS.

b) A mitral CC, unlike the loud M_1 of mitral stenosis, is sometimes louder at the left lower sternal border than at the apex [11].

5.   What extra sounds are commonly heard with a normal ball valve?

ANS.:   a) The ball often bounces and strikes the cage several times. This may produce from one up to three multiple clicks, trailing off after the major click.

Note: If the extra multiple clicks disappear, it may be a sign of early ball valve swelling or of thrombus on the cage.

b) An early systolic crunchy murmur following the OC may normally be heard when an aortic prosthesis is present.

*c) A presystolic click may be heard at the apex, due to the effect of atrial contraction, causing either eddy currents or a Bernouilli effect, which may raise the open mitral ball valve up high enough to strike the ring.

PROSTHETIC VALVE ABNORMALITIES

Aortic Prosthetic Valve Abnormalities

1.   What is meant by "ball valve variance?"

ANS.:   It refers to the deformation of a ball by swelling or cracking. The swelling is due to absorption of lipids by the plastic material. (This does not occur with the newer metallic balls.)

2.   How can you recognize aortic ball valve variance?

ANS.:   The opening click

a) Loses its high frequencies, i.e., becomes muffled [7, 8].

b) Becomes softer or disappears.

Note: a) You can easily recognize that there is aortic ball valve loss of OC amplitude by a phonocardiogram in the second right interspace. If it shows that the OC is less than 50% of the amplitude of the CC in the high-frequency range, ball valve variance should be suspected [6].

b) Occasionally, both OCs and CCs become equally muffled.

3.   Why does an expanding ball tend to decrease the OC before it affects the CC?

ANS.:   Perhaps it is because if the poppet (ball) is deformed, only a part of it contacts the cage before maximum contact occurs.

4.   What is the earliest time after surgery that an aortic ball valve may become deformed?

ANS.:   As early as 3½ months.

5.   What can mimic ball valve variance and make the OC softer in the presence of a normal ball?

ANS.:   The OC may be muffled if

a) There is a clot on the cage cushioning the poppet.

b) There is a cardiomyopathy, with poor myocardial contractility.

> *Note:* a) This is probably the cause of the nearly 15% of aortic ball valves that have an abnormal OC/CC ratio with no ball valve variance at surgery, autopsy, or on long-term follow-up [4].
>
> b) You can get an indication that the aortic OC is depressed in the presence of an aortic ejection murmur, because the frequency of vibrations of a depressed aortic OC is about the same as that of an aortic ejection murmur. This means that when they are difficult to separate, the aortic OC is probably depressed.
>
> *c) A triple valve replacement may make it impossible to tell if the aortic OC is depressed, because the delayed contraction of the right ventricle over the left ventricle may make the tricuspid OC occur simultaneously with the aortic OC. (Tricuspid prosthetic valve replacements are very rare.)

6. What can cause an aortic ball valve to become regurgitant?

   ANS.: A paravalvular (suture area) leak.

   > *Note:* a) Small aortic paravalvular leaks usually produce audible regurgitant murmurs and occur in at least 15% of such valves [12].
   >
   > b) When severe aortic regurgitation occurs after prosthetic valve replacement, there has usually been a heavily calcified valve preoperatively. The valve ring in this situation is involved in the calcific process and does not hold sutures well.
   >
   > *c) When an aortic prosthesis becomes detached and hangs only by a hinge of sutures (usually at the site of the former posterior noncoronary cusp), the rocking motion of the detached prosthesis may push up the anterior mitral leaflet and cause a relative stenosis. This can cause a mid-diastolic murmur [12].

7. What is the major difference in the OC and CC of a disc valve and those of a ball valve?

   ANS.: The OC of a disc valve is normally softer than the CC and often sounds like an abnormal ball valve.

Mitral Prosthetic Valve Abnormalities

1. How can you diagnose mitral ball valve variance or other serious interference with ball function?

   ANS.: There is a ball valve abnormality if

   a) The A_2–OC interval varies without regard to cycle length [10].

   *b) The A_2–OC interval is greater than 150 msec.

   *c) The A_2–OC is less than 70 msec. This suggests that the ball valve is too small and is producing significant stenosis [14].

   d) The OC may become muffled or disappear [9].

   e) A mitral diastolic murmur may be produced by prosthetic valve stenosis [9a].

   > *Note:* a) If the OC is less than 35% of the CC at the apex or left sternal border, and severe left ventricular failure is not present, either interference with prosthetic ball or disc movement or a paravalvular leak should be suspected [13].

          b) An OC of the mitral valve (disc or ball) can disappear with marked valve ring detachment because ventricular filling then takes place preferentially through the paravalvular leak, and flow through the prosthetic valve may not be sufficient to accelerate the ball enough to produce a sound [2].

          c) A diastolic rumble at the apex due to an Austin Flint murmur may occur even in the presence of a prosthetic mitral ball valve [9a].

2. How does the murmur of a paravalvular mitral valve leak differ from that of valvular regurgitation?

    ANS.:   a) Although a mild paravalvular leak may have the usual pansystolic apical murmur, it is often not audible even when severe [13].

          b) It may be audible only in unexpected places, such as the posterior chest wall.

          Note: The development of unexplained heart failure in a patient with a prosthetic mitral valve should always raise the suspicion of silent, severe mitral regurgitation due to a paravalvular leak.

*3. When can a mitral ball valve close even before the ventricle contracts?

    ANS.:   a) In sinus rhythm, when there is a long P—R interval. This will produce a very soft CC [3, 5].

          b) In atrial fibrillation, when there is a long R—R interval [5].

          c) In severe aortic regurgitation, when the diastolic pressure in the left ventricle exceeds left atrial pressure in mid-diastole [1].

REFERENCES

1. Agnew, T. M., and Carlisle, R. Premature valve closure in patients with a mitral Starr-Edwards prosthesis and aortic incompetence. *Br. Heart J.* 32:436, 1970.

2. Aravanis, C., Toutouzas, P., and Stavrou, S. Disappearance of opening sound of Starr-Edwards mitral valve due to valvular detachment. *Br. Heart J.* 34:1314, 1972.

3. Brown, D. F. Decreased intensity of closure sound in a normally functioning Starr-Edwards mitral valve prosthesis. *Am. J. Cardiol.* 31:93, 1973.

4. Delman, A. J. Aortic ball variance. *Am. Heart J.* 83:291, 1972.

5. Hamby, R. I., Aintablian, A., and Wisoff, G. B. Mechanism of closure of the mitral prosthetic valve and the role of atrial systole. *Am. J. Cardiol.* 31:616, 1973.

6. Hylen, J. C., Kloster, F. E., Herr, R. H., Hull, P. Q., Ames, A. W., Starr, A., and Griswold, H. E. Phonocardiographic diagnosis of aortic ball variance. *Circulation* 38:90, 1968.

7. Hylen, J. C., Kloster, F. E., Herr, R., Starr, A., and Griswold, H. E. Sound spectrographic diagnosis of aortic ball variance. *Circulation* 39:849, 1969.

8. Hylen, J. C., Kloster, F. E., Starr, A., and Griswold, H. E. Aortic ball variance: Diagnosis and treatment. *Ann. Intern. Med.* 72:1, 1970.

9. Leachman, R. D., and Cokkinos, D. V. P. Absence of opening click in dehiscence of mitral valve prosthesis. *N. Engl. J. Med.* 281:461, 1969.

9a. Schaefer, R. A., McAnulty, J. H., Starr, A., and Rahimtoola, S. H. Diastolic murmurs in the presence of Starr-Edwards mitral prosthesis. *Circulation* 51:402, 1975.

10. Schluger, J., Mannix, E. P., Jr., and Wolf, R. E. Auscultatory and phonocardiographic sign of ball variance in a mitral prosthetic valve. *Am. Heart J.* 81:809, 1971.

11. Shah, P. M., McCanon, D. M., and Luisada, A. A. Spread of the "mitral" sound over the chest: A study of five subjects with the Starr-Edwards valve. *Circulation* 28:1102, 1963.
12. Sutton, G. C., and Wright, J. E. C. Major detachment of aortic prosthetic valves. *Br. Heart J.* 32:337, 1970.
13. Willerson, J. T., Kastor, J. A., Dinsmore, R. E., Mundth, E., Buckley, M. J., Austen, G., and Sanders, C. A. Non-invasive assessment of prosthetic mitral paravalvular and intravalvular regurgitation. *Br. Heart J.* 34:561, 1972.
14. Wise, J. R., Jr., Webb-Peploe, M., and Oakley, C. M. Detection of prosthetic mitral valve obstruction by phonocardiography. *Am. J. Cardiol.* 28:107, 1971.

DEFINITIONS AND METHODS OF MEASUREMENTS

1.   What are systolic time intervals (STIs)?
     ANS.:   They are the left ventricular (LV) ejection time (ET) and the pre-ejection period
             (PEP).
2.   What is meant by the left ventricular ET? How is it measured?
     ANS.:   It is the time between the opening and closing of the aortic valve. It is measured
             between the upstroke and dicrotic notch (or incisura) of an externally derived
             carotid pulse or direct aortic pressure tracing. The externally derived carotid
             tracing is taken by applying a funnel or other pulse pickup over the artery. The
             pulse pickup goes to a pressure transducer amplifier, and recorder. (See p. 124
             for explanation of transducer.) An outward arterial movement equals an upward
             movement on the recorder.

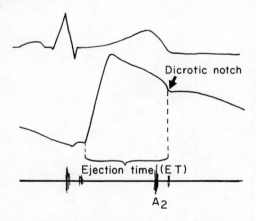

The ET is measured from the upstroke of the carotid to the dicrotic notch. A slight hump is
often seen preceding the first sharp upstroke. This probably represents isovolumic contraction
time and should not be included in the ET. The ET is often called the LVET, but the LV seems
redundant since we assume that we are dealing with left-sided events unless told otherwise.

---

*indicates material that is for electives or fellows in cardiology, or concerns rare phenomena, of interest
primarily to cardiologists.

Boldface type indicates that the term is explained in the Glossary.

3.   What is meant by the PEP? How is it measured?

ANS.:   It is the time between the beginning of electrical activation of the heart and the opening of the aortic valve. Its length is considered mostly dependent on LV **isovolumic contraction** time. It is a measure of the interval between the beginning of the QRS and the rise of pressure in the aorta. Therefore, it actually consists of three intervals:

a) Beginning of QRS to onset of left ventricular mechanical systole (electromechanical interval).

b) Onset of LV contraction to closure of mitral valve (preisovolumic contraction).

c) M_1 to onset of aortic ejection (isovolumic contraction).

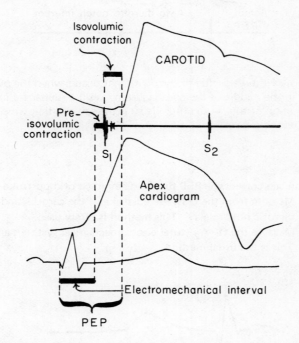

The PEP consists of 3 intervals; Q to onset of ventricular contraction, onset of ventricular contraction to M_1, and M_1 to aortic opening intervals. However, the M_1 to aortic opening (isovolumic contraction) is the major determinant of the PEP.

Note: There is a delay of 10–40 msec between the actual opening of the aortic valve and time of the upstroke of the carotid pulse. This is due to the time the pulse wave takes to travel from the aortic valve to the carotid, and from the pulse pickup on the neck through the rubber tubing to the transducer. The delay of the carotid upstroke is the same as the delay between the A_2 and the dicrotic notch [19]. The A_2 and central aortic incisura have been found to be simultaneous events when corrected for delays of transmission.

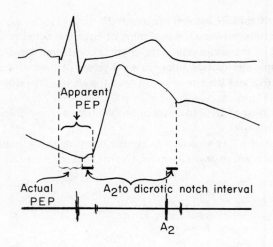

The A$_2$ to dicrotic notch interval is due to the delay that occurs when the pulse wave travels from the aortic root in the middle of the chest and through the rubber tubing of the pulse unit to the neck. The duration of the A$_2$ to notch delay is the same as that which occurs at the onset of the carotid upstroke.

You can correct the PEP for the delay in carotid upstroke by two methods:
a) Measure from the Q to the upstroke of the carotid, and subtract the A$_2$ to dicrotic notch delay. This method is rarely used.
b) Measure the Q—A$_2$ (total electromechanical systole), and subtract the ET. This is the usual method.

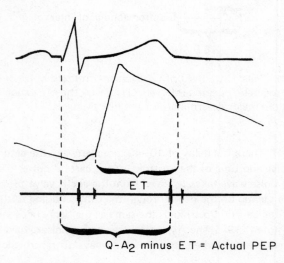

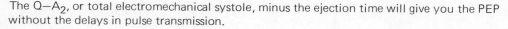

Q—A$_2$ minus E T = Actual PEP

The Q—A$_2$, or total electromechanical systole, minus the ejection time will give you the PEP without the delays in pulse transmission.

Note: Accurate measurement of STIs is only obtainable if
a) initial electrical activation is shown on the ECG lead that you use for the QRS. If multiple simultaneous leads are not obtainable, then the single lead used must show a septal vector, i.e., either a qR or an rS.
b) The upstroke of the carotid must not be measured from the beginning of any hump preceding the onset of the steepest slope. Any such hump is likely to occur during LV isovolumic contraction.

PHYSIOLOGICAL CHANGES IN SYSTOLIC TIME INTERVALS

1. How are the STIs affected by (a) heart rate, (b) sex, (c) age, and (d) active occupation?
    ANS.:   a) The faster the heart rate, the shorter the STI (both PEP and ET shorten).
    b) Women have slightly longer STIs than men mainly due to a prolongation of ET. This difference begins at puberty [12].
    c) Children have slightly shorter STIs than adults. Older subjects have slightly longer PEPs and ETs. (The ET increases by about 2 msec [0.002 sec] per decade, so that by age 80, it is about 10–20 msec [0.01–0.02 sec] longer than normal by the usual regression equation that corrects for heart rate.)
    d) People who are active have been found in one study to have shorter PEPs than those who are sedentary [34]. This, however, is controversial.

2. How can you correct the STI for heart rate and sex?
    ANS.:   Three methods are used.
    a) Read off the upper and lower limits of normal for rate and sex from graphs made from established linear regression equations. The graphs use one standard deviation as the limits [31].

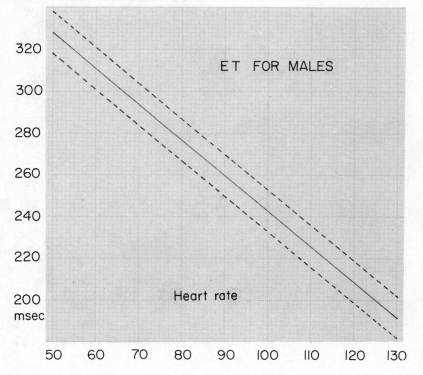

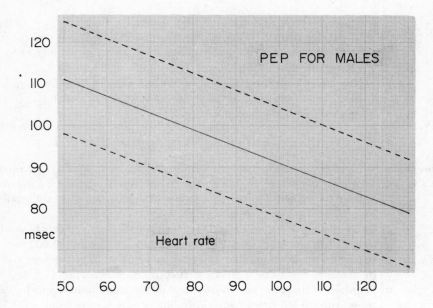

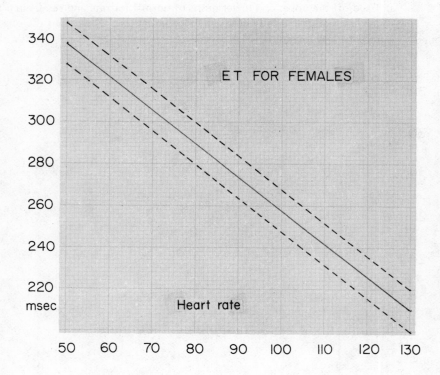

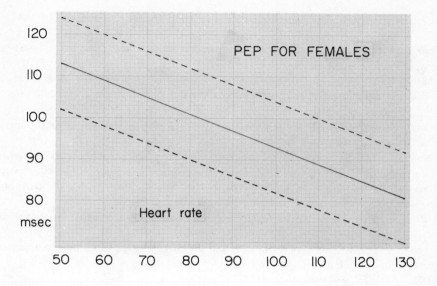

PEP FOR FEMALES

Heart rate

b) Use a single number calculated from the regression equation. This is the STI index [30].

 Note: The ET index for males is the ET plus (1.7 times the heart rate). (For females, use 1.6.) This offers a convenient expression for studying serial changes and for comparing patients.

c) Use the ratios of PEP/ET in order to ignore heart rate and sex.

Note: a) PEP/ET ratios are unrelated to age or heart rate from age 1 month to 15 years, and the mean is 0.31 (S.D. = 0.05) [27]. For adults, the mean is 0.34 (S.D. = 0.04). The upper normal should, therefore, be considered to be 0.42, i.e., two standard deviations should be used to separate normals for the purpose of any studies.

  b) These regression equations cannot be used for STIs done *during* exercise, although they can be used for the immediate postexercise state [18].

*3. How does a change in volume of the LV affect the STI?

ANS.: The increased Starling effect of an increased volume shortens the PEP, but lengthens the ET. (The $Q-S_2$ is little affected.) On the other hand, the decreased Starling effect of a decreased volume to the LV, as with diuretics or standing, lengthens the PEP and shortens the ET.

Note: a) In the seventh or eighth month of pregnancy, at the time of maximum expansion of blood volume (20–100% increase), the PEP is shortened and the ET is prolonged, as expected [24].

  b) The stroke volume has been related to ET according to the regression equation, ET = 106 + 2 SV, with a correlation coefficient (r) of 0.94 [14].

4. How does sympathetic stimulation affect the STIs?

ANS.: Both the PEP and ET shorten. Therefore, the $Q-S_2$ shortens.

EFFECT OF MYOCARDIAL DAMAGE ON THE SYSTOLIC TIME INTERVALS

1.   How does total time for contraction of a piece of muscle from a subject in heart failure compare with normal muscle?

ANS.:   Surprisingly, the total time for contraction is *unchanged*; i.e., if it took 300 msec (0.30 sec) for total contraction before failure it will take about 300 msec after heart failure [26].

2.   How has it been shown that the entire LV also takes the same time for total contraction after as before it went into failure?

ANS.:   The $Q-S_2$ (PEP + ET) is the same in patients with or without failure when the failure is due to coronary disease, hypertension, or idiopathic **cardiomyopathy**.

3.   Does the heart in failure take a longer or shorter time to raise pressure to open the aortic valve, i.e., how is isovolumic contraction time affected?

ANS.:   Isovolumic contraction is prolonged. (This is the same as saying that the PEP is prolonged.)

4.   If the PEP is prolonged in heart failure, and the total contraction time is unchanged, what must happen to the ET in heart failure?

ANS.:   The ET must shorten.

*5.   How is the PEP/ET ratio affected by heart failure?

ANS.:   Since the PEP lengthens and the ET shortens, the number increases with increasing failure. It not only encompasses changes in both intervals within one number, but also is independent of heart rate (within a range of 40–100 beats per minute).

Note: The upper normal ratio within one standard deviation is 0.38.

6.   What besides the above is the advantage of the PEP/ET ratio over the PEP and ET separately?

ANS.:   It can be used in a regression equation for **ejection fraction** in the formula

$$1.125 - (1.25 \times PEP/ET)$$

with a standard deviation of 0.08.

Note: This was done in patients with mitral valve disease (with and without atrial fibrillation), coronary and idiopathic cardiomyopathies, hypertrophic sub-aortic stenosis, aortic regurgitation, and acute pericarditis [11]. The r value was 0.90, with a p value of less than 0.01.

*HYPERTENSION AND THE SYSTOLIC TIME INTERVALS

*1.   How does chronic hypertension without failure affect the STIs?

ANS.:   a) If not severe, the STIs are normal.

b) If severe, the PEP is unchanged or prolonged, and the ET is prolonged [15].

Note: a) In the elderly, the ET increases by about 1.3 msec for each 10 mm Hg increment in systolic blood pressure [35].

b) If the PEP is prolonged in a hypertensive patient, it is due to a prolonged Q–1 and not to a prolonged isovolumic contraction time [28].

c) If the patient is young and has a hyperkinetic circulation, excess catecholamines may shorten the $Q-S_2$ despite hypertension.

*2.   With which etiology of severe hypertension is there less increase in PEP than in essential hypertension?

ANS.:   If it is due to renal artery stenosis, the PEP is shorter than in essential hypertension [28]. (This has only been studied in women.)

*3.   How are the STIs affected by a transient (a) increase in blood pressure and (b) decrease in blood pressure?

ANS.:   a) A transient increase in afterload or blood pressure prolongs the PEP and usually prolongs the ET also, but the effects on the ET are variable.

b) A transient decrease in afterload or blood pressure shortens the PEP, but lengthens the ET.

EFFECT OF CORONARY ARTERY DISEASE (WITHOUT FAILURE) ON THE SYSTOLIC TIME INTERVALS

*1.   How does coronary artery disease without heart failure affect the $Q-S_2$ (total contraction time) and STIs? Why?

ANS.:   It shortens the $Q-S_2$. This has been attributed to a hyperadrenergic state in patients with chronic coronary artery disease. One study in patients with triple coronary disease showed that this hyperadrenergic state primarily affects the ET [7], the PEP was either unchanged or only slightly increased. The isovolumic contraction time (M_1 to carotid upstroke) was prolonged but was counterbalanced by a shortening of the $Q-M_1$ interval [6]. In single or double coronary artery disease, the PEP is variable.

Note: In heart failure, the PEP is usually prolonged, not only because isovolumic contraction time is prolonged, but also because the $Q-M_1$ is also prolonged. Digitalis can then shorten the PEP, so that the STIs are almost normal, except for the short ET. In contrast, in noncoronary cardiomyopathies a long PEP will usually still be maintained despite digitalis. Thus, a top-normal PEP, together with a short ET, in a digitalized patient in failure is highly suggestive of a coronary cardiomyopathy, although I have personally seen it in a severe amyloid cardiomyopathy and in an idiopathic cardiomyopathy in which histological evidence of fibrosis was absent.

2.   How do the STIs change immediately after exercise in patients with coronary disease without failure?

ANS.:   If taken supine just after about 4 minutes of moderate exercise, the ET is prolonged [23]. The PEP is usually shortened in normal subjects and in coronary patients without failure.

Note: This prolongation of ET has identified coronary disease when the exercise ECG was negative for ischemia. However, one study showed that in a patient with coronary disease who undertakes an active exercise program three to five times a week for at least a year, the ET is not prolonged after exercise [36]. Under the influence of meperidine and diazepam (precatheterization medications), the ET may be prolonged by supine exercise even in normal subjects [20].

*3.   Why will the ET be prolonged with exercise in subjects with coronary disease?
      ANS.:   The increased volume that returns to the heart in the immediate postexercise
              state can be ejected in normal time by normal hearts because of the response of
              the LV to catecholamines. The ischemic heart presumably has a decreased ability
              to respond to catecholamines, perhaps because it is already hyperadrenergic, even
              at rest.

*4.   What happens to the STIs in the first few days of acute myocardial infarction? Why?
      ANS.:   In the first few days, all the STIs are shortened, presumably by the excess cate-
              cholamine output and drop in blood pressure [17].
              Note: a) This means that a normal PEP at this time is actually too long; i.e.,
                         under the influence of catecholamines, the PEP should be shorter than
                         one standard deviation below the mean.
                      b) The time from the onset of ventricular contraction on an apex cardio-
                         gram to the upstroke of the carotid pulse tracing should be proportional
                         to the PEP. This may be called the C-U time, and it has been found to
                         be prolonged in acute myocardial infarction [16]. The normal range
                         is 45–80 msec. In patients with old infarctions the range is 55–90 msec.
                         In acute infarction, the range is 80–130 msec. (The carotid upstroke
                         time is corrected for time delays by subtracting the A_2–dicrotic notch
                         interval.)

*5.   What STI ratio has an even better correlation with ejection fraction than PEP/ET in patients
      with coronary disease?
      ANS.:   The ejection time divided by the external isovolumic contraction time, i.e., the
              ET/EICT ratio, done immediately after exercise. The exercise should be for
              3 minutes or until angina or dyspnea develops. The external isovolumic contrac-
              tion time is calculated by subtracting the ET from the M_1–A_2 interval.
                   If the ET/EICT ratio immediately after exercise is 5.7 or less, the ejection frac-
              tion is said to be less than 50%. If the ratio is 5.8 or more, the ejection fraction
              is said to be over 50%. In normal men without angina or a history of infarction,
              the ratio after exercise is over 6 [2].

EFFECT OF VALVULAR HEART DISEASE ON THE
SYSTOLIC TIME INTERVALS

1.   How does aortic stenosis (AS) affect the STIs?
      ANS.:   The ET is prolonged. This is because the LV takes longer than normal to drop
              down to aortic valve closing pressure, due to the **gradient** between the LV and
              aorta. The PEP is shortened, i.e., becomes "supernormal." This is partly because
              the LV starts to contract from a high end-diastolic pressure.
              Note: a) In **hypertrophic subaortic stenosis** (HSS) the STIs are the same as in
                         valvular AS.
                      b) When an AS patient is in failure, the STIs may normalize, i.e., the ET
                         and PEP may be at the upper limit of normal. This means that even
                         in failure, the PEP/ET is near the low normal of about 0.30 [5].

*2.   How can HSS be diagnosed by STIs?

ANS.:   Exercise or amyl nitrite will prolong the ET.

Note: a) In valvular AS the ET may also be prolonged by exercise [9].

b) Only in HSS will a "pointed-finger" carotid be produced by exercise or amyl nitrite (midsystolic dip and late, low end-systolic shoulder). (See figure on p.39.)

3.   How does aortic regurgitation (AR) affect the STIs?

ANS.:   The increased end-diastolic volume causes a **Starling effect** that shortens the PEP. The increased volume to be ejected through only one outlet prolongs the ET.

Note: Significant AS or AR tends to make the dicrotic notch on a carotid tracing disappear, so that the ET becomes impossible to measure. You can do an ET even if the dicrotic notch is missing by using a transducer that you discarded because it developed a short time constant, thus turning it into a differential transducer that will show any change in velocity of movement as a sharp notch. The carotid first derivative upstroke onset and final nadir correlate highly with the undifferentiated carotid tracing, even though both points come slightly earlier [21] than these points on a simultaneous ordinary carotid pulse tracing.

4.   How does mitral stenosis affect the STIs?

ANS.:   If the ejection fraction is decreased, the PEP will lengthen and the ET shorten as expected.

5.   How does mitral regurgitation affect the STIs?

ANS.:   The STIs remains normal unless there is more than slight LV disease; then, the expected increase in PEP and short ET occurs. However, acute mitral regurgitation causes a prolonged PEP even with a normal myocardium.

Note: Abnormal LV function in subjects with mitral regurgitation often shows up after prosthetic valve replacement, when the STIs go from normal preoperative to abnormal postoperative intervals. As the heart shrinks over the months following the operation, the STIs tend to return to normal.

*EFFECT OF CONSTRICTION AND TAMPONADE ON THE SYSTOLIC TIME INTERVALS

*1.   How can respiratory changes in STIs help diagnose tamponade?

ANS.:   The normal maximum respiratory variation in ET is about 10 msec with slightly deeper respiration than normal. In tamponade, the ET may vary as much as 40 msec with respiration, even in the absence of any pulsus paradoxus [8].

*2.   How does chronic constrictive pericarditis (with markedly elevated venous pressure) affect the STIs?

ANS.:   The ejection fraction is usually normal by the STI formula (see p. 392). A normal cardiac index at rest is usually found in such patients. Therefore, constriction should be suspected in a patient with severe congestive failure and an ejection fraction of over 45% [1].

*3.   How can STIs differentiate constrictive pericarditis from restrictive cardiomyopathy?

ANS.:   The PEP/ET ratio in constrictive pericarditis is usually about 0.34; in restrictive cardiomyopathy, it is more likely to be about 0.70.

EFFECT OF CONDUCTION DEFECTS AND ARRHYTHMIAS ON THE SYSTOLIC TIME INTERVALS

1.   How does left bundle branch block (LBBB) affect the STIs? Why?

     ANS.:   It prolongs the PEP. The ET is not affected by LBBB. It is controversial whether the prolonged PEP is due to delay in onset of ventricular contraction or to a prolongation of isovolumic contraction. Two studies showed no delayed onset of LV contraction even with intermittent LBBB; i.e., only isovolumic contraction was prolonged [6]. In animals or human subjects with artificially induced LBBB, there *is* a delay in the onset of LBBB contraction, as was also shown in one study of chronic spontaneous LBBB [13, 33]. In a French study [4], it was found that although in some patients with LBBB the PEP was not prolonged, it was prolonged in most of the patients by a long electromechanical interval, but in some by prolonged isovolumic contraction and in others, by both [4].

*2.   How does anterior division block affect the STIs?

     ANS.:   Anterior divisional block (marked left axis deviation) may prolong the PEP slightly. If right bundle branch block is also present, the PEP is significantly prolonged, due both to a delay in the onset of LV contraction and prolongation of isovolumic contraction time [3].

*3.   How does atrial fibrillation affect the STI?

     ANS.:   As the R–R becomes shorter and shorter, the decrease in LV filling pressure prolongs the PEP and shortens the ET. However, at long R–R intervals that would give a rate of less than 75 (cycle length 80 msec or more), the STIs act much as if the patient were in sinus rhythm; you can then judge how the heart would be functioning as if the subject had been in sinus rhythm, although with the "atrial kick" absent. Therefore the STIs will show a slightly depressed myocardial function [29].

     In patients with mitral stenosis and atrial fibrillation, the ET remains linearly related to the heart rate even at rates below 75 (cycle lengths over 80 msec); i.e., as the R–R becomes longer than 80 msec, the STIs will look like those of a normal heart even if there is a low cardiac output [5, 29].

     Note: This is also true for any patient with atrial fibrillation who has either AR or severe failure due to any cause.

*4.   Why will a fast rate caused by atrial pacing not cause a short PEP, as seen in sinus tachycardias?

     ANS.:   Atrial pacing does not produce a sympathetic-outflow positive inotropic effect on the heart. It merely shortens the diastolic filling period and reduces the Starling effect on the ventricles.

     Note: Atropine acts much like atrial pacing in that the tachycardia produced causes slight or no shortening of the PEP.

EFFECT OF DRUGS, HORMONES, AND MANEUVERS ON THE SYSTOLIC TIME INTERVALS

*1.   How does 15 sec of amyl nitrite inhalation affect the STIs in normal and ischemic hearts?

ANS.:   Amyl nitrite in normal subjects produces a prolonged ET index and a short PEP index, due to the strong sympathetic outflow produced by the sudden decrease in blood pressure. In ischemic heart disease, the ET index and PEP index do not change [25].

Using the rate-corrected ETs and PEPs, it can be restated that in normal subjects the ET is unchanged or slightly shortened and the PEP is shortened, while in ischemic heart disease the ET is markedly shortened and the PEP is unchanged or only slightly shortened; i.e., the reaction of an ischemic heart patient to amyl nitrite tends to be like that of a patient in failure.

*2.   How do isoproterenol and epinephrine differ in their effects on the STIs? What is the significance of this?

ANS.:   Although they both shorten the PEP, only isoproterenol shortens the ET, suggesting that shortening of the ET is a more sensitive reflection of the positive inotropic effects of catecholamines.

Note: Phentolamine acts like epinephrine in that it shortens the PEP without shortening the ET. You may be able to tell whether or not an excess of catecholamines is the cause of a short PEP in subjects under emotional tension by giving 10 mg of propranolol intravenously (a large dose). This will prolong a normal person's PEP by only 10–15 msec; but a catecholamine-shortened PEP will be prolonged much more.

3.   How does digitalis affect the STIs of (a) normal hearts and (b) hearts in failure?

ANS.:   a) In normal hearts, both the PEP and ET are shortened.

b) In the failing heart, the PEP is shortened, while the ET can either be shortened, stay the same, or, if a marked increase in stroke volume occurs, may even be lengthened [32].

Note: The effects of heart failure are rarely completely reversed by digitalis, so that an abnormal PEP/ET ratio is usually still evident even with large doses of digitalis.

*4.   What is surprising about the effect of propranolol on the STIs of patients with moderately severe angina and normal intervals at rest?

ANS.:   The ET is slightly prolonged, and the PEP either decreases slightly or does not change with clinically effective doses. It is surprising that the negative inotropic effect of propranolol does not prolong the PEP and shorten the ET [10].

*5.   How are the STIs affected by (a) hypothyroidism and (b) hyperthyroidism?

ANS.:   a) In hypothyroidism, both the PEP and ET are prolonged.

b) In hyperthyroidism, the PEP is shortened and the ET remains normal or is only slightly shortened [22].

Note: Propranolol does not influence the PEP significantly in thyrotoxicosis.

REFERENCES

1. Armstrong, T. G., Lewis, B. S., and Gotsman, M. S. Systolic time intervals in constrictive pericarditis and severe primary myocardial disease. *Am. Heart J.* 85:6, 1973.
2. Aronow, W. S., Bowyer, A., and Kaplan, M. A. External isovolumic contraction times and left ventricular ejection time/external isovolumic contraction time ratios at rest and after exercise in coronary heart disease. *Circulation* 43:59, 1971.
3. Bache, R. J., Wang, Y., and Greenfield, J. C., Jr. Left ventricular ejection times in valvular aortic stenosis. *Circulation* 47:527, 1973.
4. Baragan, J., Fernandez-Caamano, F., Sozutek, Y., Coblence, B., and Lenègre, J. Chronic left complete bundle-branch block. *Br. Heart J.* 30:196, 1968.
5. Bonner, A. J., Jr., and Tavel, M. E. Systolic time intervals. *Arch. Intern. Med.* 132:816, 1973.
6. Braunwald, E., and Morrow, A. G. Sequence of ventricular contraction in human bundle branch block. *Am. J. Med.* 23:205, 1957.
7. Buyukozturk, K., Kimbiris, D., and Segal, B. L. Systolic time intervals. *Am. J. Cardiol.* 28:183, 1971.
8. Carter, W. H., McIntosh, H. D., and Orgain, E. S. Respiratory variation of left ventricular ejection time in patients with pericardial effusion. *Am. J. Cardiol.* 29:427, 1972.
9. Cohn, K. E., Flamm, M. D., and Hancock, E. W. Amyl nitrite inhalation as a screening test for hypertrophic subaortic stenosis. *Am. J. Cardiol.* 21:681, 1968.
10. Frankl, W. S., Smith, W. K., and Orr, P. The effect of propranolol on left ventricular function in angina pectoris as measured by systolic time intervals. *Res. Commun. Chem. Pathol. Pharmacol.* 4:77, 1972.
11. Garrard, C. L., Jr., Weissler, A. M., and Dodge, H. T. The relationship of alterations in systolic time intervals to ejection fraction in patients with cardiac disease. *Circulation* 42:455, 1970.
12. Golde, D., and Burstin, L. Systolic phases of the cardiac cycle in children. *Circulation* 42:1029, 1970.
13. Haft, J. I., Herman, M. V., and Gorlin, R. Left bundle branch block. *Circulation* 42:279, 1971.
14. Harley, A., Starmer, C. F., and Greenfield, J. C., Jr. Pressure-flow studies in man. *J. Clin. Invest.* 48:895, 1969.
15. Inoue, K., Smulyan, H., Young, G. M., Grierson, A. L., and Eich, R. H. Left ventricular function in essential hypertension. *Am. J. Cardiol.* 32:264, 1973.
16. Inoue, K., Young, G. M., Grierson, A. L., Smulyan, H., and Eich, R. H. Isometric contraction period of the left ventricle in acute myocardial infarction. *Circulation* 42:79, 1970.
17. Jain, S. R., and Lindahl, J. Apex cardiogram and systolic time intervals in acute myocardial infarction. *Br. Heart J.* 33:578, 1971.
18. Maher, J. T., Beller, G. A., Ransil, B. J., and Hartley, L. H. Systolic time intervals during submaximal and maximal exercise in man. *Am. Heart J.* 87:334, 1974.
19. Martin, C. E., Shaver, J. A., Thompson, M. E., Reddy, P. S., and Leonard, J. J. Direct correlation of external systolic time intervals with internal indices of left ventricular function in man. *Circulation* 44:419, 1971.
20. McConahay, D. R., Martin, C. M., and Cheitlin, M. D. Resting and exercise systolic time intervals. *Circulation* 45:592, 1972.

21. Nandi, P. S., and Spodick, D. H. Determination of systolic intervals utilizing the carotid first derivative. *Am. Heart J.* 80:495, 1973.

22. Parisi, A. F., Hamilton, B. P., Thomas, C. N., and Mazzaferri, E. L. The short cardiac pre-ejection period. *Circulation* 49:900, 1974.

23. Pouget, J. M., Harris, W. S., Mayron, B. R., and Naughton, J. P. Abnormal responses of the systolic time intervals to exercise in patients with angina pectoris. *Circulation* 43:289, 1971.

24. Rubler, S., Schneebaum, R., and Hammer, N. Systolic time intervals in pregnancy and the postpartum period. *Am. Heart J.* 86:182, 1973.

25. Sawayama, T., Ochiai, M., Marumoto, S., Matsuura, T., and Niki, I. Influence of amyl nitrite inhalation on the systolic time intervals in normal subjects and in patients with ischemic heart disease. *Circulation* 40:327, 1969.

26. Spann, J. F., Buccino, R. A., Sonnenblick, E. H., and Braunwald, E. Contractile state of cardiac muscle. *Circ. Res.* 21:341, 1967.

27. Spitaels, S., Arbogast, R., Fouron, J. C., and Davignon, A. The influence of heart rate and age on the systolic and diastolic time intervals in children. *Circulation* 49:1107, 1974.

28. Tarazi, R. C., Frohlich, E. D., and Dustan, H. P. Left atrial abnormality and ventricular preejection period in hypertension. *Dis. Chest* 55:214, 1969.

29. Tavel, M. E., Baugh, D. O., Feigenbaum, H., and Nasser, W. K. Left ventricular ejection time in atrial fibrillation. *Circulation* 46:744, 1972.

30. Weissler, A. M., and Garrard, C. L., Jr. Systolic time intervals in cardiac disease (1). *Mod. Concepts Cardiol. Dis.* 40:1, 1971.

31. Weissler, A. M., Harris, W. S., and Schoenfeld, C. D. Systolic time intervals in heart failure in man. *Circulation* 37:149, 1968.

32. Weissler, A. M., and Schoenfeld, C. D. Effect of digitalis on systolic time intervals in heart failure. *Am. J. Med. Sci.* 259:4, 1970.

33. Wennemark, J. R., Blake, D. F., and Keyde, P. Cardiodynamic effects of experimental bundle branch block in the dog. *Circ. Res.* 10:280, 1962.

34. Whitsett, T. L., and Naughton, J. The effect of exercise on systolic time intervals in sedentary and active individuals and rehabilitated patients with heart disease. *Am. J. Cardiol.* 27:352, 1971.

35. Willems, J. L., Roelandt, J., DeGeest, H., Kesteloot, H., and Joossens, J. V. The left ventricular ejection time in elderly subjects. *Circulation* 42:37, 1970.

36. Winter, W. G., Leaman, D. M., and Anderson, R. A. The effect of exercise on intrinsic myocardial performance. *Circulation* 48:50, 1973.

19

Summary of Clinical Findings in the
Most Important Cardiac Abnormalities

THE COMMON CONGENITAL HEART LESIONS

Uncomplicated and Moderately Severe Atrial Septal Defect

Inspection and Palpation

1. Hyperkinetic, nonsustained right ventricular rock and absent left ventricular apex impulse.
2. Jugulars with a Y descent larger than expected (i.e., an exaggerated V wave with the Y descent almost as large as the X').
   Note: If with a large V wave and other signs of an ASD cyanosis is present, then, in the absence of signs of severe pulmonary hypertension, a common atrium or total anomalous pulmonary venous drainage is probably present.

Auscultation

1. S_2 with a relatively fixed wide split and accentuated P_2, even heard at the apex.
2. Tricuspid inflow murmur and occasionally a presystolic murmur.
3. Pulmonary ejection murmur with scratchy, crunchy character.
4. Tricuspid opening snap common.
5. Peripheral pulmonary artery flow murmur occasionally heard in posterior or lateral chest.

Eisenmenger Atrial Septal Defect

Inspection and Palpation

1. Clubbing and cyanosis (beginning in adulthood).
2. Sustained, marked parasternal right ventricular rock.
3. Jugular vessels probably have a regurgitant V wave.

Auscultation

1. S_2 is still moderately widely split and fixed, with very loud P_2 that is also heard at the apex.
2. Tricuspid regurgitation murmur.
3. Pulmonary ejection click and murmur.
4. Graham Steell murmur.

Ventricular Septal Defect

Inspection and Palpation

1. Easily palpable, enlarged area apex beat which is not sustained.
2. Moderate left lower sternal border right ventricular movement, with a systolic thrill.

Auscultation

1. S_2 is split slightly widely and may be relatively fixed. P_2 is slightly accentuated but not heard at the apex.
2.   Harsh pansystolic lower sternal border murmur grade 4/6 to 6/6.
3.   Apical S_3 and possible flow murmur following it.

Eisenmenger Ventricular Septal Defect

Inspection and Palpation

1.   Clubbing and cyanosis (since childhood).
2.   Left parasternal movement sustained. Left ventricular apex beat is still palpable. It may be displaced.

Auscultation

1. S_2 is single and loud.
2.   Pulmonary ejection click and murmur.
3.   Graham Steell murmur.

Patent Ductus Arteriosus

Inspection and Palpation

1.   Apex beat is displaced, slightly enlarged, and hyperkinetic, i.e., not sustained.

Auscultation

1. S_2 is single or paradoxically split.
2.   Continuous murmur, loudest at the second left interspace and next loudest in the first left interspace. The systolic component is crescendo to the S_2. The diastolic component may end in mid-diastole.
3. S_3 at the apex with perhaps a diastolic flow murmur following it.

Eisenmenger Patent Ductus Arteriosus

Inspection and Palpation

1.   Differential cyanosis (toes, and perhaps the fingers of the left hand, more cyanotic and clubbed than the fingers of the right hand).
2.   Sustained left parasternal movement grade 2/4–4/4.
3.   Large or even giant jugular A wave.

Auscultation

1. S_2 is normally split in both movement and width.
2.   Graham Steell murmur.
3.   Pulmonary ejection click and systolic ejection murmur.

Valvular Pulmonary Stenosis

Inspection and Palpation

1. Sustained but slight left parasternal movement with no left ventricular apex beat.
2. Thrill at the mid- or high left parasternal area.
3. Jugulars have exaggerated A waves.

Auscultation

1. S_2 is widely split, with a soft P_2.
2. Pulmonary ejection click (increasing on expiration) may or may not be present.
3. Pulmonary ejection murmur grade 3/6–5/6 at high left parasternal area, increasing on inspiration at the left lower sternal border.
4. S_4 at left lower sternal border or epigastrium during inspiration or after exercise.

Tetralogy of Fallot

Inspection and Palpation

1. Palpable S_2 at the second or third left interspace.
2. Cyanosis and clubbing (since infancy).
3. Left parasternal movement slight but sustained and without a left ventricular apex beat.

Auscultation

1. Ejection murmur grade 2/6–4/6, loudest at the third or fourth left interspace, increasing with inspiration.
2. The S_2 is single.

Coarctation of the Aorta[1]

Inspection and Palpation

1. Carotid vessels have large volume.
2. Either no femoral pulse or, if present, its peak is delayed over the radial pulse peak.
3. Blood pressure is much lower in the lower extremities than in the brachial vessels.
4. Apex beat is hyperkinetic and slightly enlarged.
5. Posterior intercostal artery movement is visible and palpable.

Auscultation

1. S_2 is single or narrowly split, with a loud A_2.
2. Aortic ejection sound, followed by a grade 2/6–3/6 ejection murmur.
3. Continuous murmur over the posterior intercostal spaces.

---

[1]Usually with bicuspid aortic valve.

Hypertrophic Subaortic Stenosis

Inspection and Palpation

1.   Arterial pulses with brisk rate of rise, occasionally slightly bisferiens.
2.   Apex beat sustained, with double or triple outward movement of atrial hump plus mid-systolic dip.

Auscultation

1. S_2 is single or with narrowly reversed split.
2.   Harsh ejection murmur, loudest either at the left lower sternal border or apex, increases with the Valsalva maneuver and standing, and decreases with handgrip and squatting.

TAMPONADE (AND HOW CONSTRICTIVE PERICARDITIS DIFFERS)

Inspection and Palpation

1.   Jugular pulsations elevated. Larger X prime than Y descent, even with atrial fibrillation. (Constrictive pericarditis has larger Y descent than X prime.)
2.   Impalpable apex impulse or an unexpected systolic retraction.
3.   Inspiratory fall of blood pressure over 6 mm Hg on quiet respiration. (Constrictive pericarditis may have no abnormal fall of blood pressure on inspiration.)

Auscultation

1.   Wide split of S_2 on inspiration.
2.   Absent S_4.
3. S_3 may not be present. (Constrictive pericarditis has loud, early S_3.)

RHEUMATIC HEART DISEASE

Valvular Aortic Stenosis

Inspection and Palpation

1.   Slowly rising pulses, often with carotid thrill.
2.   Apex beat sustained and enlarged in area, with possible palpable atrial hump.

Auscultation

1. S_2 is either single or with a narrowly reversed split. It may be soft or absent.
2.   Aortic ejection click.
3.   Harsh ejection murmur is loudest anywhere in a sash area from the second right interspace to apex.
4. S_4.

Aortic Regurgitation

Inspection and Palpation

1. Pulses rise rapidly, slapping and with large volume.
2. Positive Hill's sign.
3. Apex beat is displaced, enlarged, and sustained, with marked medial retraction of all the left parasternal area.

Auscultation

1. S_2 is single and slightly sharp or slapping and loud.
2. Pandiastolic medium- and high-frequency murmur, loudest over the sternum and left lower sternal border.
3. Austin Flint murmur at the apex.
4. Aortic ejection sound and murmur.

Uncomplicated Mitral Stenosis with Only Mild to Moderate Pulmonary Hypertension

Inspection and Palpation

1. Grade 2/4–3/4 left parasternal sustained movement.
2. May be a diastolic thrill at the apex in the left lateral decubitus position.
3. S_2 may be palpable.
4. M_1 may be palpable at the apex.

Auscultation

1. Slightly exaggerated P_2, with a normal split.
2. Opening snap is loudest between the apex and left lower sternal border.
3. Closing snap (M_1) at the apex.
4. Apical diastolic murmur with presystolic crescendo.

Mitral Regurgitation

Inspection and Palpation

1. Brisk pulse.
2. Sustained left parasternal movement grade 2/4–3/4.
3. Sustained, enlarged-area, displaced apical movement, with possible systolic thrill and good medial retraction.

Auscultation

1. S_2 is widely split, with normal movement on respiration.
2. Pansystolic murmur loudest at the apex.
3. S_3 at the apex, often followed by an inflow murmur.

IDIOPATHIC OR CORONARY CARDIOMYOPATHY WITH DECREASED OUTPUT EVEN AT REST

Inspection and Palpation

1. Apex beat is displaced, large, and sustained, with a palpable atrial hump and medial retraction.
2. Jugulars may be elevated to above 4.5 cm at 45 degrees; if not, they will rise with abdominal compression.

Auscultation

1. S_3 and S_4.
2. Mitral regurgitation due to papillary muscle dysfunction, i.e., usually either pansystolic or crescendo to the S_2.

THE PHYSICAL SIGNS OF PULMONARY HYPERTENSION[2]

Inspection and Palpation

1. Giant A wave in the jugular pulse if the patient is in normal sinus rhythm; a large tricuspid regurgitant systolic wave with a pulsating liver in the presence of atrial fibrillation.
2. Large, sustained left parasternal right ventricular movement, often with a right ventricular rock.
3. Palpable pulmonary artery movement in the second left interspace.
4. Palpable S_2.

Auscultation

1. Loud P_2 heard also at the apex and second right interspace. (The split S_2 may have a normal width and movement or be widely split and relatively fixed.)
2. Pulmonary ejection sound.
3. S_4 gallop that increases on inspiration in the right ventricular area.
4. Tricuspid regurgitation murmur.
5. Pulmonary ejection murmur, grade 1/6 to 2/6 and slightly crunchy in quality.
6. Graham Steell murmur.

[2]See Index under Hypertension, Pulmonary for details of physical findings in pulmonary hypertension secondary to specific lesions.

aneurysm Localized dilatation of either a blood vessel or a heart chamber. The commonest cause of an arterial aneurysm is atherosclerosis. In the aorta, an atherosclerotic aneurysm may be found in any part of the vessel where atrophy of the media (muscular layer) deep to an atherosclerotic plaque results in either a saccular or sharply demarcated fusiform (spindle-shaped) dilatation. The commonest site is in the abdomen distal to the renal arteries. Syphilis (lues) used to be the commonest cause of thoracic aortic aneurysms, usually in the ascending aorta. Aortic aneurysms cause death by rupture. When infection destroys a local area of any artery, a mycotic aneurysm may form.

    dissecting aneurysm Localized aortic dilatation that results from stripping of the layers of the aortic wall by hemorrhage into the media secondary to degeneration of the media (cystic medial necrosis). In some patients, it may begin with an intimal tear. It usually dissects distally, but when it dissects proximally, it may involve the aortic valve and produce aortic regurgitation, or it may involve the pericardial space and produce a fatal tamponade.

    ventricular aneurysm A dilated segment of LV. It is commonly caused by myocardial infarction, but trauma has also caused it. These aneurysms vary in size from a few centimeters in diameter to a size one-half that of the left ventricle. They rarely ever rupture, but are likely to be the cause of mild to severe heart failure or to become the source of an embolus, due to thrombus formation that may completely fill the aneurysm. If the aneurysm pouch is empty, it will usually bulge during systole (paradoxical motion or dyskinesis). Sometimes, a large area of damaged myocardium fails to show any motion during systole, and this also is sometimes called an aneurysm. However, it is better to call it an area of akinesis, and, if the movement is slight but normal in direction, it may be called an area of hypokinesis.

anomalous pulmonary venous connection or drainage Drainage of one or more pulmonary veins, usually into the right atrium, superior vena cava, or inferior vena cava. In partial anomalous pulmonary venous return, one (or more) of the pulmonary veins from the right lung empties into any one of the following: azygos vein, superior or inferior vena cava, or right atrium. More rarely, a vein (or veins) from the left lung empties into the innominate vein, a left vertical vein, or the coronary sinus. The anomalous connection results in a left-to-right shunt with the same chambers overloaded as in an **atrial septal defect.** In *total anomalous pulmonary venous return,* all of the pulmonary veins may enter any one of the following: a left vertical vein, the innominate vein, the coronary sinus, the right atrium, the superior or inferior vena cava, or the portal vein. An atrial septal defect is essential for survival. The hemodynamics are similar to that of a large atrial septal defect.

aortic sclerosis   See **calcific aortic sclerosis.**

aortic stenosis   Obstruction to LV outflow. This can occur at valvular, supravalvular, or subvalvular levels. The subvalvular obstruction may be due to a congenital fibrous ring just below the aortic valve (discrete subvalvular AS), or it may be due to a hypertrophied septum impinging on the anterior leaflet of the mitral valve during systole (hypertrophic subaortic stenosis). See figure on p. 277. The supravalvular type is associated with a characteristic facies. See p. 30.

Pure aortic valvular stenosis is almost always congenital, and about half of the congenital ones are due to calcification of a bicuspid aortic valve. The acquired ones are usually due to rheumatic valvulitis and are associated with some mitral valve disease. Over age 70, degenerative calcification of the aortic valve may be the commonest cause of aortic stenosis, especially in women.

arteriosclerosis   1. Atherosclerosis (the progressive laying down of lipid in the intima of an artery, starting with a fatty streak and ending with fibrosis and calcium and finally in a plaque). 2. Medial sclerosis (fibrosis of the media or muscular layer of arteries, which may end in "pipestem" arteries). Medial sclerosis affects only the large arteries; i.e., coronary arteries are subject to atherosclerosis and not to medial sclerosis. Arterioles are not affected either by medial sclerosis or by atherosclerosis.

atrial myxoma   Tumor made up of soft, loose, friable tissue that is usually on a pedicle (pedunculated) attached to the atrial septum in the region of the fossa ovalis. It is almost twice as common in the left as in the right atrium. It can protrude through its respective atrioventricular valve in diastole to produce a partial obstruction that imitates mitral or tricuspid stenosis and occasionally causes syncope. It may merely prevent closure of the valve and various degrees of mitral or tricuspid regurgitation. If the tumor becomes calcified, it may act as a wrecking ball, and completely destroy the atrioventricular valve, to produce severe systolic regurgitation. Emboli from the friable tumor are among the commonest causes of clinical manifestations. For unknown reasons, the tumor acts as an inflammatory agent and commonly produces a high sedimentation rate and intermittent fevers, which, together with the occasional **clubbing,** mimics infective endocarditis. It may even produce reactions of an allergic type, resulting in puzzling skin and joint manifestations.

atrial septal defect   Opening between the atria, which may occur at three possible levels. The lower one is called a *primum* defect, the middle one is a *secundum* defect, and the upper one is called a *sinus venosus* defect. By far the commonest is the secundum, or fossa ovalis defect.

primum defect   An atrial septal defect that is part of a possible spectrum of abnormalities caused by maldevelopment of the endocardial cushions, which are the dorsal and ventral tissues in the center of the fetal

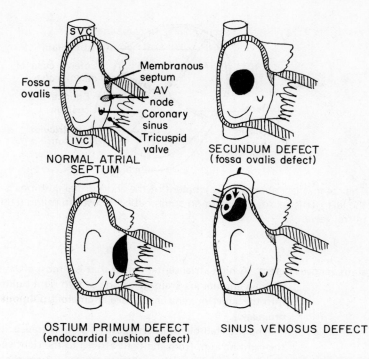

NORMAL ATRIAL SEPTUM

SECUNDUM DEFECT (fossa ovalis defect)

OSTIUM PRIMUM DEFECT (endocardial cushion defect)

SINUS VENOSUS DEFECT

The three levels of atrial septal defects are, in general, low, middle, and high. It may help your memory if you think of the lower two levels as the "first floor," or primum defect, and the "second floor," or secundum defect. The sinus venosus defect then remains and thus must be the "top floor," or high defect. The sinus venosus is the embryological site of the pacemaker of the heart, or the sinoatrial node. If you keep in mind that the sinoatrial node is at the junction of the superior vena cava and right atrium, it will be easy for you to remember that the sinus venosus defect is the high one.

When the inferior wall of the fossa ovalis acts like a flap valve, it is called a patent foramen ovale. There will then be flow from the right to the left atrium only if the pressures rises abnormally high in the right atrium. The flap is normally closed by the higher pressure in the left atrium relative to that in the right atrium. Note that in the sinus venosus defect, pulmonary veins are shown draining into the superior vena cava.

heart that give rise to
a) The inferior part of the atrial septum above.
b) The upper part of the ventricular septum below.
c) The medial cusp of the mitral valve to the left.
d) The medial cusp of the tricuspid valve to the right.
Any permutation or combination of endocardial cushion defects may occur. When defects in all four of the above structures are present, the condition is called a *complete atrioventricular canal.*

A left axis deviation on ECG is so common with endocardial cushion defects and so rare with atrial septal defects at higher levels that clinical differentiation of the primum from the secundum and sinus venosus defects by the electrocardiogram is quite helpful.

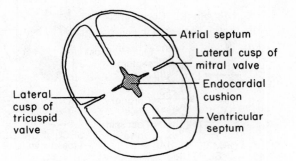

The commonest aborted development of the endocardial cushions is upward and to the left. This causes the common combination of ostium primum defect and cleft mitral valve.

sinus venosus defect A high atrial septal defect that is almost always associated with an anomalous drainage of one or two right pulmonary veins into the superior vena cava. (See **anomalous pulmonary venous drainage.**)

    The shunted blood in atrial septal defects travels from the left to the right atrium, from the right atrium to the right ventricle, from the right ventricle to the pulmonary artery, from the pulmonary artery to the pulmonary arterioles and veins, and from the pulmonary veins to the left atrium. Therefore, the right atrium, right ventricles, and pulmonary vessels all have a volume overload. The left atrium, however, serves only as a conduit and does not become enlarged except under exceptional circumstances.

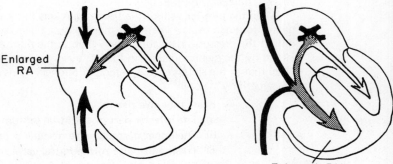

Note that with an atrial septal defect, the right atrium and ventricle receive blood from two sources. They are volume-overloaded at the expense of blood to the left ventricle. An increase in total blood volume is the compensatory mechanism by which the left ventricle receives a normal volume for average physiological needs. When an atrial septal defect or any other left-to-right shunt is closed surgically, the total blood volume of the body decreases.

atrioventricular block (AV block)   Conduction delay anywhere from the AV node to the ending of the bundle branches in the ventricle; i.e., the delay may occur in the AV node, bundle of His, or bundle branches. A first-degree AV block is recognized on an ECG by seeing a long P-R interval. Second-degree AV block refers to intermittent complete AV block so that a dropped QRS occurs periodically. If the AV block is complete, the atria and ventricles are dissociated and an independent pacemaker for the ventricles occurs either at or below the bundle of His. To use the term "heart block" to refer specifically to AV block should be avoided since all conduction defects are heart blocks. Also, "heart block" is a terrifying term to a patient.

atrioventricular dissociation   A condition in which the atria and ventricles have independent pacemakers. The lower pacemaker may be in the junctional area or deep in the ventricle. AV dissociation implies that atrial contraction has varying relationships to ventricular contraction; i.e., if the atria are in sinus rhythm, the P-R interval will be continually changing in a haphazard manner.

base of the heart   The upper part of the heart, or **semilunar valve** area. The term implies that the heart looks like a cone placed upside down in the chest. The base of the cone is in the upper chest area.

beriberi heart disease   The effect on the heart of total body capillary dilatation caused by a deficiency of vitamin B_1 (thiamine). In order to fill the enlarged vascular bed, a marked hyperkinetic state is produced, with a high venous pressure, tachycardia, cardiomegaly, peripheral edema, and rapid **circulation time.** In the Occident, it is seen almost entirely in alcoholic persons who resort to an enormous intake of beer. An acute fulminant, nonedematous form characterized by cardiovascular collapse and death within hours or days has been called Shoshin beriberi. (*Sho* is Japanese for "acute damage" and *shin* means "heart.")

Bernheim effect   Encroachment on the right ventricular cavity by the interventricular septum, which is bowed to the right by a dilated left ventricle, as described by the pathologist Bernheim in 1915 [1]. The enlargement of the left ventricle in diastole prevents diastolic filling of the right ventricle, but does not interfere with right ventricular outflow; i.e., it is not a kind of infundibular outflow obstruction, but an obstruction to inflow. Such a large left ventricle is usually due to severe, chronic mitral regurgitation.

Bernoulli effect   The drop in pressure on the surface of any structure that is caused by a flow over that structure. This tends to pull the structure toward the stream. An instrument utilizing the Bernoulli effect to measure flow is called a Venturi meter. The Bernoulli effect on the wings of an airplane raises it and keeps it off the ground.

calcific aortic sclerosis or aortic sclerosis   The infiltration of the aortic valve with fibrous tissue and often also with enough calcium to stiffen it and create turbulent flow but not enough to produce a significant pressure gradient across the valve. It is due to an unknown aging process. The term may also refer to atherosclerotic plaques in the aortic root, possibly responsible for some ejection murmurs in the elderly. Without calcium it is simply aortic sclerosis.

carcinoid heart disease Accumulation of grossly whitish-yellow fibrous tissue on the inner surface of the ventricles or atrium, as well as on the undersurface of the tricuspid and pulmonary valves (rarely, of the mitral valve). It can hold the tricuspid or pulmonary valve in the semiclosed position and so cause tricuspid or pulmonary stenosis and regurgitation. Carcinoid heart disease is usually associated with a carcinoid

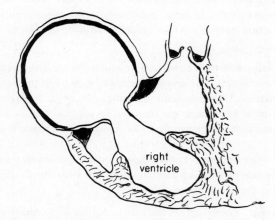

right
ventricle

Carcinoid deposits tend to form on the undersurface of the tricuspid valves and the upper surface of the pulmonary valves and so hold them in a rigid, semiclosed position. The **compliance** of the right atrium can be reduced by a lining of carcinoid material, thus raising its pressure conspicuously.

tumor of the bowel and with metastases to the liver. Bronchospasm, diarrhea, and various types of flushing (general redness, bright red patches or violaceous cyanosis) are all part of the carcinoid syndrome.

cardiomyopathy Myocardial damage from any cause. Therefore, it should have an adjective preceding it, e.g., idiopathic cardiomyopathy (often called primary myocardial disease), amyloid cardiomyopathy, and coronary or ischemic cardiomyopathy [3, 4, 10]. In the past, the term meant specifically only an idiopathic cardiomyopathy or primary myocardial disease. Some prefer "myocardiopathy" instead of "cardiomyopathy" to distinguish idiopathic types from other causes of reduced ejection fraction. How you arrange *myo-* and *cardio-* neither changes the meaning nor helps to clarify the situation.

Cheyne-Stokes respiration The periodic breathing characterized by a gradually increasing depth of respiration, culminating in a period of apnea that may last from a few seconds to as long as a minute. The commonest associated condition for the cardiologist is severe low output heart failure. The neurologist more commonly sees it as a result of cerebral disease. Since it is exaggerated when dozing, and the hyperpneic phase can cause enough cerebral stimulation to prevent sleep, it is a possible cause of insomnia in a patient with heart failure.

circulation time The time it takes for a marker material to travel from the site of injection to the site of appearance, usually after it passes through the lungs or lesser circulation.

When the time of appearance is dependent on a subjective sensation such as taste, the test becomes unreliable. It has fallen into disuse in most centers because the usual injected materials, such as 5 ml of 20% Decholin (dehydrocholic acid) or 20% calcium gluconate, have caused occasional serious reactions, and because comparison with objective methods (fluorescein) has shown many false prolongations of circulation time [12]. The poor correlation coefficient (about 0.63) with cardiac output is sometimes due to dilution of the test material in dilated cardiac chambers, which can falsely prolong the circulation time [14]. The normal range is 10—18 sec.

clubbing A condition in which soft tissue of the terminal phalanges of the fingers or toes becomes hypertrophied and the nail finally curves excessively, to give a drumstick appearance. (See p. 27 for method of eliciting.) In cardiac patients, clubbing is usually associated with **cyanosis,** but if not, it should suggest the presence of acute **infective endocarditis** that has been present for a few weeks, suppurative lung lesions, anoxic **cor pulmonale,** or metastatic lung cancer. More rarely, it is caused by chronic diarrhea with ulcerative colitis or may even be familial. In cardiac patients, the commonest causes of clubbing are tetralogy of Fallot and transposition of the great vessels. When clubbing and cyanosis are greater in the toes than in the hands, the condition is called differential cyanosis (see p. 27) and clubbing. (See figure on p. 27.)

Note: Since the flow rate through clubbed digits is higher than normal, and their venous blood from the arm appears brighter than the blood of a normal person, one of the possible causes of clubbing is patent arteriovenous anastomoses that bypass the capillaries, resulting in oxygen deficit and tissue hypertrophy [15].

coarctation Localized or diffuse narrowing of the aorta. The degree of constriction varies from slight to severe; rarely, it is complete. It is usually seen around the isthmus which is the area just beyond both the left subclavian artery and the ductus arteriosus.

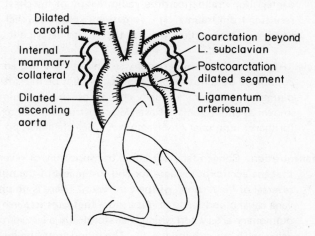

Localized narrowing of the aorta most often occurs at the junction of the aortic arch and the descending aorta distal to the ductus arteriosus. When on rare occasions it occurs proximal to the ductus, the narrowing is often diffuse and for some unknown reason associated with severe pulmonary hypertension and therefore with differential cyanosis.

It can occur proximal to the left subclavian artery and occasionally even in the abdominal aorta. Collateral circulation to the vessels beyond the coarcted site is from arteries proximal to the coarctation, so that with the usual site of coarctation, collateral vessels develop via the internal mammary and shoulder girdle arteries to the intercostal arteries and can become very large and even palpable. In all the vessels proximal to the coarctation, there is hypertension and increased pulse pressure, as well as dilatation. There is a low systolic pressure and pulse pressure beyond the coarctation.

The aortic valve is commonly bicuspid and regurgitant, but is occasionally stenotic.

Preductal coarctation is commonly associated with diffuse narrowing of the aortic arch, pulmonary hypertension, and an **Eisenmenger syndrome,** as well as with differential cyanosis (see p. 329). This is sometimes known as the infantile type.

compliance   Elastic resistance or stiffness of a structure, e.g., the stiffer the left ventricle, the less the compliance. To physicists it is change of volume/change of pressure. Generally, a thick ventricle is a noncompliant or stiff ventricle. Chronically volume-overloaded ventricles due to shunt or regurgitant flows are generally compliant. Pressure overloaded ventricles are noncompliant.

constrictive pericarditis   Thickening of the pericardium by a dense, fibrous tissue that may calcify. It results primarily in restriction of expansion of the heart, but also often causes a slight restriction of systole as well, especially if the duration of the con- striction is long enough to allow much infiltration of the epicardium by the fibrous tissue. Although both ventricles and atria are almost always simultaneously involved, inflow into the atria is not affected. The commonest cause is idiopathic, but the commonest *known* cause is tuberculosis. It has occasionally followed bacterial or viral pericarditis, radiotherapy of the chest, and the hemopericardium resulting from trauma. It is sometimes known as "Pick's disease" for no very good reason, since Pick was not the first to describe it.

cor pulmonale   Right ventricular hypertrophy secondary to a lung abnormality. The term *cor pulmonale* does not require that the patient be in right ventricular failure. The pulmonary problem is usually chronic obstructive pulmonary disease (formerly known as emphysema) or arteriolar obstruction due to emboli or idiopathic (primary) pulmonary hypertension. (See checklist, pp. 7 and 11, for clinical picture.)

corrected transposition   Congenitally corrected transposition, or reversal of the great vessels so that the aortic root is anterior and to the left of the pulmonary artery, but with reversal or "inversion" of the ventricles. There is no physiological disturbance since vena caval blood feeds a right atrium that goes to a ventricle that gives off the pulmonary artery and which is anatomically a left ventricle, i.e., it has a mitral valve and a smooth inner wall. The blood from the lungs flows into a left atrium, which passes through a tricuspid valve to a systemic ventricle that is anatomically a right ventricle (trabeculated and with an **infundibulum,** or outflow tract).

Corrigan's pulse   Large-volume carotid pulsations seen in patients with severe aortic regurgitation. It refers to what is seen and not to what is felt [5].

cor triatriatum Congenital cardiac anomaly in which all the pulmonary veins join together to form a common chamber and empty into the left atrium via a small opening; i.e., it is a kind of supravalvular mitral stenosis. The common chamber is usually situated inside the left atrium. Its major complication is secondary pulmonary hypertension, and the occasional patient who lives to adulthood will present as a possible case of **primary pulmonary hypertension.**

cyanosis Bluish or purplish color imparted to the skin and mucous membranes, usually as a result of at least 5 gm of reduced hemoglobin per 100 ml of blood in the surface capillaries, but occasionally due to the presence in the blood of an abnormal pigment derived from hemoglobin such as sulfmethemoglobin or methemoglobin. Cyanosis is usually visible in patients whose arterial oxygen has dropped to between 80 and 85%. There is normally already about 2.25 gm of reduced hemoglobin per 100 ml of blood in capillaries. The higher the absolute level of circulatory hemoglobin, the more easily will cyanosis be apparent. For example, an 80% saturation in a child who has 10 gm of hemoglobin per 100 ml of blood would produce 2 gm of reduced hemoglobin; whereas the same percentage of saturation in a person with 15 gm of hemoglobin would produce 3 gm of reduced hemoglobin and thus more definite cyanosis.

> **central cyanosis** A condition in which the arterial blood is unsaturated with oxygen as a result of either a cardiac or a pulmonary lesion or a combination of both. When it is severe and chronic, polycythemia and digital clubbing accompany it. It can be seen in the warm areas, such as the tongue and inner surface of the lips.

> **differential cyanosis** See pp. 27, 329–330.

> **peripheral cyanosis** Cyanosis associated with normally saturated arterial blood, seen in cold areas such as the nose, ears, cheeks, and fingers. It is due to excessive extraction of oxygen in these tissues, usually resulting from low flow secondary to heart failure.

Down's syndrome (mongolism or trisomy 21) Syndrome in which the outstanding findings are mental retardation, hypotonia, medial epicanthus, large (often protruding) fissured tongue, small orbits, gray-white specks in the iris (Brushfield's spots), and a hand with short fingers, a distally displaced axial triradius, and a horizontal side-to-side palmar crease (simian crease). The major cardiac abnormalities are some form of endocardial cushion defect (see **atrial septal defect**).

ductus arteriosus See **patent ductus arteriosus.**

Ebstein's anomaly Congenital downward displacement of the tricuspid valve into the right ventricle [7]. The tricuspid valve is deformed to various degrees, so that there is commonly tricuspid regurgitation. Even though you would expect the right ventricle to be small since part of it is in the right atrium, tricuspid regurgitation can enlarge the remainder of the right ventricle, which consists largely of **outflow tract.** The right atrium may be so large that it dominates the ECG and x-ray picture. A right-to-left shunt through an **atrial septal defect** or patent foramen ovale with resultant cyanosis is very likely. Arrhythmias or heart failure are the most common complications.

Eisenmenger syndrome or reaction   Severe pulmonary hypertension due to fixed pulmonary arteriolar resistance, causing right-to-left shunting through an ASD, VSD, or PDA. When a VSD is the cause of the pulmonary hypertension, it is often called an Eisenmenger *complex,* because this is the original lesion described by Eisenmenger in 1897 [8]. The right-to-left shunt may be dominant or it may be a balanced shunt, i.e., as much left-to-right as right-to-left.

Eisenmenger syndromes begin in infancy when a PDA or VSD is responsible; it begins in the teens or later when the shunt is at ASD level. The pulmonary hypertension of the Eisenmenger syndrome is irreversible and prohibits surgical closure of the defect. The patient with the irreversible pathological changes in the lung vessels due to an Eisenmenger reaction is often said to have pulmonary vascular disease.

ejection fraction   Relationship between stroke volume (volume ejected) and end-diastolic volume (volume at the moment of greatest filling of the ventricle at the end of diastole). A low normal ejection fraction is about 55%; i.e., at least 55% of what is in the ventricle when it is full should be ejected into the aorta. Usually, about 60—80% is ejected.

endocardial cushion defect   See **atrial septal defect.**

endocarditis   See **infective endocarditis.**

Fallot's tetralogy   See **tetralogy of Fallot.**

filling pressure   Pressure in the ventricle that distends it, especially toward the end of diastole, so that it is most relevant to the end-diastolic pressure in the ventricle and is called the preload. It is controlled on the right side by venous pressure and, in sinus rhythm, also by the power of the right atrial contraction. On the left side it is controlled by the left atrial pressure and, in sinus rhythm, also by the power of left atrial contraction or the "atrial kick."

frequency   Number of oscillations per second made by a vibrating or sound-producing structure. Pitch is the highness or lowness of sound heard by the ear. High-pitched sounds are produced by high frequencies, and vice versa. The words frequency and pitch are often used interchangeably.

gradient   Difference in pressure along a conduit that results in flow from highest to lowest pressure. In cardiology, it usually refers to a difference in pressure across an obstruction; i.e., it is generally caused by a drop in pressure across an obstruction (usually a stenotic artery or valve), so that the pressure is higher proximal than distal to the obstruction. (See figure on p. 263.)

Hurler's syndrome (gargoylism)   A rare autosomal recessive metabolic disorder in which abnormal glycoproteins are deposited in most of the organs to produce a progressive disease resulting in dwarfism, mental retardation, deafness, and **cardiomyopathy.** The heart valves may be thickened.

hypertelorism   Widely set eyes found in such syndromes as pulmonary stenosis with **atrial septal defect,** and supravalvular aortic stenosis.

hypertrophic subaortic stenosis Disproportionate hypertrophy of the septum, which causes obstruction in midsystole as the septum draws toward the anterior or septal mitral leaflet in systole. (See figure on p. 277 for hemodynamics.) The disproportionate septal hypertrophy has engendered the term *asymmetric septal hypertrophy.* Originally, it was called idiopathic hypertrophic subaortic stenosis in the first extensive report [2] ; but the term *idiopathic* seems an unnecessary appendage. *Asymmetric septal hypertrophy* (commonly called ASH) does not necessarily imply obstruction to outflow, since ASH can occur without obstruction. Therefore, *hypertrophic subaortic stenosis* should be used when referring to a patient with obstruction due to asymmetric septal hypertrophy.

infective endocarditis Infection of the heart valves or of certain congenital defects, usually those that cause regurgitant or retrograde flows, such as **ventricular septal defect** or **patent ductus arteriosus.**

In former years, the infection was nearly always bacterial and thus the condition was called bacterial endocarditis. Since it could last for as long as two years before the diagnosis was made, it was known as subacute bacterial endocarditis. Today, fungi and *Rickettsia* are the causative organisms in a significant proportion of infections. Therefore, *infective* is a more embracing term.

The diagnosis used to be considered when there was fever and "changing murmurs." Since a regurgitant murmur is the only murmur likely to develop when a valve is destroyed, the term *changing* should be modified to mean a new or increasing *regurgitant* valvular murmur. (See checklist, p. 6, for clinical details.)

inflow and outflow tract of the left ventricle The inflow tract of the left ventricle is the area just below the mitral valve. The outflow tract is made up of the septum anteromedially and the anteromedial or septal leaflet of the mitral valve, plus their chordae laterally. (See figure on p. 282.)

infundibulum Outflow tract of the right ventricle, made up mostly of muscle called the crista supraventricularis. It is much like the spout of a teapot, the body of the right ventricle being the pot. (See figure on p. 282.)

intermittent claudication Pain in ischemic working muscle produced by certain metabolites, classically, pain in the legs due to inadequate arterial supply during walking. If the obstruction is high in the aortoiliac area, the pain may be in the hip or buttocks. However, the pain may be felt in unusual sites, such as in the thighs or the arch of the foot. When the **ischemia** is due to thrombosis of the lower aorta (chronic aortoiliac occlusion), impotence and leg weakness may occur as well (Leriche's syndrome) [11]. If the celiac or mesenteric arteries are involved, the pain after meals is called "abdominal angina."
Note: Intermittent claudication is not related to the nocturnal leg or foot muscle cramps that occur in bed.

ischemia Inadequate blood supply to a part of the body. (Pronounced "is-kē-mi-a.")

isovolumic contraction The rise in LV pressure between closure of the mitral valve and opening of the aortic valve. This used to be called isometric contraction, but since the measurements of the ventricle change while the volume does not, the term *isovolumic* is more accurate. In much of the cardiological literature the period from the beginning of ventricular contraction to the opening of the aortic valve is considered to be isovolumic. This is not the physiologists' definition, and it is not really a proper use of *isovolumic,* since the volume is still changing until the mitral valve closes.

isovolumic relaxation   The fall in LV pressure between closure of the aortic valve and opening of the mitral valve. If the opening of the mitral valve is audible as in the presence of mitral stenosis or a prosthetic mitral valve, the A2 — opening snap, or A2 — opening click interval represents isovolumic relaxation time. (See figure on p. 343.)

left lateral decubitus position   Body position in which the subject is horizontal and lying on his left side. (See figure on p. 233.)

malpositions of the heart   Abnormal placement of the cardiac chambers. The three commonest cardiac malpositions are situs inversus, dextroversion, and levoversion. *Situs solitus (solitus* means "usual") is the term used to denote a normal position of all chambers and vessels of the heart, and, when used alone, it implies that the viscera are also normally placed. It specifically means that the descending aorta, left atrium, cardiac apex, and stomach are all on the left. In *situs inversus,* the descending aorta, left atrium, apex, and stomach are all on the right. This is also known as mirror-image dextrocardia. In *dextroversion,* the aorta and stomach are the same as in situs solitus, but the heart is rotated so that the apex is on the right. In *levoversion,* the aorta and stomach are the same as in dextrocardia, but the heart has rotated so that the apex is on the left. The term *levocardia* has been used for situs solitus of the heart, but with the viscera inverted (stomach on the right). Levoversion and levocardia are almost always associated with other congenital anomalies.
Note: Kartagener's syndrome is situs inversus with sinusitis and bronchiectasis.

Marfan's syndrome   See pp. 24 and 29.

medial sclerosis   See **arteriosclerosis.**

Mueller maneuver   An inspiratory effort against a closed mouth and nose or glottis, that decreases intrathoracic pressure. It is the opposite to a Valsalva maneuver.

neurocirculatory asthenia   Syndrome occurring in some patients with anxiety neurosis, and consisting of palpitations and tachycardias, nondescript chest pains, shortness of breath, chronic fatigue, and other signs of sympathetic overactivity. It has been called "soldier's heart," "effort syndrome," "Da Costa's syndrome," and "neurotic heart syndrome." If these patients are chronic hyperventilators, their breath-holding time will be less than 20 sec.

Noonan's syndrome   Condition in which the physical characteristics of Turner's syndrome are present, but there are no known chromosomal abnormalities (called Ullrich's syndrome in Europe). It has been referred to as "male Turner syndrome," which is a poor term because it ignores the condition in females [13] . (See **Turner's syndrome** for physical and cardiac characteristics.)

outflow tract   See **inflow and outflow tract.**

patent ductus arteriosus Opening between the aorta and pulmonary artery in which flow
normally occurs between the higher pressure aorta and the lower pressure pulmonary
artery. Thus some of the blood ejected by the LV into the aorta will pass into
the pulmonary artery resulting in a left-to-right shunt. The volume overload occurs
where the shunted blood circulates, i.e., in the pulmonary artery, pulmonary
veins, left atrium, and LV. Therefore, you should expect dilatation of all the
vessels and chambers that lead from the pulmonary artery to the LV, but normal
right-sided chambers.

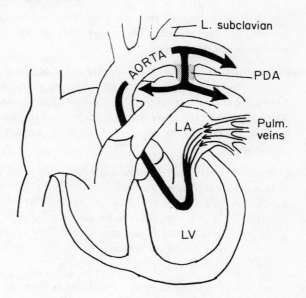

The patent ductus arteriosus is a slightly left-sided structure that usually connects
the junction of the main and pulmonary artery to the aorta just distal to the
origin of the left subclavian artery. Since normal aortic pressure (120/80 mm Hg)
is usually higher than pulmonary artery pressure (25/10 mm Hg), the shunt flow
is normally from aorta to pulmonary artery in both systole and diastole.

A patent ductus arteriosus represents persistence of the patency of the fetal
ductus arteriosus, designed to bypass the lungs in fetal life; i.e., the high pulmonary
artery pressure in the fetus forces blood into the aorta through the ductus.

In patent ductus arteriosus, severe pulmonary hypertension may develop if the
fetal arterioles do not involute, and when pulmonary hypertension does develop,
its onset is early in infancy or childhood. Then the right ventricle will remain or
become more hypertrophied and result in an **Eisenmenger syndrome or reaction,**
with right-to-left shunting. If a patient with a large patent ductus reaches adulthood without pulmonary hypertension having developed in infancy, then he may
go into heart failure with acute pulmonary edema. **Infective endocarditis** can
occur as one of the complications of a small patent ductus arteriosus. (See p. 329
for explanation of differential cyanosis, which is one of the characteristics of the
Eisenmenger reaction in patent ductus arteriosus.)

pectus excavatum   Posterior displacement of the lower sternum. It can be slight or so severe that it not only displaces the heart to the left but also may interfere with cardiac function by raising right ventricular diastolic pressure, and can cause palpitations and dyspnea on strenuous exertion [16]. It is commonly seen in Marfan's syndrome (see p. 29) and in patients with the straight back syndrome (see p. 270). The three degrees of severity have been described as the "saucer," "cup," and "funnel." If the anteroposterior measurement of the adult chest is measured by obstetric calipers and is less than 6½ inches (about 16 cm), the heart is very likely to be compressed. If the anteroposterior measurement is less than 5 inches (about 11 cm), the entire heart will usually be displaced to the left, but without compression. The apex beat is almost always displaced to the left, even in saucer depressions.

postextrasystolic potentiation   Increased contractility that occurs in the beat following a premature electrical depolarization of the heart. Although a pause after a premature beat can increase contractility by the long diastole, causing more filling and a **Starling effect,** premature depolarization itself produces increased contractility, i.e., independent of the length of diastole. The cause of this increased inotropism is unknown.

postmyocardial infarction syndrome   Syndrome consisting of fever, pneumonitis, and painful pericarditis and pleuritis that may occur from about 2 – 11 weeks after a myocardial infarction and is probably an autoimmune response to myocardial necrosis. It is only dangerous in the presence of anticoagulants, when it may produce a bloody effusion and **tamponade.** The syndrome closely resembles the postcardiotomy syndrome and may be recurrent for as long as two years. Also called Dressler's syndrome [6].

pressure load   Load on a ventricle caused by a resistance to ejection. An increased pressure load may result from such conditions as hypertension, coarctation of the aorta, or aortic stenosis. Also called a systolic load or afterload.

primary pulmonary hypertension   Irreversible pulmonary hypertension of unknown etiology, usually progressing to severe degrees, producing more and more right ventricular hypertrophy and dilatation, as well as main pulmonary artery dilatation and atherosclerosis. The age and sex incidence strongly favors females under age 40. Histologically, the small pulmonary arteries and arterioles usually show intimal fibrosis and proliferation, as well as medial thickening.

pulse pressure or volume   Amplitude of a pulse. In palpation, it refers to how far your fingers are moved between the least and the greatest expansion of a vessel. On an arterial pulse tracing, it refers to the difference between systolic and diastolic pressure.

Raynaud's phenomenon   Intermittent constriction of small arteries and arterioles of the fingers, resulting in a change in color, usually produced by cooling but also by sympathetic stimulation of any kind. It begins with blanching, progresses to cyanosis, and often ends with a reactive redness (reactive hyperemia) that may be very painful. It is occasionally a precursor of a collagen or other connective-tissue disease.

It is called Raynaud's *disease* when it is not secondary to trauma or to neurogenic lesions or other systemic diseases.

Note: Acrocyanosis, which is a persistent blueness and coldness of the distal parts of the extremities, probably due to an abnormality of the small vessels, should not be confused with Raynaud's phenomenon.

right ventricular failure   Usually, a condition in which there is high venous pressure and peripheral edema due to low cardiac output. It does not mean that the right ventricular muscle has necessarily "failed." The right ventricle may be perfectly healthy, but is most often responding to the low output of a damaged left ventricle. The right ventricle cannot put out more than it receives from the left ventricle. If a damaged left ventricle puts out only 30 ml (instead of a normal 60 ml) with each systole, the right ventricle will receive, and therefore also eject, 30 ml per systole. If the right ventricle did more than this, pulmonary edema would quickly follow. Since the fibers of the left ventricle are intertwined with those of the right ventricle, the output of the latter is usually mechanically dependent on the action of the LV. Therefore if the left ventricle is in failure, the right ventricle will act the same way in terms of **ejection fraction** and stroke volume. To call this "right ventricular failure" is placing the blame on the wrong ventricle.

True right ventricular failure is rare, but can occur chronically with severe obstruction to right ventricular outflow, such as in very severe pulmonary stenosis or pulmonary hypertension. Acutely, it can occur with a massive pulmonary embolism.

The high venous pressure and peripheral edema caused by left ventricular failure is better called "peripheral congestive failure." (See checklist, p. 4.) When the left ventricle fails, the high venous pressure is caused as much by the high venous tone and increased blood volume secondary to its low output as it is by the secondary response of the right ventricle. The peripheral edema is caused by the salt retention and high venous pressure, both of which can be blamed on the low output of the left ventricle.

semilunar valves   Aortic or pulmonary valves whose leaflets are half-moon-shaped (semilunar).

sinus arrhythmia   Increase in heart rate with inspiration and decrease with expiration due to vagal inhibition during inspiration. (Remember "in" for "*in*crease" on inspiration.)

sinuses of Valsalva   The three bulges or sinuses at the root of the aorta, two of which give rise to the coronary arteries. They help to prevent the open aortic valves from occluding the orifice of the coronary arteries. Occasionally, they may be congenitally weak and rupture into adjacent chambers; or they may become aneurysmal, especially in Marfan's syndrome (see p. 29), and produce any degree of aortic regurgitation. (See illustration on next page.)

Starling effect   The effect of the Frank-Starling law of the heart, which states that if the heart muscle is stretched before it contracts, it will contract with more energy. This is equivalent to a bow-and-arrow effect; i.e., the more taut the bow, the farther the arrow will go.

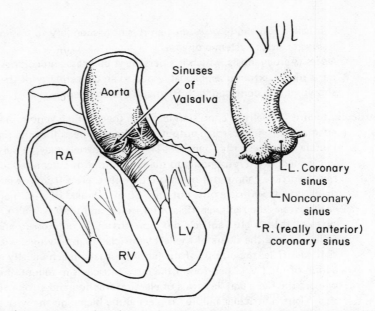

The right coronary sinus is anterior when viewed from above, but it is called the right coronary sinus probably because it gives rise to the right coronary artery.

sternal angle, or angle of Louis (pronounced Loo-ee) The first protuberance or hump on the sternum below the suprasternal notch. It is at the junction of the manubrium and body of the sternum. It marks the point where the second costal cartilage joins the sternum. Below this cartilage is the second intercostal space.

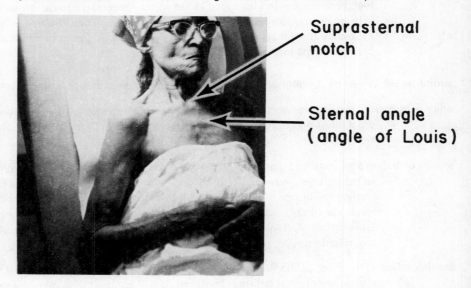

The sternal angle is one of the most important landmarks in cardiology, not only because it is the zero level for jugular pressures but also because it is the only accurate way to find the fourth right interspace in order to place the V_1 electrode for an ECG.

Stokes-Adams attack or **Adams-Stokes attack**   An episode of syncope secondary to complete AV block (see p. 411 of Glossary). Any cerebral symptom secondary to complete AV block may probably also be considered to be a minor degree of Stokes-Adams attack since it may presage syncope and death. Syncope secondary to any other arrhythmia should probably be called cardiac syncope and not a Stokes-Adams attack.

subclavian steal   Use of a vertebral artery as collateral circulation to feed a subclavian artery beyond an obstruction (usually on the left). Blood from a vertebral artery flows retrogradely into the distal subclavian, thus "stealing" blood from the brain. (See checklist, p. 14, for symptoms.)

tamponade   Restriction of cardiac diastole caused by fluid in the pericardium. Since the pressure in the pericardium is equal to venous pressure, the patient with tamponade must of necessity have a high venous pressure and usually also has peripheral edema when the tamponade becomes severe. Pericardial effusion without a high venous pressure should not be called tamponade. A combination of fluid and solid pericardial material causing constriction is called "effusive-constrictive pericarditis."

tetralogy of Fallot   Classically it refers to a large ventricular septal defect (VSD), pulmonary stenosis, an overriding aorta, and right ventricular hypertrophy (RVH) [9]. Since pulmonary stenosis will always lead to RVH, the latter is a necessary result of the other congenital lesions and not really part of the basic abnormality.

The pulmonary stenosis may be either valvular, infundibular, or both and is the cause of the murmur. The overriding of the aorta is probably the result of the high level of the VSD which is contiguous with the aortic root so that the aorta hangs freely over the septal defect. The enlargement of the aorta by virtue of receiving blood from both ventricles may contribute to the overriding.

Tetralogy of Fallot is the commonest form of congenital cyanotic heart disease.

thrill   Vibratory sensation similar to what is felt when touching the head and neck of a purring cat. A long thrill is merely a palpable murmur and signifies that the murmur is at least grade 4/6 in loudness. A short thrill on the chest wall may be a juxtaposition of split heart sound vibrations. A short thrill felt on a carotid artery may be due to a midsystolic dip or minor degree of bisferiens pulse.

transposition of the great vessels   Often called "complete" transposition of the great vessels, this term means that the anteroposterior relationships of the aorta and pulmonary arteries are reversed, i.e., instead of the aorta being posterior to the pulmonary artery it is anterior (and often to the right). This results in the RV giving rise to the aorta and the LV to the pulmonary artery. One or more abnormal communications between the systemic and pulmonary circulations must exist for the patient to survive. Mixing may occur through either an atrial septal defect, a ventricular septal defect, a patent ductus, or large bronchial arteries.

Cyanosis is usually present either from birth or within a few days of birth. The commonest cause of cyanosis combined with shunt vascularity in the lungs on x-ray is transposition of the great vessels, especially if accompanied by congestive failure in infancy.

Turner's syndrome   Female phenotype consisting of short stature, receding chin, webbed neck, low hairline over the back of the neck, broad shield chest resulting in widely separated nipples, exaggerated carrying angle, sparse axillary and pubic hair, lymphedema of the lower extremities (in infancy), and a short fourth metacarpal. It is sometimes simply described as short stature, neck webbing, and sexual infantilism in a female with a sex chromosome abnormality (absence of one of the two sex chromosomes). Coarctation of the aorta is the commonest associated cardiovascular lesion. When patients with such an appearance have normal sex chromosomes and also have hypertelorism with a slight antimongoloid slant to the eyes as well as ptosis of the upper lids and exophthalmos, especially if the above physical characteristics are found in a male, they are likely to have pulmonary stenosis and are said to have **Noonan's syndrome** [14]. Hypertrophic cardiomyopathies and patent ductus arteriosus have also been associated with Noonan's syndrome.

Valsalva maneuver   A forced expiration against a closed glottis. It is used as a simple way to raise intrathoracic pressure. The patient is asked either to blow up a column of mercury to as close to 50 mm Hg as possible or to push his abdomen up against your hand for about 10 sec. The rise in intrathoracic pressure (phase 1) decreases venous return to the heart despite a marked rise in venous pressure, thus causing a gradual decrease in heart size, stroke volume, and pulse pressure. Despite a reflex tachycardia, the blood pressure falls (phase 2). On release of the strain there is a further sudden drop of blood pressure for a few beats because most of the blood in the RV is used to fill the almost empty pulmonary venous reservoir (phase 3). There now occurs a slowing of the heart rate and an excessive rise in blood pressure for a few beats that may be due either to reflex sympathetic stimulation caused by the strain that takes a few seconds to get "turned off," or to the effect of a sudden increase in volume distending the carotid baroreceptors.

ventricular aneurysm   See **aneurysm**.

ventricular septal defect   Opening or hole in the ventricular septum. This is the commonest of all congenital lesions and is most usually found in the membranous portion of the ventricle, i.e., in the translucent area, a few centimeters below the aortic valve. It may, however, be in the muscular septum, in the supracristal area, leading directly into the pulmonary artery (rare), or posterior and superior to the attachment of the tricuspid valve to the membranous septum and therefore may lead directly into the right atrium (Gerbode defect). (See figure on p. 318.) Ventricular septal defect shunts that occur during systole are normally from left to right, i.e., left to right ventricle, and produce volume overloads in the right ventricle, pulmonary artery, pulmonary veins, left atrium, and left ventricle.

The defect usually varies from pinpoint size to slightly more than a centimeter in diameter. When it involves the entire septum, a single ventricle is produced. When multiple muscular defects are present, it is known as a *Swiss cheese defect*.

No matter how large the shunt flow in infancy, the hole may close in the first few years of life, often with a membranous septal pouch or **aneurysm**.

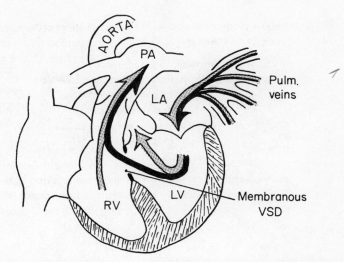

In most ventricular septal defects, only the right atrium is spared the volume over-load caused by the left-to-right shunt. In the rare left ventricle-to-right atrium type of ventricular septal defect, however, all cardiac chambers are volume-overloaded.

In this figure, the black portion of the arrow represents the shunt flow, and the dotted portion represents the normal flow that comes from the venae cavae.

A dreaded complication of large defects is severe pulmonary hypertension, which may become irreversible. When it becomes severe enough to reverse the shunt, this is known as an Eisenmenger complex (see **Eisenmenger syndrome)**, which usually occurs within the first year or two of life.

water-hammer pulse   A brisk, sharp, rapidly rising arterial pulse. A water-hammer was a Victorian toy consisting of a tube in which a vacuum was produced and containing water that dropped like a rock with the unopposed gravity when the tube was turned. When the water struck against the vessel, it produced a noise similar to that of a hammer.

Wolff-Parkinson-White (W-P-W) preexcitation   Electrocardiographic phenomenon in which an abnormal conduction pathway between atrium and ventricle bypasses the atrio-ventricular node, thus shortening the P-R interval and producing a wide QRS. When this pathway is used to produce a circular reentry passageway for a tachy-cardia, it is called a *Wolff-Parkinson-White syndrome.*

xanthelasma   Flat xanthoma found on or around the eyelid. It is a yellowish, cholesterol-filled plaque, and is often, but not invariably, associated with hypercholesteremia.

xanthoma   Cholesterol-filled nodule found either subcutaneously or over a tendon. *Tuberous xanthomas* — subcutaneous xanthomas on extensor surfaces of the extremities. They are associated with an increase in serum levels of both cholesterol and triglycerides. They are most commonly found in patients with type III hyper-lipoproteinemia, but it may be predominately type II or IV. They are associated with coronary disease, even before puberty. Since they are under the skin, their yellow pigment is visible. Tendon xanthomas are too deep to impart any change of color to the skin.

eruptive xanthomas   Tiny yellowish nodules, 1–2 mm in diameter, on an erythematous base and found all over the body. They are often transient and vary with the degree of hypertriglycerdemia, with which they are associated. They are found in patients with high triglycerides, whatever the cause, whether diabetes or pure type I hyperlipoproteinemia. There is some correlation with coronary disease.

planar xanthomas   Very small xanthomas found in the palmar creases and probably representing an early state of the tuberous type.

REFERENCES

1. Bernheim, P. De la stenose ventriculaire droite. *Rev. Gen. Clin. Therap.* (or *J. Pract.*) 29:721, 1915.
2. Braunwald, E., Lambrew, C. T., Rockoff, S. D., Ross, J., Jr., and Morrow, A. G. Idiopathic hypertrophic subaortic stenosis: Description based on analysis of 64 patients. *Circulation* 29 (Suppl. IV):1, 1964.
3. Burch, G. E. Ischemic cardiomyopathy. *Am. Heart J.* 79:291, 1970.
4. Burch, G. E., Giles, T. D., and Colcolough, H. L. Ischemic cardiomyopathy. *Br. Heart J.* 79:291, 1970.
5. Corrigan, D. J. On permanent patency of the mouth of the aorta, or inadequacy of the aortic valves. *Edin. Med. Surg. J.* 37:229, 1832.
6. Dressler, W. The post-myocardial infarction syndrome. *Arch. Intern. Med.* 103:28, 1959.
7. Ebstein, W. Über einem sehr seltenen Fall von Insufficienz der Valvula Tricuspidalis. *Arch. f. Anat. Physiol. u. wissensch Med.* January, 1866.
8. Eisenmenger, V. Die angeborenen Defect de Kammerscheidewand des Herzens. *Ztschr. f. Klin. Med.* 32:1, 1897.
9. Fallot, A. Contribution a l'anatomie pathologique de la maladie bleu (cyanose cardiaque). *Marseille Med.* 25:77, 1888.
10. Gould, K. L., Lipscomb, K., Hamilton, G. W., and Kennedy, J. W. Left ventricular hypertrophy in coronary artery disease. *Am. J. Med.* 55:595, 1973.
11. Leriche, R., and Morel, A. The syndrome of thrombotic obliteration of the aortic bifurcation. *Ann. Surg.* 127:193, 1948.
12. Mahl, M. M., and Lange, K. Reliability of subjective circulation time determinations. *Circulation* 17:922, 1958.
13. Noonan, J. A., and Ehmke, D. A. Associated noncardiac malformations in children with congenital heart disease. *J. Pediatr.* 63:468, 1963.
14. Selzer, A. Circulation time and venous pressure: Routine tests? *Am. Heart J.* 80:142, 1970.
15. Takaro, T., and Hines, E. A., Jr. Digital arteriography in occlusive arterial disease and in clubbing of the fingers. *Circulation* 35:682, 1967.
16. vanBuchem, F. S. P., and Nieveen, J. Findings with funnel chest. *Acta Med. Scand.* 174:657, 1963.

The following abbreviations, although explained in the text, are listed here for easy reference.

A_2	aortic component of second sound
ACG	apex cardiogram
AR	aortic regurgitation
AS	aortic stenosis
ASD	atrial septal defect
AV	atrioventricular
A-V	arteriovenous
HSS	hypertrophic subaortic stenosis
LBBB	left bundle branch block
LV	left ventricle, left ventricular
LVH	left ventricular hypertrophy
M_1	mitral component of first sound
MR	mitral regurgitation
MS	mitral stenosis
OS	opening snap
P_2	pulmonary component of second sound
PDA	patent ductus arteriosus
PR	pulmonary regurgitation
PS	pulmonary stenosis
RBBB	right bundle branch block
RV	right ventricle, right ventricular
S_1	first heart sound
S_2	second heart sound
S_3	third heart sound
S_4	fourth heart sound
TR	tricuspid regurgitation
TS	tricuspid stenosis
VSD	ventricular septal defect

Numbers in italics refer to illustrations.